B-Vitamins and Human Health

B-Vitamins and Human Health

Editor: Douglas Haywood

AMERICAN
MEDICAL PUBLISHERS
www.americanmedicalpublishers.com

AMERICAN
MEDICAL PUBLISHERS
www.americanmedicalpublishers.com

Cataloging-in-Publication Data

B-vitamins and human health / edited by Douglas Haywood.
p. cm.
Includes bibliographical references and index.
ISBN 978-1-63927-609-7
1. Vitamin B complex. 2. Vitamin B complex--Physiological effect.
3. Vitamin B in human nutrition. 4. Vitamin B complex--Therapeutic use.
5. Dietary supplements. I. Haywood, Douglas.
QP772.V52 B56 2023
612.399--dc23

American Medical Publishers,
41 Flatbush Avenue,
1st Floor, New York,
NY 11217, USA

ISBN 978-1-63927-609-7 (Hardback)

Contents

Preface

I am honored to present to you this unique book which encompasses the most up-to-date data in the field. I was extremely pleased to get this opportunity of editing the work of experts from across the globe. I have also written papers in this field and researched the various aspects revolving around the progress of the discipline. I have tried to unify my knowledge along with that of stalwarts from every corner of the world, to produce a text which not only benefits the readers but also facilitates the growth of the field.

B-vitamins are a group of water soluble vitamins that play significant roles in cell metabolism and synthesis of red blood cells. There are eight B-vitamins, namely, B1 (thiamin), B2 (riboflavin), B3 (niacin), B5 (pantothenic acid), B6 (pyridoxine), B7 (biotin), B9 (folate [folic acid]), and B12 (cobalamin). Vitamin B9 and vitamin B12 are essential water-soluble vitamins that perform pivotal function in the maintenance of one-carbon metabolism. The one carbon metabolism is a set of interconnected metabolic pathways driven by folate and methionine. It generates methyl groups for use in DNA synthesis, amino acid homeostasis, antioxidant generation, and epigenetic regulation. Developmental defects, impaired cognitive function, or blocked normal blood production are some of the possible outcomes associated with a diet deficient in vitamins B9 and B12. It has been observed in certain studies that higher levels of these vitamins may lead to immune dysfunction, cancer, or increased mortality. Research in B-vitamins is now primarily focused on developing specific therapies that target one-carbon metabolism for managing cancer and immune diseases. This book includes some of the vital pieces of works being conducted across the world, on various topics related to B-vitamins and their role in human health. Students, researchers, experts and all associated with this area of study will benefit alike from this book.

Finally, I would like to thank all the contributing authors for their valuable time and contributions. This book would not have been possible without their efforts. I would also like to thank my friends and family for their constant support.

Editor

1

B Vitamins and One-Carbon Metabolism: Implications in Human Health and Disease

Peter Lyon [1,2], Victoria Strippoli [1,2], Byron Fang [1,2] and Luisa Cimmino [1,2,*]

1 Department of Biochemistry and Molecular Biology, Miller School of Medicine, University of Miami, Miami, FL 33136, USA; peterlyon@med.miami.edu (P.L.); vfs15@miami.edu (V.S.); b.fang1@umiami.edu (B.F.)

2 Sylvester Comprehensive Cancer Center, Miller School of Medicine, University of Miami, Miami, FL 33136, USA

* Correspondence: luisa.cimmino@med.miami.edu

Abstract: Vitamins B9 (folate) and B12 are essential water-soluble vitamins that play a crucial role in the maintenance of one-carbon metabolism: a set of interconnected biochemical pathways driven by folate and methionine to generate methyl groups for use in DNA synthesis, amino acid homeostasis, antioxidant generation, and epigenetic regulation. Dietary deficiencies in B9 and B12, or genetic polymorphisms that influence the activity of enzymes involved in the folate or methionine cycles, are known to cause developmental defects, impair cognitive function, or block normal blood production. Nutritional deficiencies have historically been treated with dietary supplementation or high-dose parenteral administration that can reverse symptoms in the majority of cases. Elevated levels of these vitamins have more recently been shown to correlate with immune dysfunction, cancer, and increased mortality. Therapies that specifically target one-carbon metabolism are therefore currently being explored for the treatment of immune disorders and cancer. In this review, we will highlight recent studies aimed at elucidating the role of folate, B12, and methionine in one-carbon metabolism during normal cellular processes and in the context of disease progression.

Keywords: folate; Vitamin B12; methionine; one-carbon metabolism

---

1. Introduction

The B vitamins comprise a group of eight water-soluble vitamins (B1, B2, B3, B5, B6, B7, B9, and B12) that act as cofactors, precursors, and substrates for numerous biological processes (Table 1). Dietary intake of these B vitamins is essential for the maintenance of human health and deficiencies can have severe health consequences. Almost all of the B vitamins are either directly or tangentially involved in one-carbon metabolism. One-carbon metabolism plays a central role in the generation of methyl donors in the form of S-adenosylmethionine (SAM), the sole methyl donor utilized by DNA, RNA, histone, and protein methyltransferases [1–5]. Methylation is essential for many cellular processes, including protein–protein interactions and epigenetic regulation, which have important roles in embryonic development, cognitive function, and hematopoiesis [6,7]. Furthermore, perturbations in the uptake and homeostasis of B vitamins, which results in deficiency or excess of one-carbon metabolism intermediates, can lead to neurological defects, anemia, aberrant immune responses, and cancer [8–10]. Given the central role of vitamin B9 (folate) and vitamin B12 (B12) as direct participants of one-carbon metabolism, this review will focus on their biological roles in human health.

Table 1. Biological roles of the B vitamins.

Vitamin	Biological Function
B1 (thiamine)	cofactor for enzymes in glucose metabolism, amino acid catabolism, nucleotide synthesis, and fatty acid synthesis [11]
B2 (riboflavin)	precursor for flavin mononucleotide (FMN) and flavin adenine dinucleotide (FAD) for cellular respiration [12]
B3 (nicotinamide)	precursor for nicotinamide adenine dinucleotide (NAD) utilized in biosynthetic pathways, energy metabolism, and protection from reactive oxygen species [13]
B5 (pantothenic acid)	precursor for coenzyme A (coA), an acyl-carrier required for the activity of many enzymes [14]
B6 (pyridoxine)	cofactor for over 150 enzymes involved mainly in amino acid synthesis and degradation [15]
B7 (biotin)	plays an essential role in carboxylation reactions [16] and also has many applications in laboratory research
B9 (folate)	substrate for nucleotide synthesis and methyl-donors in the one-carbon metabolism pathway [12]
B12 (cobalamin)	cofactor for enzymes in one-carbon metabolism and the propionate catabolic pathway [12]

2. Key Regulators of One-Carbon Metabolism

One-carbon metabolism is driven by the folate and methionine cycles that together regulate DNA synthesis and methylation reactions (Figure 1). These two cycles are linked by methionine synthase (MS), the rate-limiting enzyme in one-carbon metabolism that converts homocysteine (Hcy) to methionine (Met) using 5-methyltetrahydrofolate (5-mTHF) as a methyl donor and B12 as an essential cofactor [8,17]. The key regulators of one carbon metabolism are all essential dietary requirements: Methionine, Folate (B9), and Vitamin B12.

2.1. *Methionine*

Methionine (Met) is one of nine essential amino acids and plays a critical role in multiple biological processes, including the initiation of all eukaryotic peptide synthesis, lipid biosynthesis, and as the primary source of methyl groups utilized by DNA, RNA, histone, and protein methyltransferases [18,19]. Adequate methionine levels are required for normal growth and development and the maintenance of healthy skin, hair, and nails [20]. After protein digestion, methionine is absorbed in the small intestine through sodium-dependent amino acid transporters that are involved in the transport of several amino acids [21]. Methionine is then excreted into the serum through L-type amino acid transporter 4, which also excretes other neutral amino acids [21].

2.2. *Folate*

Folate (Vitamin B9) is an essential micronutrient that is naturally and most commonly found in dark leafy green vegetables. Due to its hydrophilicity, folate and its derivatives depend on highly specific transporters for its absorption in the intestinal tract and other systemic tissues [22]. The reduced folate carrier (RFC) is expressed on most mammalian cells and is the primary mode of transport for reduced folate uptake into systemic tissues at a neutral pH. In addition to RFC, there are folate receptors α and β (FRα/β) that are highly tissue-specific, membrane-bound receptors that bind reduced folates, allowing them to enter cells via endocytosis [23].

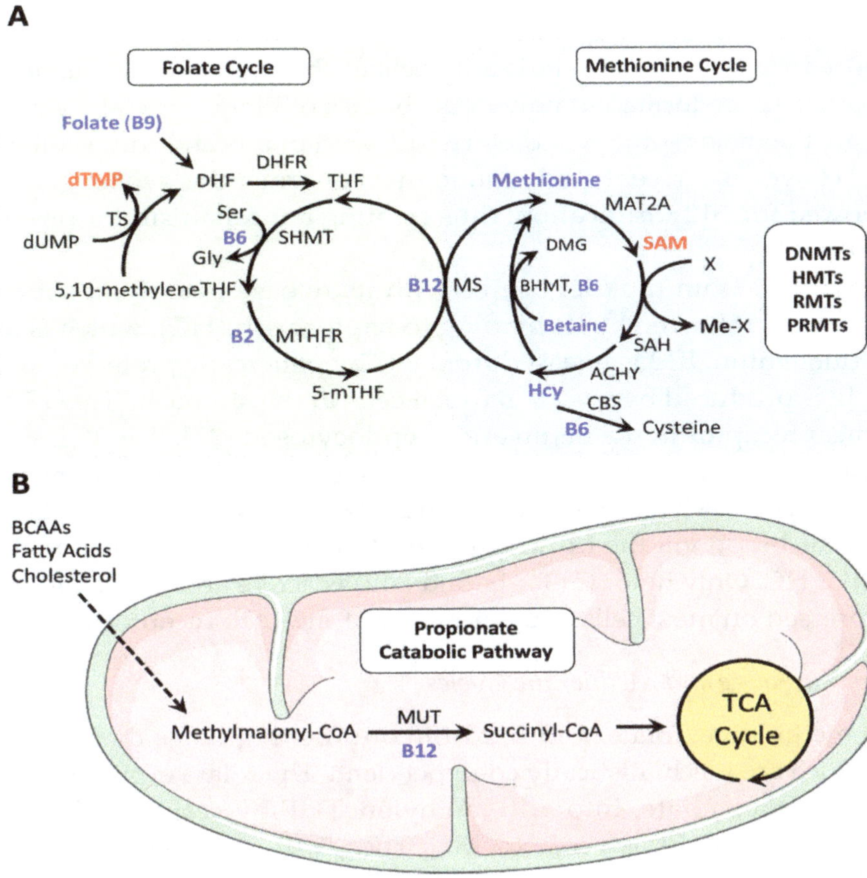

Figure 1. The regulation of metabolism by B vitamins. (**A**) B vitamins in one-carbon metabolism. The folate cycle begins with the conversion of dietary folate (B9) into dihydrofolate (DHF), which is then reduced to tetrahydrofolate (THF) by the enzyme dihydrofolate reductase (DHFR). THF is next converted to 5,10-methyleneTHF by serine hydroxymethyltransferase (SHMT), a reaction that is coupled with the hydroxylation of serine (Ser) to glycine (Gly) and requires B6 as a cofactor. Thymidylate synthase (TS) uses 5,10-methyleneTHF as a methyl donor to methylate deoxyuridine monophosphate (dUMP), creating deoxythymidine monophosphate (dTMP). This step regenerates DHF for continued cycling. Alternatively, 5,10-methyleneTHF can be reduced by methylenetetrahydrofolate reductase (MTHFR) to 5-methytetrahydrofolate (5-mTHF) using B2 as a cofactor. As part of the methionine cycle, 5-mTHF donates a methyl group to regenerate methionine from homocysteine (Hcy), which is catalyzed by methionine synthase (MS) and requires B12, in the form of methylcobalamin, as a cofactor. To generate the methyl donor S-adenosylmethionine (SAM) for use by multiple methyltransferases (MTs) specific for RNA (RMT), DNA (DNMT), histones (HMT), and protein (PRMT) methylation reactions, an adenosine is transferred to methionine by methionine adenosyltransferase 2A. SAM is demethylated during the methyltransferase reactions to form S-adenosylhomocysteine (SAH) that is then hydrolysed by S-adenosylhomocysteine hydrolase (AHCY) to form Hcy. Hcy can also enter the transsulfuration pathway catalyzed by cystathionine beta synthase (CBS) and vitamin B6 to create cysteine. In the liver, betaine from the diet can act as a methyl donor for betaine-homocysteine S-methyltransferase (BHMT), using B6 as a cofactor, to make methionine and dimethylglycine (DMG) as a byproduct. Important dietary micronutrients and metabolite intermediates are highlighted in blue. Items in red are important byproducts of one-carbon metabolism. (**B**) B12 and propionate metabolism. The propionate catabolic pathway breaks down branched-chain amino acids (BCAAs), odd-chain fatty acids, and cholesterol to be used in the tricarboxylic acid (TCA) cycle in the mitochondria. Methylmalonyl-CoA mutase (MUT) converts methylmalonyl-CoA into succinyl-CoA using B12, in the form of adenosylcobalamin, as a cofactor. Succinyl-CoA then enters the TCA cycle.

2.3. Vitamin B12

Vitamin B12 is produced solely by bacteria and archaea through aerobic or anaerobic pathways [24]. Bacteria that synthesize B12 are located mainly in the bodies of higher predatory organisms, thus meat, milk, eggs, and fish are the major sources of dietary B12, with plants and fungi contributing little B12 to the human diet [25]. However, a recent study found that co-fermenting wheat germ with two different bacterial species allowed for B12 fortification, thus creating a mechanism for producing B12 fortified plant-origin products [26].

The absorption of B12 from the diet begins with its release from food sources by gastric acid and pepsin in the stomach, followed by its binding to haptocorrin (HC), which is found in saliva and gastric fluid. In the duodenum, B12 is released from HC by pancreatic proteases and is then bound by intrinsic factor (IF). IF is produced by gastric parietal cells in the stomach. This IF-B12 complex binds the cubulin-amnionless receptor in the ileum and is endocytosed [27]. The IF is degraded and B12 is released in the lysosome and enters the cytoplasm. How B12 exits the lysosome is currently unclear, but some groups have hypothesized that LMBD1 and ABCD4 play a role in B12's export [28,29]. B12 is then released into the blood via the Multidrug resistance protein 1 (MRP1) where it is bound by transcobalamin (TC) or HC. Only holoTC (TC-bound B12) is active and available for uptake by CD320, the B12 receptor expressed on most cells and a member of the LDL receptor family [30].

2.4. Co-Dependence of the Folate and Methionine Cycles

The balance of methionine, folate, and B12 from our diet regulates the activity of the folate and methionine cycles, which are mechanistically co-dependent. The folate cycle converts tetrahydrofolate (THF), sourced from dietary folate, into 5,10-methyleneTHF by serine hydroxymethyltransferase (SHMT), an enzyme that requires B6 as a cofactor [31]. Then, 5,10-methyleneTHF acts as a methyl-donor for thymidylate synthase (TS) to synthesize deoxythymidine monophosphate (dTMP) from deoxyuracil monophosphate (dUMP) or for methylenetetrahydrofolate reductase (MTHFR) to generate 5-mTHF [31] (Figure 1).

In the methionine cycle, Met is converted to SAM by methyl-adenosyl transferase 2A (MAT2A) and SAM then acts as a substrate used by a diverse group of methyltransferases. The product of these methylation reactions is S-adenosylhomocysteine (SAH), which can be hydrolysed into homocysteine (Hcy) by S-adenosylhomocysteine hydrolase (AHCY), then resynthesized into Met by MS using 5-mTHF as a methyl donor and B12 as an essential cofactor [8,17,32]. Occasionally, the cobalt group of B12 becomes oxidized to Co(II) during its reaction [33]. Methionine synthase reductase (MTRR) reduces Co(II) back to Co(I), thereby regenerating this essential cofactor for MS activity. Methionine can also be recycled from Hcy using betaine, which is derived from dietary choline, as a methyl donor [7] or directly from SAM through polyamine synthesis and the methionine salvage pathway. Using B6 as a cofactor, Hcy can also be converted to cysteine via transsulfuration for use in glutathione synthesis [34] (Figure 1).

In addition to the role of B12 as a cofactor in the recycling of Hcy to Met, it also acts as an important cofactor for another metabolic enzyme, methyl-malonyl CoA mutase (MUT). MUT is located in the mitochondria and utilizes B12 in the form of adenosylcobalamin to convert L-methylmalonyl-CoA to succinyl-CoA, which can then enter the tricarboxylic acid (TCA) cycle. Genetic loss of MUT activity can disrupt TCA cycle function [35] and mitochondrial redox function [36,37], suggesting that B12 levels can influence both one-carbon metabolism, energy metabolism, and redox metabolism.

3. Methionine, Folate, and B12 Deficiency on One-Carbon Metabolism: Causes and Consequences

3.1. Causes of Deficiency

Given the importance of one-carbon metabolism in cell proliferation and survival, it is not surprising that folate and B12 deficiencies can have severe biological consequences. Reduced levels of the micronutrients involved in one-carbon metabolism would logically cause defects in the production of SAM and nucleotide synthesis. Methionine, folate, or B12 deprivation reduces cell proliferation due to blocks in cell cycling [38–41], and deficiencies in one of these metabolites, either through deprivation or genetic alterations, has been shown to cause global DNA hypomethylation [41–44]. Methionine deprivation can cause a global decrease in histone methylation [41,45] and models of B12 deficiency have also been shown to decrease the methylation level of proteins [46,47] (Figure 2A).

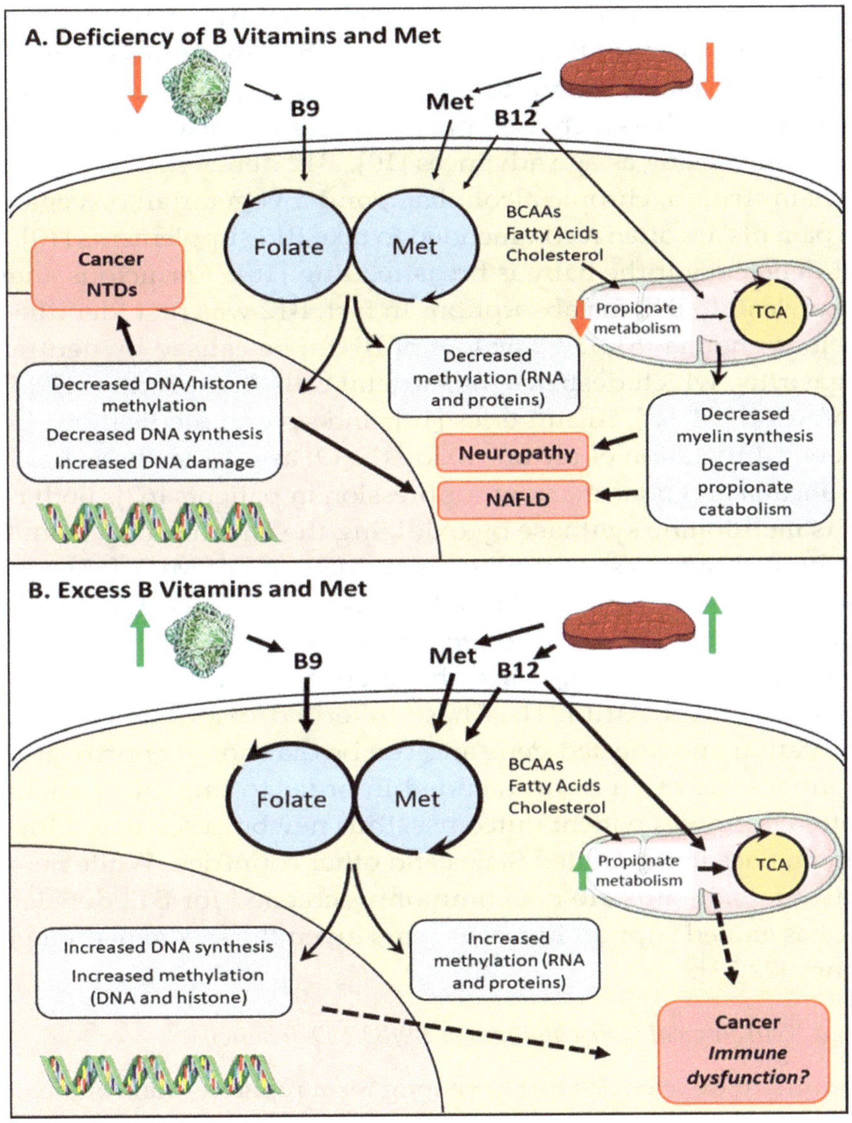

Figure 2. Systemic effects of altered micronutrients in one-carbon metabolism. (**A**) Reduced folate, methionine, or B12 can cause a decrease in one-carbon metabolism output, leading to decreased DNA synthesis, increased genomic instability, and decreased methylation potential. This can promote the development of neural tube defects (NTDs), non-alcoholic fatty liver disease (NAFLD), and cancer (specifically colorectal cancer). Reduced B12 also decreases activity of the propionate catabolic pathway through decreased methylmalonyl-CoA mutase (MUT) enzymatic activity, leading to decreased myelin synthesis, increased cellular stress, and disrupted tricarboxylic acid (TCA) cycling. These factors influence the development of neuropathies and promote NAFLD. (**B**) Effects of excess folate, methionine, and B12 are less understood, but increases can promote cell proliferation and can increase SAM (S-adenosylmethionine) levels, which allow cells to maintain their methylated states. This could lead to the development of cancers as maintenance of methylation is important for some malignancies. Excessive folate also disrupts normal hematopoiesis, possibly through increased one-carbon metabolism.

In normal adults, deficiencies in a sole amino acid like methionine would be rare with adequate nutrition, though a methionine-deficient diet that reduces serum methionine can be achieved in patients [48]. B9 deficiency can occur during pregnancy [49] as pregnant women need to support an immense amount of rapid cell division and tissue growth, and the epigenome also dynamically changes during embryonic development to regulate gene expression at discrete stages of differentiation. Folate deficiency is also associated with malnutrition and lower socioeconomic status.

B12 deficiency presenting with clinical manifestations, hematologic and/or neurologic, is relatively uncommon in the general US population, however, low serum B12 status can be seen in 10.6% of the US population [50]. Global studies of B12 status find much higher rates of deficiency in developing countries [10], possibly due to malnutrition. B12 deficiency is also more prevalent in the elderly, due to a diverse number of factors, such as increased prevalence of pernicious anemia and dietary changes, with rates of deficiency increasing as age advances [10]. B12 deficiency can be the result of a myriad of causes. General malnutrition, chronic alcoholism, and a vegetarian or vegan diet can cause B12 deficiency and these patients are often recommended to take B12 supplements [10]. Maternal deficiency may result in infant deficiency if the baby is breastfeeding [10]. Pernicious anemia, the absence of intrinsic factor (IF), can lead to B12 malabsorption. In fact, B12 was first identified from the liver as a treatment for pernicious anemia [51,52]. The loss of IF can be caused by neutralizing antibodies to IF or autoimmune gastritis, which destroys the parietal cells that produce IF [53]. Gastrointestinal (GI) diseases [10], infection [54–57], GI surgeries [10], and several medications [58–61] are all known causes of B12 deficiency. Inhalation of nitrous oxide (N_2O) as an anesthetic has long been known to cause megaloblastic anemia and bone marrow suppression in patients [62]. Both nitric oxide [63] (NO) and N_2O [64] inhibits methionine synthase by oxidizing the cobalt group from Co(I) to Co(II). This oxidation of B12 has been shown to specifically inhibit MS and not MUT [65].

Polymorphisms in genes related to B12 uptake have also been correlated with decreased serum B12 [66–68]. Similarly, polymorphisms in folate uptake genes can cause a folate deficiency [69,70]. Genetic errors in intracellular B12 metabolism have been extensively studied and are excellently reviewed by Froese and Gravel 2010 [71]. These inherited disorders can have varying severity depending on the mutation and affected gene and can be diagnosed shortly after infancy or later in life. Dietary interventions are often recommended in order to improve patient quality of life and early intervention often improves patient outcomes, thus newborn screening for inherited metabolic disorders is common practice in the United States and other countries. While newborn screenings can expose metabolic disorders, infants are not commonly screened for B12 deficiency at birth, though serum B12 screening has gained support in recent years given the severe neurological consequences of infantile B12 deficiency [72,73].

3.2. *Developmental and Neurological Consequences of B9/B12 Deficiency*

Maternal micronutrient deficiencies can have long term repercussions on health of offspring. Both B9 and B12 deficiencies have been linked to adverse pregnancy outcomes, such as low birthweight, preterm delivery, and abruptio placentae [49]. Correlation between low folate or B12 levels and risk of neural tube defects (NTDs) has been well documented [74,75] and periconceptional vitamin supplements containing folic acid (FA) have been shown to significantly reduce NTDs [76–78]. FA supplementation reduces NTDs in mothers who had a previously affected pregnancy and in a double-blind prevention trial, oral supplementation with 4 mg of FA per day was shown to reduce recurrent risk of NTDs by 72% [79]. The Centers for Disease Control and Prevention (CDC) in the United States recommends that women who previously experienced NTDs in pregnancy supplement 4 mg of FA per day [80], equivalent to 10 times the recommended daily allowance (400 μg) for women of reproductive years [81].

While previous studies have observed correlations between increased serum folate and red blood cell folate levels with a decreased risk of NTDs [78], the mechanism of action of how FA prevents NTDs is not fully known. There have been studies describing several ways in which NTDs are driven by abnormal epigenetic modifications. Proper closure of the neural tube depends on gene silencing induced by DNA methylation and inadequate DNA methyl transferase (DNMT) activity and methylation cycle inhibitors can hinder this process [82]. Since B9 and B12 are linked to both NTDs and one-carbon metabolism, it has been hypothesized that defective one-carbon metabolism is the cause of the NTDs (Figure 2A). Environmental and maternal dietary factors play a crucial role in ensuring normal DNA methylation in the developing embryo, suggesting that folate and B12, key factors in one-carbon metabolism, are instrumental in preventing NTDs through their effects on methylation [82]. Novel discoveries also point to aberrant epigenetic modifications during neural tube development that directly link folate deficiency to NTDs. Inhibiting folate transport and metabolism causes DNA hypomethylation of the *Sox2* locus, leading to neural crest associated defects [83]. In addition, polymorphisms in one-carbon metabolism genes *MTHFR, MTR,* and *MTRR* have been implicated in the risk of developing NTDs [84,85]. However, a recent study found that an alternate mechanism may also be involved in the development of NTDs independently of one-carbon metabolism. Kim et al. found that folate and B12 are competitive antagonists of the aryl hydrocarbon receptor (AhR), a nuclear receptor that binds hydrocarbon compounds, like the poison dioxin, and induces expression not only of detoxifying enzymes, but also of homeostatic and developmental genes [86]. Loss of AhR antagonism by folate or B12 due to deficiency or activation of AhR by known agonists increases AhR activity and mimics symptoms of B9 and B12 deficiency [86]. This research generates a novel causative mechanism for NTDs that could have clinical implications.

B12 deficiency, in addition to NTDs, also affects adult brain function and is associated with other neurological consequences, including myelopathy, neuropathy, and nerve atrophy. These symptoms have been linked to MUT, the other enzyme that relies on B12 as a cofactor. B12 deficiency can lead to defective myelin synthesis due to decreased MUT activity, which causes incorporation of abnormal fatty acids into neuronal lipids [87]. The ensuing demyelination can lead to subacute combined degeneration (SCD) in the spinal cord, resulting in loss of sensation of vibration and proprioception. B12 deficiency has also been reported to cause some neuropsychiatric syndromes, including psychosis, mania, depression, and chronic fatigue syndrome [87]. In healthy elderly individuals and Alzheimer's patients, low B12 levels have also been correlated with decreased cognitive function [88]. The underlying mechanisms of these neuropsychiatric symptoms associated with B12 deficiency are unclear.

3.3. *Hematological Consequences of B9/B12 Deficiency*

The classical hematological symptom of folate or B12 deficiency is megaloblastic anemia. This anemia is macrocytic, in which the mean corpuscular volume of the erythrocytes is >100 fL and erythrocytes often exhibit anisocytosis. Neutrophils can also have hyper-segmented nuclei and leukopenia and thrombocytopenia may be present. In bone marrow, megaloblastic changes can be observed, with larger erythroblasts with granular nuclei and large granulocyte precursors [89]. This blastic change can even lead to the misdiagnosis of leukemia in B12-deficient patients [90,91] and is most often attributed to a maturation arrest of cells due to impaired DNA synthesis from altered one-carbon metabolism [89]. However, activation of the aryl hydrocarbon receptor, potentially from loss of antagonism due to B12 or folate deficiency, can also cause megaloblastic anemia [86], so this alternate mechanism must not be ruled out and can be explored further in clinical studies.

3.4. *One-Carbon Metabolism Defiencies and Colorectal Cancer*

Disruption of one-carbon metabolism can lead to decreased DNA synthesis, genomic instability, and decreased methyl donor production. Colorectal cancer (CRC) is associated with genomic instability and DNA hypomethylation [92]. Folate and B12 deficiency are also known to increase uracil incorporation into DNA, leading to DNA damage, which can result in the development of CRC [93,94] (Figure 2A). Clinical studies suggest an inverse relationship between folate or methionine intake and CRC risk [93,95,96]. One study found that colonic DNA hypomethylation in patients with CRC correlated with lower folate status, leading to the notion that low folate levels and DNA hypomethylation may be a risk factor in CRC [97]. Another study showed that higher genomic DNA methylation in their leukocytes was associated with a lower risk of colorectal adenomas, which are pre-cancerous lesions, but DNA methylation levels were not associated with folate intake [98]. Both studies provide evidence that hypomethylation could be an important factor in early colorectal carcinogenesis. However, there is not enough conclusive evidence to confirm whether DNA hypomethylation due to folate or B12 deficiency is a direct causal factor in the development of CRC. In addition, it has been shown that 5-azacitidine (5-aza), a DNA hypomethylating agent, has synergistic effects when given with a topoisomerase 1 inhibitor, irinotecan, for the treatment of CRC [99], further complicating the role of DNA methylation in CRC.

3.5. Non-Alcoholic Fatty Liver Diseases and One-Carbon Metabolism

The liver plays an important role in the absorption and storage of nutrients and proper liver function is essential for glucose, amino acid, and lipid metabolism. Alterations of dietary nutrients, such as B vitamins, could foreseeably impair proper liver physiology. In fact, altered one-carbon metabolism has been associated with the pathogenesis of nonalcoholic fatty liver disease (NAFLD). NAFLD affects nearly 30% of the population [100] and is characterized by lipid accumulation in the liver, causing increased inflammatory cytokine recruitment, altered resident macrophage function [101], oxidative stress, and even genetic and epigenetic alterations [102,103].

A methionine-choline deficient (MCD) diet has been a well-established model for inducing the full spectrum of NAFLD in rodent studies as methionine, folate, and B12 deficiency all have been linked to NAFLD [104,105] (Figure 2A). MCD mice display altered expression of genes involved in lipid metabolism, as well as elevated SAH and homocysteine levels [104,106] and even impaired mitochondrial function [102]. These studies suggest that disruptions in one-carbon metabolism may trigger the progression of NAFLD to non-alcoholic steatohepatitis (NASH) and eventually liver fibrosis by impairing very low density lipoproteins (VLDL) secretions from the liver [100]. One study in humans found that a choline-deficient diet led to the development of liver dysfunction in as little as 3 weeks [107], while another study showed that choline deficiency was associated with increased fibrosis amongst postmenopausal women [108]. Dietary supplementation of methyl-donors was found to halt progression of NAFLD in mice [109], emphasizing that proper one-carbon metabolism is essential for liver health.

While deficiencies of nutrients essential for one-carbon metabolism may be causing NAFLD due to decreased methyl-donor production or decreased DNA synthesis, other hypotheses are possible. Decreased levels of methyl donors, methionine, and choline could lead to monopolization of B12 by one-carbon metabolism-mediated recycling of methionine to compensate for the lack of these nutrients in the diet. The bias towards methionine recycling would limit the availability of B12 to activate MUT. The MUT enzyme is part of the propionate catabolic pathway, which controls the breakdown of branched-chain amino acids (isoleucine, methionine, threonine, and valine), odd-chain fatty acids, and cholesterol into succinyl-CoA for use by the TCA cycle. Both increased propionyl-CoA, a propionate pathway intermediate, and decreased MUT enzymatic activity have been linked to increased production of odd-chain fatty acid from BCAAs in adipocytes [110]. In fact, one study suggests that B12 deficiency can promote odd-chain fatty acid synthesis through accumulation of methyl-malonic acid, the substrate of MUT [111], and another found that B12 deficiency increases serum cholesterol and triglycerides and increases adiposity in mice [112]. These biological changes may impact the development of NAFLD and underline the importance of both B12 sufficiency and intact one-carbon metabolism for proper liver health.

3.6. Fortification and Supplementation for the Treatment of B9/B12 Deficiency

Folate and B12 deficiency have several detrimental effects in children, adults, and developing fetuses. NTDs are often untreatable, so in a preventative effort, the United States Food and Drug Administration (FDA) mandated the fortification of grain and flour products with FA, effective on

1 January 1998 [113]. Over 50 countries now have regulations for mandatory FA fortification, however, not all these programs have been implemented yet [114]. Dietary folates predominantly exist in polyglutamated forms and must undergo hydrolysis to monoglutamated forms for absorption in the jejunum. For this reason, FA is preferred for supplementation, because it does not require this conversion step [115]. After evaluating the impact of fortification on NTDs, specifically on spina bifida and anencephaly, one study found a 19% overall reduction in prevalence [116]. Another study reported a reduction of about 30% in NTDs for Hispanic and non-Hispanic white births [117].

While there is no mandatory fortification of grains and flour with B12, some foods and energy drinks are supplemented with B12. As a treatment for deficiency, B12 supplementation is achieved either via 1 mg oral dosing or 1 mg intramuscular injection. B12 is generally supplemented in the form of cyanocobalamin, but hydroxycobalamin is also used. These forms of B12 are converted intracellularly to the active forms methylcobalamin and adenosylcobalamin for the enzymes MS and MUT, respectively. Intramuscular injection results in much higher B12 serum levels than oral dosing [118], though even in situations of B12 malabsorption, oral supplementation with 1 mg can be sufficient to restore normal B12 levels [89].

FA or B12 supplementation can reverse megaloblastic anemia entirely depending on the deficiency, however, for some neurological changes associated with deficiency, the effects can be permanent. Furthermore, for those patients with neurological symptoms associated with deficiency, high doses of FA should be clinically assessed with caution [119] as FA supplementation can mask a B12 deficiency and a risk of long-term neurological damage if lack of folate was not the initial cause [80]. This is potentially due to competition of one-carbon metabolism and MUT for B12: if increased FA causes increased B12 demand for use in one-carbon metabolism, this could disrupt MUT enzymatic function, which is known to cause neurological symptoms.

4. The Role of Methionine, Folate, and B12 Excess in Disease Progression

The role of one-carbon metabolism deficiency has been widely studied in human health, however, the implications of excessive levels of these metabolites is less well known. In the case of folate and B12, there are no reports of direct toxicity of either excess folate or B12 consumption [12], however, there are growing concerns about an upper limit of supplementation. Analyses of FA-fortified foods have reported higher than expected levels of folate compared to the mandated amount by federal regulation and the amount listed on the nutrition labels, some even reaching 300% of reported levels [120]. After the mandatory fortification of foods with folate, a study found that serum levels of folate in the population were double what was predicted, leading to the hypothesis that many people were overconsuming folate-fortified foods [121]. Similarly, the average B12 intake in Americans is almost double the recommended daily intake, though increased intakes are recommended for pregnant women, elderly individuals, and those with potential or known B12 absorption issues [12]. Some multivitamins and energy drinks and supplements contain amounts of B12 greater than 1000 times the daily recommended intake. B12 administration is also available at certain "wellness" clinics around the United States (where intramuscular injections of B12 can cause serum level concentrations that exceed 10X the normal range [118]). A recent study by Arendt and Nexo showed that approximately 15% of hospitalized patients that had B12 measurements taken exhibited high serum levels of B12 [122]. In a separate study of 5771 patients, those with increased serum B12 levels (above 455 pg/mL or 336 pmol/L) had increased all-cause mortality upon follow-up [123]. Whether high B12 serum levels are causative or correlative with morbidity and mortality requires further investigation.

4.1. High Serum B9/B12 Levels and Cancer

Altered metabolism is a hallmark of cancer and targeting one-carbon metabolism has recently gained attention for the treatment of various malignancies. Increased folate serum levels may be associated with a higher risk of lung cancer [124], breast cancer [125], and even CRC [126], where low levels are also associated with increased CRC risk. Elevated B12 serum levels have also been associated with an increased risk of cancer within 1 year of follow-up in two large population-based studies [127,128]. Hypercobalaminemia has been observed in both solid and hematological malignancies at diagnosis [129] and is associated with an increased risk of prostate cancer [130] (Figure 2B).

In the previously mentioned large population studies, elevated serum B12 conveyed the highest risk of hematologic malignancies within 1 year of patient follow-up compared to all other cancers [127,128]. In fact, B12 levels have been known to be increased upon diagnosis in hematological malignancies for over 60 years [131–135]. This may be partially attributed to increased production of HC from cancer cells, leading to increased B12 binding in the serum and decreased cellular uptake [135–137]. Increased HC or TC production is also seen in hepatic and pancreatic cancers [138–140]. HC expression was recently found to be a negative prognostic biomarker in colon cancer and HC expression decreased after neoadjuvant chemotherapy [141]. Overexpression of HC is also associated with adverse outcomes and poor therapeutic response in rectal cancer [142]. Overall, increased HC levels may be falsely inflating B12 serum levels and could even be depriving tumors and normal tissues of sufficient B12. Future studies assessing B12 levels in cancer patients should include serum holoTC measurements as this is the only protein-bound B12 available for cellular uptake.

Since some cancers are associated with higher levels of serum micronutrients, it is relevant to address the influence of vitamin supplementation on cancer risk. B12 supplement intake is associated with increased lung cancer risk in men (not women), especially in smokers [143,144]. In a randomized trial, FA supplementation was associated with increased prostate cancer risk [145]. Supplementation with B12 and FA for 2–3 years has also been shown to increase the overall risk of cancer and risk of colorectal cancer in a randomized study [146]. This increase in cancer risk may be associated with increased folate-cycle driven metabolism, such as increasing nucleotide synthesis, to the benefit of rapidly dividing cancer cells. One could hypothesize a similar effect for methionine, but a recent meta-analysis comparing high plant protein intake to high animal protein intake found no change in cancer-associated mortality, though there was an increase in all-cause mortality with a high animal protein diet [147].

4.2. *Excess One-Carbon Metabolites in Immunity and Organ Function*

One-carbon metabolism controls DNA synthesis and methyl donor availability, which are essential for the normal function of cells in the immune system. Altered levels of one-carbon micronutrients, B9 and B12, are observed in both normal immune cells and hematological cancers. A study found that un-metabolized FA in the plasma was associated with a decrease in natural killer (NK) cell toxicity, suggesting that excess FA may be associated with immune dysfunction [148] (Figure 2B). Another recent study in mice found that both high and low FA levels impair hematopoiesis, resulting in DNA damage and compromised production of lymphocytes [149]. Rheumatoid arthritis (RA) and other inflammatory diseases have also been associated with hypercobalaminemia, potentially through increased TC in acute inflammation [129]. Conversely, Systemic Lupus Erythmatosus, another inflammatory condition, has recently been linked to lower B12 levels in a meta-analysis [150]. Whether excess of B12 in inflammatory diseases causes immune dysfunction as seen with excess folate requires further investigation.

Preservation of one-carbon cycling is important for solid organ function, as previously noted with the liver and NAFLD. The liver is involved in homeostasis of nutrients like B12, and both the liver and kidney store and excrete B12. Several clinical studies have found increased amounts of serum B12 in patients with liver diseases due to varying mechanisms. Acute hepatitis can lead to the release of stored B12 and decreased TC synthesis [151]. Cirrhosis is thought to cause decreased uptake of HC-bound B12 for excretion in bile and the severity of cirrhosis has been positively correlated to serum B12 levels [151]. Alcoholic liver disease is thought to increase the levels of HC and decrease levels of TC, leading to simultaneously decreased uptake of B12 and increased serum B12 levels [152]. High B12 levels have been associated with reduced kidney function [153], chronic kidney disease [154], and renal failure [155] due to unknown mechanisms. Further studies into the underlying mechanisms and effects of this increased B12 on disease initiation and progression are needed.

5. Targeting One-Carbon Metabolism for the Treatment of Disease

While the above research suggests that supplementation with FA and B12 could potentially be harmful, B12 supplementation, even in patients with normal serum B12 levels, has been explored to counteract certain neurological defects, given that B12 deficiency can cause neurological symptoms. B12 treatment does have potential as a therapy for peripheral neuropathic pain [156] and acute herpetic neuralgia [157,158]. This may be due to the restoration of MUT enzymatic activity, which is inversely associated with neuronal damage. However, excessive and prolonged B12 treatment, like in patients with B12 deficiency, can lead to antibodies against TC [159]. These antibodies permit B12 binding to TC, but limit cellular uptake of holoTC [159], ultimately raising serum B12 levels.

Since adequate B12 is vital for properly-functioning one-carbon metabolism, B12 supplementation has been hypothesized to impact DNA, RNA, and protein methylation. Indeed, administration of B12 has been shown to alter DNA methylation patterns in patients [160]. B12 supplementation has also been shown to promote DNA methylation changes and affect the antidepressant response in a mouse model [161]. Supplementation also restores hippocampal DNA methylation levels in rats with bacterial meningitis [162]. These studies suggest that B12 supplementation could be explored in scenarios where increased methylation potential is required, analogous to the FA supplementation of pregnant women to prevent NTDs.

5.1. *Folate and Methionine-Cycle Targeted Therapies*

One-carbon metabolism has an essential role in nucleic acid synthesis pathways, making it a powerful therapeutic target to slow down cellular proliferation in the treatment of cancer. In fact, some of the first chemotherapies were folate antagonists, known as anti-folates, which act as antiproliferative agents by inhibiting DHFR and disrupting DNA synthesis [163]. The anti-folate aminopterin was the first anti-folate shown to significantly reduce tumor burden in humans [164]. In 1948, the temporary remission of 10 out of 16 children with acute lymphoblastic leukemia (ALL) was observed after treatment with this drug [164]. Since this seminal study, folate antagonists have been used to treat an array of neoplasms, including various types of leukemia, Hodgkin's disease, lymphosarcoma, breast cancer, and prostate cancer [165]. The most successful anti-folate in chemotherapy to date is methotrexate (MTX), formerly known as a-methopterin. MTX used in high doses remains one of the most effective therapies for treatment of childhood ALL [166]. However, high-dose MTX treatment has been associated with hematological, gastrointestinal, and hepatic toxicity [167–169]. Because of these adverse effects, correct dosage and timing is essential in therapy. Further, 5-fluorouracil (5-FU), a uracil analog that inhibits TS, also disrupts the folate cycle and DNA synthesis and is used to treat several types of cancers [170]. Leucovorin, also known as folinic acid, is a derivative of the metabolically active THF that is often administered with MTX as it has been shown to mitigate toxicity and increase efficacy by providing a substrate to restore the folate cycle [169,171].

While high-dose MTX is commonly used in cancer treatment, low doses have been shown to be beneficial for the treatment of autoimmune disorders. RA patients treated with low-dose MTX exhibit a significant decrease in the number of tender or painful joints, the duration of morning stiffness, and an overall reduction in disease activity [172]. The mechanism of action of theses anti-inflammatory effects of MTX are not fully understood [173]. Studies have shown that one potential role for MTX in RA treatment could be through its ability to promote demethylation and increased expression of the FOXP3 gene. FOXP3 is an important transcriptional regulator for the differentiation of regulatory T cells, which are known to suppress inflammatory responses in RA patients [174,175]. Being a folate antagonist, MTX acts directly upstream of both nucleic acid synthesis and methionine recycling and therefore has the potential to influence methyltransferase activity and alter the epigenome.

Targeting the methionine cycle within one-carbon metabolism also has demonstrative therapeutic potential. Further, 5-aza and 5-aza-2′deoxycitidine (decitibine) are methylated cytadine analogs that act as DNMT1 inhibitors, which cause DNA hypomethylation and are used in MDS/AML patients. SAM analogs have been developed, which interfere with the enzymatic activity of histone methyltransferases and these drugs may also act as inhibitors of DNMTs and other protein or lipid methyltransferases or affect DNA repair mechanisms [176,177]. Compounds that block the conversion of methionine to SAM are currently being developed in order to disrupt the influence of one-carbon metabolism on the epigenome. However, in light of the myriad of studies describing a link between methionine deficiency and NAFLD, side-effects of interventions targeting the methionine cycle for long-term methionine deprivation should perhaps be approached with caution. In addition, the effects of over-/under-consumption of dietary folate and B12 as it affects one-carbon metabolism targeted therapies, such as 5-azacitidine or 5-FU, should also be explored.

Targeting B12, the cofactor for the rate limiting reaction of the folate- and methionine-cycles, appears an opportune strategy as high serum levels are associated with increased cancer risk. However, it is still not known whether these high serum levels are causative or correlative with disease. Expression levels of MTRR, the gene responsible for reducing B12 to its active form for use by MS, are increased in ovarian carcinoma and targeting MTRR using RNA interference has been shown to inhibit growth and cisplatin resistance in both in vitro and in vivo models, making it a potential target for therapy [178].

5.2. Dietary Interventions of One-Carbon Metabolism

Recently, there has been much interest in the influence of diet and lifestyle on human health and disease states. Nutritional deficits of micronutrients can alter cellular metabolism and cause phenotypic changes in humans, thus adjusting the intake of these nutrients could be exploited for therapeutic benefit. Cancer cells are known to have altered metabolism and increasing metabolic stress through nutrient deficiencies could be a suitable addition to current cancer therapies.

Studies in animal models have shown a therapeutic benefit to maintaining a methionine restricted (MR) diet, including an overall extension of lifespan [179–182]. The earliest reports from the Orentreich group showed that reducing dietary levels of methionine in rats increased longevity by 30–40% [179,181]. Other benefits include improved metabolism [181], decreased adiposity [183,184], and decreased inflammation and oxidative stress [180,185–191].

A reduction in dietary methionine has also been shown to influence the epigenome in mice due to changes in methyltransferase activity [45,192]. Aberrant DNA and histone methylation patterns are a hallmark of cancer [193–195] and many genetic and epigenetic functional studies have identified methyltransferases to be frequently mutated in all types of malignancies [196–201]. Recent studies highlight a potential therapeutic role for MR in cancer metabolism as many tumors exhibit a higher requirement for exogenous methionine, either due to an increased metabolic need for this amino acid in the maintenance of accelerated tumor growth or due to poor methionine recycling from homocysteine [202,203]. This enhanced metabolic need for methionine in cancer cells can be targeted by restricting methionine availability in the diet or by specifically targeting enzymes and cofactors of the methionine cycle. Sugimura et al. was the first to report anti-tumor effects of an MR diet [204] in 1959 and since then, the field has exploded with different potential interventional avenues. In vitro cell culture models using numerous cancer cell lines or primary patient tumor cells showed that many were intrinsically sensitive to low methionine levels [205–207]. Studies using patient-derived xenografts (PDX) models of colorectal cancer [48], prostate cancer [208,209], and pre-malignant breast cancer [210] have all shown that MR also suppressed tumor growth *in vivo*. In a PDX model of colorectal cancer, it was found that the beneficial effect of MR may be through alteration of one-carbon metabolism flux, specifically in regard to redox and nucleotide balance that in combination with antimetabolite or radiation therapy, inhibits tumor growth [48]. MR has also been effective in reducing metastasis in animal models of breast cancer [211] and melanoma [212]. Clinical studies investigating the role of MR in diseases such as cancer are still limited. However, it has been shown that short-term MR in patients with gastric tumors in conjunction with 5-FU has a synergistic effect on reducing TS activity, tumor volume, and weight [213].

While FA fortification has been successful in the prevention of NTDs, studies suggest that both low and high FA may negatively alter immune function. Therefore, consumption of FA should be approached with caution, especially since fortified foods contain more folate than reported levels [120] and people are consuming more than expected [121]. High levels of FA supplementation may be necessary for women of reproductive years, however, monitoring folate levels in blood cell maintenance and malignancy may also be necessary. The influence of folate on the epigenome, specifically DNA methylation in cancer, highlights the need for closely monitoring folate levels in cancer patients. Other than CRC, it is not yet clear whether folate levels can influence cancer initiation or progression in other lineages.

In the case of B12, dietary intervention studies are currently lacking, which warrants investigation. A limited amount of studies have reported no significant reduction in cancer mortality in vegans and vegetarians [214], who likely have decreased B12 serum levels due to lack of meat consumption. However, many vegan and vegetarian individuals take B12 supplements to maintain B12 serum levels. Interestingly, the G allele of a polymorphism in MTRR (A66G) decreases its enzymatic activity and reduces conversion of homocysteine to methionine [215,216], effectively mimicking the effect of reduced B12 availability on one-carbon metabolism. The GG genotype is associated with decreased leukemia risk in Caucasians and children, especially for acute lymphoblastic leukemia [217]. Pooled data from 85 studies show that the homozygosity for the G allele in this MTRR A66G polymorphism is associated with increased overall cancer susceptibility [218]. These genetic studies strengthen the need for more exploration into the effects of B12-deficient diets on cancer outcomes.

6. Conclusions and Future Directions

One-carbon metabolism is essential for cellular function and relies on B vitamins to drive and coordinate the generation of methyl groups for a myriad of biological outcomes. Alterations in one-carbon metabolism can be caused by B vitamin deficiencies, leading to developmental, neurological, and hematological consequences. The importance of one-carbon metabolism and the epigenome has been given renewed attention, given that epigenetic dysregulation is a hallmark of many types of cancer, including solid tumors and blood cell malignancies. B vitamins can also influence other diseases that involve aberrant immune responses, as evidenced by the epigenetic block observed in regulatory T cell maturation in patients with arthritis, which can be overcome by inhibiting the folate cycle. The production of methyl donors from the methionine cycle that maintains histone methylation patterns specific to cancer cells also provides the opportunity to target these essential metabolic components specifically for the treatment of cancer [219]. However, the systemic bioavailability of these micronutrients needs to be considered when targeting one-carbon metabolism. For instance, tumor cell-intrinsic effects may be at odds with effects on the tumor microenvironment, as is potentially the case for colon cancer, where DNA hypomethylation is observed in the cancerous colonic epithelia while the surrounding immune cells of these tumors exhibit DNA hypermethylation. In the context of tumor immunology, the levels of these micronutrients could therefore have important implications and complicate treatment strategies. Both dietary and pharmacological interventions should also be explored in future studies to determine the impact of B vitamins and methionine on disease initiation and progression in order to fully understand how one-carbon metabolism plays a role in human health.

Author Contributions: Conceptualization, L.C.; writing—original draft preparation, P.L., V.S., and B.F.; writing—review and editing, P.L., V.S., B.F., and L.C. All authors have read and agreed to the published version of the manuscript.

References

1. Chen, C.; Nott, T.J.; Jin, J.; Pawson, T. Deciphering arginine methylation: Tudor tells the tale. *Nat. Rev. Mol. Cell Biol.* **2011**, *12*, 629–642. [CrossRef] [PubMed]
2. Landgraf, B.J.; McCarthy, E.L.; Booker, S.J. Radical S-Adenosylmethionine Enzymes in Human Health and Disease. *Annu. Rev. Biochem.* **2016**, *85*, 485–514. [CrossRef] [PubMed]
3. Teperino, R.; Schoonjans, K.; Auwerx, J. Histone methyl transferases and demethylases; can they link metabolism and transcription? *Cell Metab.* **2010**, *12*, 321–327. [CrossRef] [PubMed]
4. Yang, Y.; Bedford, M.T. Protein arginine methyltransferases and cancer. *Nat. Rev. Cancer* **2013**, *13*, 37–50. [CrossRef] [PubMed]
5. Zeisel, S. Choline, Other Methyl-Donors and Epigenetics. *Nutrients* **2017**, *9*, 445. [CrossRef] [PubMed]
6. Lanouette, S.; Mongeon, V.; Figeys, D.; Couture, J.-F. The functional diversity of protein lysine methylation. *Mol. Syst. Biol.* **2014**, *10*, 724. [CrossRef] [PubMed]
7. Chiuve, S.E.; Giovannucci, E.L.; Hankinson, S.E.; Zeisel, S.H.; Dougherty, L.W.; Willett, W.C.; Rimm, E.B. The association between betaine and choline intakes and the plasma concentrations of homocysteine in women. *Am. J. Clin. Nutr.* **2007**, *86*, 1073–1081. [CrossRef]
8. Guéant, J.-L.; Oussalah, A.; Zgheib, R.; Siblini, Y.; Hsu, S.B.; Namour, F. Genetic, epigenetic and genomic mechanisms of methionine dependency of cancer and tumor-initiating cells: What could we learn from folate and methionine cycles. *Biochimie* **2020**, *173*, 123–128. [CrossRef]
9. Guillamot, M.; Cimmino, L.; Aifantis, I. The Impact of DNA Methylation in Hematopoietic Malignancies. *Trends Cancer* **2016**, *2*, 70–83. [CrossRef]
10. Green, R.; Allen, L.H.; Bjørke-Monsen, A.-L.; Brito, A.; Guéant, J.-L.; Miller, J.W.; Molloy, A.M.; Nexo, E.; Stabler, S.; Toh, B.-H.; et al. Vitamin B12 deficiency. *Nat. Rev. Dis. Primers* **2017**, *3*, 17040. [CrossRef]
11. Kerns, J.C.; Gutierrez, J.L. Thiamin. *Adv. Nutr.* **2017**, *8*, 395–397. [CrossRef] [PubMed]
12. Institute of Medicine (US) Standing Committee on the Scientific Evaluation of Dietary Reference Intakes and its Panel on Folate, Other B Vitamins, and Choline. The National Academies Collection: Reports funded by National Institutes of Health. In *Dietary Reference Intakes for Thiamin, Riboflavin, Niacin, Vitamin B6, Folate, Vitamin B12, Pantothenic Acid, Biotin, and Choline*; National Academies Press (US): Washington, DC, USA, 1998. [CrossRef]
13. Sauve, A.A. NAD^+ and vitamin B3: From metabolism to therapies. *J. Pharmacol. Exp. Ther.* **2008**, *324*, 883–893. [CrossRef] [PubMed]
14. Plesofsky-Vig, N.; Brambl, R. Pantothenic acid and coenzyme A in cellular modification of proteins. *Annu. Rev. Nutr.* **1988**, *8*, 461–482. [CrossRef] [PubMed]
15. Ueland, P.M.; Ulvik, A.; Rios-Avila, L.; Midttun, Ø.; Gregory, J.F. Direct and Functional Biomarkers of Vitamin B6 Status. *Annu. Rev. Nutr.* **2015**, *35*, 33–70. [CrossRef]
16. McMahon, R.J. Biotin in metabolism and molecular biology. *Annu. Rev. Nutr.* **2002**, *22*, 221–239. [CrossRef]
17. Tong, X.; Zhao, F.; Thompson, C.B. The molecular determinants of de novo nucleotide biosynthesis in cancer cells. *Curr. Opin. Genet. Dev.* **2009**, *19*, 32–37. [CrossRef]
18. Deberardinis, R.J.; Sayed, N.; Ditsworth, D.; Thompson, C.B. Brick by brick: Metabolism and tumor cell growth. *Curr. Opin. Genet. Dev.* **2008**, *18*, 54–61. [CrossRef]
19. Vander Heiden, M.G.; Lunt, S.Y.; Dayton, T.L.; Fiske, B.P.; Israelsen, W.J.; Mattaini, K.R.; Vokes, N.I.; Stephanopoulos, G.; Cantley, L.C.; Metallo, C.M.; et al. Metabolic pathway alterations that support cell proliferation. *Cold Spring Harb. Symp. Quant. Biol.* **2011**, *76*, 325–334. [CrossRef]
20. Methionine in National Center for Biotechnology Information. PubChem Database. Available online: https://pubchem.ncbi.nlm.nih.gov/compound/6137 (accessed on 15 September 2020).
21. Mastrototaro, L.; Sponder, G.; Saremi, B.; Aschenbach, J.R. Gastrointestinal methionine shuttle: Priority handling of precious goods. *IUBMB Life* **2016**, *68*, 924–934. [CrossRef]
22. Zhao, R.; Matherly, L.H.; Goldman, I.D. Membrane transporters and folate homeostasis: Intestinal absorption and transport into systemic compartments and tissues. *Expert Rev. Mol. Med.* **2009**, *11*, e4. [CrossRef]
23. Antony, A.C. Folate receptors. *Annu. Rev. Nutr.* **1996**, *16*, 501–521. [CrossRef] [PubMed]
24. Watanabe, F.; Bito, T. Vitamin B12 sources and microbial interaction. *Exp. Biol. Med.* **2018**, *243*, 148–158. [CrossRef] [PubMed]

25. Watanabe, F. Vitamin B12 sources and bioavailability. *Exp. Biol. Med.* **2007**, *232*, 1266–1274. [CrossRef] [PubMed]
26. Xie, C.; Coda, R.; Chamlagain, B.; Varmanen, P.; Piironen, V.; Katina, K. Co-fermentation of Propionibacterium freudenreichii and Lactobacillus brevis in Wheat Bran for in situ Production of Vitamin B12. *Front. Microbiol.* **2019**, *10*, 1541. [CrossRef] [PubMed]
27. Kozyraki, R.; Cases, O. Vitamin B12 absorption: Mammalian physiology and acquired and inherited disorders. *Biochimie* **2013**, *95*, 1002–1007. [CrossRef] [PubMed]
28. Gailus, S.; Höhne, W.; Gasnier, B.; Nürnberg, P.; Fowler, B.; Rutsch, F. Insights into lysosomal cobalamin trafficking: Lessons learned from cblF disease. *J. Mol. Med.* **2010**, *88*, 459–466. [CrossRef] [PubMed]
29. Coelho, D.; Kim, J.C.; Miousse, I.R.; Fung, S.; du Moulin, M.; Buers, I.; Suormala, T.; Burda, P.; Frapolli, M.; Stucki, M.; et al. Mutations in ABCD4 cause a new inborn error of vitamin B12 metabolism. *Nat. Genet.* **2012**, *44*, 1152–1155. [CrossRef]
30. Alam, A.; Woo, J.-S.; Schmitz, J.; Prinz, B.; Root, K.; Chen, F.; Bloch, J.S.; Zenobi, R.; Locher, K.P. Structural basis of transcobalamin recognition by human CD320 receptor. *Nat. Commun.* **2016**, *7*, 12100. [CrossRef]
31. Cai, X.C.; Kapilashrami, K.; Luo, M. Synthesis and Assays of Inhibitors of Methyltransferases. *Methods Enzymol.* **2016**, *574*, 245–308. [CrossRef]
32. Chaturvedi, S.; Hoffman, R.M.; Bertino, J.R. Exploiting methionine restriction for cancer treatment. *Biochem. Pharmacol.* **2018**, *154*, 170–173. [CrossRef]
33. Koutmos, M.; Datta, S.; Pattridge, K.A.; Smith, J.L.; Matthews, R.G. Insights into the reactivation of cobalamin-dependent methionine synthase. *Proc. Natl. Acad. Sci. USA* **2009**, *106*, 18527–18532. [CrossRef] [PubMed]
34. Lu, S.C. Glutathione synthesis. *Biochim. Biophys. Acta* **2013**, *1830*, 3143–3153. [CrossRef] [PubMed]
35. Wongkittichote, P.; Cunningham, G.; Summar, M.L.; Pumbo, E.; Forny, P.; Baumgartner, M.R.; Chapman, K.A. Tricarboxylic acid cycle enzyme activities in a mouse model of methylmalonic aciduria. *Mol. Genet. Metab.* **2019**, *128*, 444–451. [CrossRef] [PubMed]
36. Costanzo, M.; Caterino, M.; Cevenini, A.; Jung, V.; Chhuon, C.; Lipecka, J.; Fedele, R.; Guerrera, I.C.; Ruoppolo, M. Proteomics Reveals that Methylmalonyl-CoA Mutase Modulates Cell Architecture and Increases Susceptibility to Stress. *Int. J. Mol. Sci.* **2020**, *21*, 4998. [CrossRef]
37. Costanzo, M.; Cevenini, A.; Marchese, E.; Imperlini, E.; Raia, M.; Del Vecchio, L.; Caterino, M.; Ruoppolo, M. Label-Free Quantitative Proteomics in a Methylmalonyl-CoA Mutase-Silenced Neuroblastoma Cell Line. *Int. J. Mol. Sci.* **2018**, *19*, 3580. [CrossRef] [PubMed]
38. Huang, R.-F.S.; Ho, Y.-H.; Lin, H.-L.; Wei, J.-S.; Liu, T.-Z. Folate Deficiency Induces a Cell Cycle-Specific Apoptosis in HepG2 Cells. *J. Nutr.* **1999**, *129*, 25–31. [CrossRef]
39. Yang, Y.; Li, X.; Sun, Q.; He, B.; Jia, Y.; Cai, D.; Zhao, R. Folate deprivation induces cell cycle arrest at G0/G1 phase and apoptosis in hippocampal neuron cells through down-regulation of IGF-1 signaling pathway. *Int. J. Biochem. Cell Biol.* **2016**, *79*, 222–230. [CrossRef]
40. Battaglia-Hsu, S.F.; Akchiche, N.; Noel, N.; Alberto, J.M.; Jeannesson, E.; Orozco-Barrios, C.E.; Martinez-Fong, D.; Daval, J.L.; Gueant, J.L. Vitamin B12 deficiency reduces proliferation and promotes differentiation of neuroblastoma cells and up-regulates PP2A, proNGF, and TACE. *Proc. Natl. Acad. Sci. USA* **2009**, *106*, 21930–21935. [CrossRef]
41. Shiraki, N.; Shiraki, Y.; Tsuyama, T.; Obata, F.; Miura, M.; Nagae, G.; Aburatani, H.; Kume, K.; Endo, F.; Kume, S. Methionine Metabolism Regulates Maintenance and Differentiation of Human Pluripotent Stem Cells. *Cell Metab.* **2014**, *19*, 780–794. [CrossRef]
42. Choi, S.W.; Friso, S.; Ghandour, H.; Bagley, P.J.; Selhub, J.; Mason, J.B. Vitamin B-12 deficiency induces anomalies of base substitution and methylation in the DNA of rat colonic epithelium. *J. Nutr.* **2004**, *134*, 750–755. [CrossRef]
43. Fernandez-Roig, S.; Lai, S.C.; Murphy, M.M.; Fernandez-Ballart, J.; Quadros, E.V. Vitamin B12 deficiency in the brain leads to DNA hypomethylation in the TCblR/CD320 knockout mouse. *Nutr. Metab.* **2012**, *9*, 41. [CrossRef] [PubMed]
44. Jacob, R.A.; Gretz, D.M.; Taylor, P.C.; James, S.J.; Pogribny, I.P.; Miller, B.J.; Henning, S.M.; Swendseid, M.E. Moderate folate depletion increases plasma homocysteine and decreases lymphocyte DNA methylation in postmenopausal women. *J. Nutr.* **1998**, *128*, 1204–1212. [CrossRef] [PubMed]

45. Mentch, S.J.; Mehrmohamadi, M.; Huang, L.; Liu, X.; Gupta, D.; Mattocks, D.; Gomez Padilla, P.; Ables, G.; Bamman, M.M.; Thalacker-Mercer, A.E.; et al. Histone Methylation Dynamics and Gene Regulation Occur through the Sensing of One-Carbon Metabolism. *Cell Metab.* **2015**, *22*, 861–873. [CrossRef] [PubMed]
46. Battaglia-Hsu, S.F.; Ghemrawi, R.; Coelho, D.; Dreumont, N.; Mosca, P.; Hergalant, S.; Gauchotte, G.; Sequeira, J.M.; Ndiongue, M.; Houlgatte, R.; et al. Inherited disorders of cobalamin metabolism disrupt nucleocytoplasmic transport of mRNA through impaired methylation/phosphorylation of ELAVL1/HuR. *Nucleic Acids Res.* **2018**, *46*, 7844–7857. [CrossRef] [PubMed]
47. Ghemrawi, R.; Arnold, C.; Battaglia-Hsu, S.F.; Pourié, G.; Trinh, I.; Bassila, C.; Rashka, C.; Wiedemann, A.; Flayac, J.; Robert, A.; et al. SIRT1 activation rescues the mislocalization of RNA-binding proteins and cognitive defects induced by inherited cobalamin disorders. *Metabolism* **2019**, *101*, 153992. [CrossRef] [PubMed]
48. Gao, X.; Sanderson, S.M.; Dai, Z.; Reid, M.A.; Cooper, D.E.; Lu, M.; Richie, J.P., Jr.; Ciccarella, A.; Calcagnotto, A.; Mikhael, P.G.; et al. Dietary methionine influences therapy in mouse cancer models and alters human metabolism. *Nature* **2019**, *572*, 397–401. [CrossRef]
49. Molloy, A.M.; Kirke, P.N.; Brody, L.C.; Scott, J.M.; Mills, J.L. Effects of folate and vitamin B12 deficiencies during pregnancy on fetal, infant, and child development. *Food Nutr. Bull.* **2008**, *29*, S101–S111, discussion S112–S115. [CrossRef]
50. Bailey, R.L.; Carmel, R.; Green, R.; Pfeiffer, C.M.; Cogswell, M.E.; Osterloh, J.D.; Sempos, C.T.; Yetley, E.A. Monitoring of vitamin B-12 nutritional status in the United States by using plasma methylmalonic acid and serum vitamin B-12. *Am. J. Clin. Nutr.* **2011**, *94*, 552–561. [CrossRef]
51. Rickes, E.L.; Brink, N.G.; Koniuszy, F.R.; Wood, T.R.; Folkers, K. Crystalline Vitamin B12. *Science* **1948**, *107*, 396. [CrossRef]
52. Smith, E.L. Purification of Anti-pernicious Anæmia Factors from Liver. *Nature* **1948**, *161*, 638–639. [CrossRef]
53. Lahner, E.; Annibale, B. Pernicious anemia: New insights from a gastroenterological point of view. *World J. Gastroenterol.* **2009**, *15*, 5121–5128. [CrossRef] [PubMed]
54. Vuylsteke, P.; Bertrand, C.; Verhoef, G.E.; Vandenberghe, P. Case of megaloblastic anemia caused by intestinal taeniasis. *Ann. Hematol.* **2004**, *83*, 487–488. [CrossRef] [PubMed]
55. Cordingley, F.T.; Crawford, G.P. Giardia infection causes vitamin B12 deficiency. *Aust. N. Z. J. Med.* **1986**, *16*, 78–79. [CrossRef]
56. Quigley, E.M.; Murray, J.A.; Pimentel, M. AGA Clinical Practice Update on Small Intestinal Bacterial Overgrowth: Expert Review. *Gastroenterology* **2020**. [CrossRef] [PubMed]
57. Premkumar, M.; Gupta, N.; Singh, T.; Velpandian, T. Cobalamin and folic Acid status in relation to the etiopathogenesis of pancytopenia in adults at a tertiary care centre in north India. *Anemia* **2012**, *2012*, 707402. [CrossRef] [PubMed]
58. Aroda, V.R.; Edelstein, S.L.; Goldberg, R.B.; Knowler, W.C.; Marcovina, S.M.; Orchard, T.J.; Bray, G.A.; Schade, D.S.; Temprosa, M.G.; White, N.H.; et al. Long-term Metformin Use and Vitamin B12 Deficiency in the Diabetes Prevention Program Outcomes Study. *J. Clin. Endocrinol. Metab.* **2016**, *101*, 1754–1761. [CrossRef]
59. Bauman, W.A.; Shaw, S.; Jayatilleke, E.; Spungen, A.M.; Herbert, V. Increased intake of calcium reverses vitamin B12 malabsorption induced by metformin. *Diabetes Care* **2000**, *23*, 1227–1231. [CrossRef]
60. Lam, J.R.; Schneider, J.L.; Zhao, W.; Corley, D.A. Proton pump inhibitor and histamine 2 receptor antagonist use and vitamin B12 deficiency. *JAMA* **2013**, *310*, 2435–2442. [CrossRef]
61. Andersen, K.J.; Schjønsby, H. Intrinsic factor-mediated binding of cyanocobalamin to cholestyramine. *J. Pharm. Sci.* **1978**, *67*, 1626–1627. [CrossRef]
62. Amess, J.A.; Burman, J.F.; Rees, G.M.; Nancekievill, D.G.; Mollin, D.L. Megaloblastic haemopoiesis in patients receiving nitrous oxide. *Lancet* **1978**, *2*, 339–342. [CrossRef]
63. Danishpajooh, I.O.; Gudi, T.; Chen, Y.; Kharitonov, V.G.; Sharma, V.S.; Boss, G.R. Nitric oxide inhibits methionine synthase activity in vivo and disrupts carbon flow through the folate pathway. *J. Biol. Chem.* **2001**, *276*, 27296–27303. [CrossRef] [PubMed]
64. Drummond, J.T.; Matthews, R.G. Nitrous oxide degradation by cobalamin-dependent methionine synthase: Characterization of the reactants and products in the inactivation reaction. *Biochemistry* **1994**, *33*, 3732–3741. [CrossRef] [PubMed]

65. Deacon, R.; Lumb, M.; Perry, J.; Chanarin, I.; Minty, B.; Halsey, M.J.; Nunn, J.F. Selective inactivation of vitamin B12 in rats by nitrous oxide. *Lancet* **1978**, *2*, 1023–1024. [CrossRef]
66. Hu, Y.; Raffield, L.M.; Polfus, L.M.; Moscati, A.; Nadkarni, G.; Preuss, M.H.; Zhong, X.; Wei, Q.; Rich, S.S.; Li, Y.; et al. A common TCN1 loss-of-function variant is associated with lower vitamin B12 concentration in African Americans. *Blood* **2018**, *131*, 2859–2863. [CrossRef] [PubMed]
67. Namour, F.; Olivier, J.-L.; Abdelmouttaleb, I.; Adjalla, C.; Debard, R.; Salvat, C.; Guéant, J.-L. Transcobalamin codon 259 polymorphism in HT-29 and Caco-2 cells and in Caucasians: Relation to transcobalamin and homocysteine concentration in blood. *Blood J. Am. Soc. Hematol.* **2001**, *97*, 1092–1098. [CrossRef]
68. Guéant, J.-L.; Chabi, N.W.; Guéant-Rodriguez, R.-M.; Mutchinick, O.M.; Debard, R.; Payet, C.; Lu, X.; Villaume, C.; Bronowicki, J.-P.; Quadros, E.V.; et al. Environmental influence on the worldwide prevalence of a 776C→G variant in the transcobalamin gene (*TCN2*). *J. Med Genet.* **2007**, *44*, 363. [CrossRef]
69. Serrano, M.; Pérez-Dueñas, B.; Montoya, J.; Ormazabal, A.; Artuch, R. Genetic causes of cerebral folate deficiency: Clinical, biochemical and therapeutic aspects. *Drug Discov. Today* **2012**, *17*, 1299–1306. [CrossRef]
70. Steele, J.W.; Kim, S.-E.; Finnell, R.H. One-carbon metabolism and folate transporter genes: Do they factor prominently in the genetic etiology of neural tube defects? *Biochimie* **2020**, *173*, 27–32. [CrossRef]
71. Froese, D.S.; Gravel, R.A. Genetic disorders of vitamin B_{12} metabolism: Eight complementation groups—Eight genes. *Expert Rev. Mol. Med.* **2010**, *12*, e37. [CrossRef]
72. Sarafoglou, K.; Rodgers, J.; Hietala, A.; Matern, D.; Bentler, K. Expanded Newborn Screening for Detection of Vitamin B_{12} Deficiency. *JAMA* **2011**, *305*, 1198–1200. [CrossRef]
73. Gramer, G.; Fang-Hoffmann, J.; Feyh, P.; Klinke, G.; Monostori, P.; Mütze, U.; Posset, R.; Weiss, K.H.; Hoffmann, G.F.; Okun, J.G. Newborn Screening for Vitamin B_{12} Deficiency in Germany Strategies, Results, and Public Health Implications. *J. Pediatr.* **2020**, *216*, 165–172.e4. [CrossRef]
74. Smithells, R.W.; Sheppard, S.; Schorah, C.J. Vitamin deficiencies and neural tube defects. *Arch. Dis. Child.* **1976**, *51*, 944–950. [CrossRef] [PubMed]
75. Crider, K.S.; Bailey, L.B.; Berry, R.J. Folic acid food fortification-its history, effect, concerns, and future directions. *Nutrients* **2011**, *3*, 370–384. [CrossRef] [PubMed]
76. Smithells, R.W.; Sheppard, S.; Schorah, C.J.; Seller, M.J.; Nevin, N.C.; Harris, R.; Read, A.P.; Fielding, D.W. Possible prevention of neural-tube defects by periconceptional vitamin supplementation. *Lancet* **1980**, *1*, 339–340. [CrossRef]
77. Laurence, K.M.; James, N.; Miller, M.H.; Tennant, G.B.; Campbell, H. Double-blind randomised controlled trial of folate treatment before conception to prevent recurrence of neural-tube defects. *Br. Med. J. (Clin. Res. Ed.)* **1981**, *282*, 1509–1511. [CrossRef] [PubMed]
78. Czeizel, A.E.; Dudas, I. Prevention of the first occurrence of neural-tube defects by periconceptional vitamin supplementation. *N. Engl. J. Med.* **1992**, *327*, 1832–1835. [CrossRef]
79. MRC Vitamin Study Research Group. Prevention of neural tube defects: Results of the Medical Research Council Vitamin Study. *Lancet* **1991**, *338*, 131–137. [CrossRef]
80. Centers for Disease Control. Use of folic acid for prevention of spina bifida and other neural tube defects—1983–1991. *MMWR Morb. Mortal. Wkly. Rep.* **1991**, *40*, 513–516.
81. Centers for Disease Control. Recommendations for the Use of Folic Acid to Reduce the Number of Cases of Spina Bifida and Other Neural Tube Defects. *MMWR Recomm. Rep.* **1992**, *41*, 1–7.
82. Greene, N.D.; Stanier, P.; Moore, G.E. The emerging role of epigenetic mechanisms in the etiology of neural tube defects. *Epigenetics* **2011**, *6*, 875–883. [CrossRef]
83. Alata Jimenez, N.; Torres Pérez, S.A.; Sánchez-Vásquez, E.; Fernandino, J.I.; Strobl-Mazzulla, P.H. Folate deficiency prevents neural crest fate by disturbing the epigenetic Sox2 repression on the dorsal neural tube. *Dev. Biol.* **2018**, *444*, S193–S201. [CrossRef] [PubMed]
84. Botto, L.D.; Yang, Q. 5,10-Methylenetetrahydrofolate reductase gene variants and congenital anomalies: A HuGE review. *Am. J. Epidemiol.* **2000**, *151*, 862–877. [CrossRef]
85. Imbard, A.; Benoist, J.-F.; Blom, H.J. Neural tube defects, folic acid and methylation. *Int. J. Environ. Res. Public Health* **2013**, *10*, 4352–4389. [CrossRef]
86. Kim, D.J.; Venkataraman, A.; Jain, P.C.; Wiesler, E.P.; DeBlasio, M.; Klein, J.; Tu, S.S.; Lee, S.; Medzhitov, R.; Iwasaki, A. Vitamin B_{12} and folic acid alleviate symptoms of nutritional deficiency by antagonizing aryl hydrocarbon receptor. *Proc. Natl. Acad. Sci. USA* **2020**, *117*, 15837–15845. [CrossRef] [PubMed]

87. Briani, C.; Dalla Torre, C.; Citton, V.; Manara, R.; Pompanin, S.; Binotto, G.; Adami, F. Cobalamin deficiency: Clinical picture and radiological findings. *Nutrients* **2013**, *5*, 4521–4539. [CrossRef] [PubMed]
88. Whyte, E.M.; Mulsant, B.H.; Butters, M.A.; Qayyum, M.; Towers, A.; Sweet, R.A.; Klunk, W.; Wisniewski, S.; DeKosky, S.T. Cognitive and behavioral correlates of low vitamin B12 levels in elderly patients with progressive dementia. *Am. J. Geriatr. Psychiatry* **2002**, *10*, 321–327. [CrossRef] [PubMed]
89. Green, R. Vitamin B12 deficiency from the perspective of a practicing hematologist. *Blood* **2017**, *129*, 2603–2611. [CrossRef] [PubMed]
90. Konda, M.; Godbole, A.; Pandey, S.; Sasapu, A. Vitamin B_{12} deficiency mimicking acute leukemia. *Proceedings (Bayl. Univ. Med. Cent.)* **2019**, *32*, 589–592. [CrossRef]
91. Singh, N.; Qayyum, S.; Wasik, M.A.; Luger, S.M. Combined B12 and folate deficiency presenting as an aggressive hematologic malignancy. *Am. J. Hematol.* **2015**, *90*, 964–965. [CrossRef]
92. Feinberg, A.P.; Gehrke, C.W.; Kuo, K.C.; Ehrlich, M. Reduced genomic 5-methylcytosine content in human colonic neoplasia. *Cancer Res.* **1988**, *48*, 1159–1161.
93. Friso, S.; Choi, S.W. The potential cocarcinogenic effect of vitamin B_{12} deficiency. *Clin. Chem. Lab. Med.* **2005**, *43*, 1158–1163. [CrossRef] [PubMed]
94. Duthie, S.J. Folate and cancer: How DNA damage, repair and methylation impact on colon carcinogenesis. *J. Inherit. Metab. Dis.* **2011**, *34*, 101–109. [CrossRef] [PubMed]
95. Kim, Y.I. Folate and colorectal cancer: An evidence-based critical review. *Mol. Nutr. Food Res.* **2007**, *51*, 267–292. [CrossRef] [PubMed]
96. Zhou, Z.-Y.; Wan, X.-Y.; Cao, J.-W. Dietary Methionine Intake and Risk of Incident Colorectal Cancer: A Meta-Analysis of 8 Prospective Studies Involving 431,029 Participants. *PLoS ONE* **2013**, *8*, e83588. [CrossRef]
97. Pufulete, M.; Al-Ghnaniem, R.; Leather, A.J.; Appleby, P.; Gout, S.; Terry, C.; Emery, P.W.; Sanders, T.A. Folate status, genomic DNA hypomethylation, and risk of colorectal adenoma and cancer: A case control study. *Gastroenterology* **2003**, *124*, 1240–1248. [CrossRef]
98. Lim, U.; Flood, A.; Choi, S.W.; Albanes, D.; Cross, A.J.; Schatzkin, A.; Sinha, R.; Katki, H.A.; Cash, B.; Schoenfeld, P.; et al. Genomic methylation of leukocyte DNA in relation to colorectal adenoma among asymptomatic women. *Gastroenterology* **2008**, *134*, 47–55. [CrossRef] [PubMed]
99. 99. Sharma, A.; Vatapalli, R.; Abdelfatah, E.; Wyatt McMahon, K.; Kerner, Z.; Guzzetta, A.; Singh, J.; Zahnow, C.; Baylin, S.B.; Yerram, S.; et al. Hypomethylating agents synergize with irinotecan to improve response to chemotherapy in colorectal cancer cells. *PLoS ONE* **2017**, *12*, e0176139. [CrossRef]
100. Radziejewska, A.; Muzsik, A.; Milagro, F.I.; Martínez, J.A.; Chmurzynska, A. One-Carbon Metabolism and Nonalcoholic Fatty Liver Disease: The Crosstalk between Nutrients, Microbiota, and Genetics. *Lifestyle Genom.* **2020**, *13*, 53–63. [CrossRef]
101. Stahl, E.C.; Haschak, M.J.; Popovic, B.; Brown, B.N. Macrophages in the Aging Liver and Age-Related Liver Disease. *Front. Immunol.* **2018**, *9*, 2795. [CrossRef]
102. Eudy, B.J.; McDermott, C.E.; Fernandez, G.; Mathews, C.E.; Lai, J.; da Silva, R.P. Disruption of hepatic one-carbon metabolism impairs mitochondrial function and enhances macrophage activity in methionine-choline-deficient mice. *J. Nutr. Biochem.* **2020**, *81*, 108381. [CrossRef]
103. Kim, S.H.; Lim, Y.; Park, J.B.; Kwak, J.-H.; Kim, K.-J.; Kim, J.-H.; Song, H.; Cho, J.-Y.; Hwang, D.Y.; Kim, K.S.; et al. Comparative study of fatty liver induced by methionine and choline-deficiency in C57BL/6N mice originating from three different sources. *Lab. Anim. Res.* **2017**, *33*, 157–164. [CrossRef] [PubMed]
104. Aissa, A.F.; Tryndyak, V.; de Conti, A.; Melnyk, S.; Gomes, T.D.; Bianchi, M.L.; James, S.J.; Beland, F.A.; Antunes, L.M.; Pogribny, I.P. Effect of methionine-deficient and methionine-supplemented diets on the hepatic one-carbon and lipid metabolism in mice. *Mol. Nutr. Food Res.* **2014**, *58*, 1502–1512. [CrossRef] [PubMed]
105. Mahamid, M.; Mahroum, N.; Bragazzi, N.L.; Shalaata, K.; Yavne, Y.; Adawi, M.; Amital, H.; Watad, A. Folate and B_{12} Levels Correlate with Histological Severity in NASH Patients. *Nutrients* **2018**, *10*, 440. [CrossRef] [PubMed]
106. Martínez-Uña, M.; Varela-Rey, M.; Cano, A.; Fernández-Ares, L.; Beraza, N.; Aurrekoetxea, I.; Martínez-Arranz, I.; García-Rodríguez, J.L.; Buqué, X.; Mestre, D.; et al. Excess S-adenosylmethionine reroutes phosphatidylethanolamine towards phosphatidylcholine and triglyceride synthesis. *Hepatology* **2013**, *58*, 1296–1305. [CrossRef] [PubMed]

107. Zeisel, S.H.; Da Costa, K.-A.; Franklin, P.D.; Alexander, E.A.; Lamont, J.T.; Sheard, N.F.; Beiser, A. Choline, an essential nutrient for humans. *FASEB J.* **1991**, *5*, 2093–2098. [CrossRef]

108. Guerrerio, A.L.; Colvin, R.M.; Schwartz, A.K.; Molleston, J.P.; Murray, K.F.; Diehl, A.; Mohan, P.; Schwimmer, J.B.; Lavine, J.E.; Torbenson, M.S.; et al. Choline intake in a large cohort of patients with nonalcoholic fatty liver disease. *Am. J. Clin. Nutr.* **2012**, *95*, 892–900. [CrossRef] [PubMed]

109. Dahlhoff, C.; Worsch, S.; Sailer, M.; Hummel, B.A.; Fiamoncini, J.; Uebel, K.; Obeid, R.; Scherling, C.; Geisel, J.; Bader, B.L.; et al. Methyl-donor supplementation in obese mice prevents the progression of NAFLD, activates AMPK and decreases acyl-carnitine levels. *Mol. Metab.* **2014**, *3*, 565–580. [CrossRef]

110. Crown, S.B.; Marze, N.; Antoniewicz, M.R. Catabolism of Branched Chain Amino Acids Contributes Significantly to Synthesis of Odd-Chain and Even-Chain Fatty Acids in 3T3-L1 Adipocytes. *PLoS ONE* **2015**, *10*, e0145850. [CrossRef]

111. Green, C.R.; Wallace, M.; Divakaruni, A.S.; Phillips, S.A.; Murphy, A.N.; Ciaraldi, T.P.; Metallo, C.M. Branched-chain amino acid catabolism fuels adipocyte differentiation and lipogenesis. *Nat. Chem. Biol.* **2016**, *12*, 15–21. [CrossRef]

112. Ghosh, S.; Sinha, J.K.; Putcha, U.K.; Raghunath, M. Severe but Not Moderate Vitamin B_{12} Deficiency Impairs Lipid Profile, Induces Adiposity, and Leads to Adverse Gestational Outcome in Female C57BL/6 Mice. *Front. Nutr.* **2016**, *3*, 1. [CrossRef]

113. U.S. Food and Drug Administration. *Food Standards: Amendment of Standards of Identity for Enriched Grain Products to Require Addition of Folic Acid; Correction*; Department of Health and Human Services: Washington, DC, USA, 1996; Volume 61.

114. Centers for Disease Control and Prevention. CDC Grand Rounds: Additional opportunities to prevent neural tube defects with folic acid fortification. *MMWR Morb. Mortal. Wkly. Rep.* **2010**, *59*, 980–984.

115. Liu, J.J.; Ward, R.L. Folate and one-carbon metabolism and its impact on aberrant DNA methylation in cancer. *Adv. Genet.* **2010**, *71*, 79–121. [CrossRef] [PubMed]

116. Honein, M.A.; Paulozzi, L.J.; Mathews, T.J.; Erickson, J.D.; Wong, L.Y. Impact of folic acid fortification of the US food supply on the occurrence of neural tube defects. *JAMA* **2001**, *285*, 2981–2986. [CrossRef] [PubMed]

117. Williams, L.J.; Rasmussen, S.A.; Flores, A.; Kirby, R.S.; Edmonds, L.D. Decline in the prevalence of spina bifida and anencephaly by race/ethnicity: 1995–2002. *Pediatrics* **2005**, *116*, 580–586. [CrossRef] [PubMed]

118. Glass, G.B.J.; Skeggs, H.R.; Lee, D.H.; Jones, E.L.; Hardy, W.W. Hydroxocobalamin. I. Blood Levels and Urinary Excretion of Vitamin B12 in Man After a Single Parenteral Dose of Aqueous Hydroxocobalamin, Aqueous Cyanocobalamin and Cyanocobalamin Zinc-Tannate Complex. *Blood* **1961**, *18*, 511–521. [CrossRef]

119. Beck, W.S. Diagnosis of megaloblastic anemia. *Annu. Rev. Med.* **1991**, *42*, 311–322. [CrossRef]

120. Rader, J.I.; Weaver, C.M.; Angyal, G. Total folate in enriched cereal-grain products in the United States following fortification. *Food Chem.* **2000**, *70*, 275–289. [CrossRef]

121. Quinlivan, E.P.; Gregory, J.F., 3rd. Effect of food fortification on folic acid intake in the United States. *Am. J. Clin. Nutr.* **2003**, *77*, 221–225. [CrossRef]

122. Arendt, J.F.B.; Nexo, E. Cobalamin related parameters and disease patterns in patients with increased serum cobalamin levels. *PLoS ONE* **2012**, *7*, e45979. [CrossRef]

123. Flores-Guerrero, J.L.; Minović, I.; Groothof, D.; Gruppen, E.G.; Riphagen, I.J.; Kootstra-Ros, J.; Muller Kobold, A.; Hak, E.; Navis, G.; Gansevoort, R.T.; et al. Association of Plasma Concentration of Vitamin B12 With All-Cause Mortality in the General Population in the Netherlands. *JAMA Netw. Open* **2020**, *3*, e1919274. [CrossRef]

124. Yang, J.; Li, H.; Deng, H.; Wang, Z. Association of One-Carbon Metabolism-Related Vitamins (Folate, B6, B12), Homocysteine and Methionine With the Risk of Lung Cancer: Systematic Review and Meta-Analysis. *Front. Oncol.* **2018**, *8*, 493. [CrossRef] [PubMed]

125. Essén, A.; Santaolalla, A.; Garmo, H.; Hammar, N.; Walldius, G.; Jungner, I.; Malmström, H.; Holmberg, L.; Van Hemelrijck, M. Baseline serum folate, vitamin B_{12} and the risk of prostate and breast cancer using data from the Swedish AMORIS cohort. *Cancer Causes Control.* **2019**, *30*, 603–615. [CrossRef] [PubMed]

126. Mason, J.B.; Dickstein, A.; Jacques, P.F.; Haggarty, P.; Selhub, J.; Dallal, G.; Rosenberg, I.H. A Temporal Association between Folic Acid Fortification and an Increase in Colorectal Cancer Rates May Be Illuminating Important Biological Principles: A Hypothesis. *Cancer Epidemiol. Biomark. Prev.* **2007**, *16*, 1325. [CrossRef] [PubMed]

127. Arendt, J.F.; Pedersen, L.; Nexo, E.; Sorensen, H.T. Elevated plasma vitamin B12 levels as a marker for cancer: A population-based cohort study. *J. Natl. Cancer Inst.* **2013**, *105*, 1799–1805. [CrossRef] [PubMed]
128. Arendt, J.F.H.; Sorensen, H.T.; Horsfall, L.J.; Petersen, I. Elevated Vitamin B12 Levels and Cancer Risk in UK Primary Care: A THIN Database Cohort Study. *Cancer Epidemiol. Biomark. Prev.* **2019**, *28*, 814–821. [CrossRef] [PubMed]
129. Andrès, E.; Serraj, K.; Zhu, J.; Vermorken, A.J.M. The pathophysiology of elevated vitamin B12 in clinical practice. *QJM Int. J. Med.* **2013**, *106*, 505–515. [CrossRef] [PubMed]
130. Collin, S.M.; Metcalfe, C.; Refsum, H.; Lewis, S.J.; Zuccolo, L.; Smith, G.D.; Chen, L.; Harris, R.; Davis, M.; Marsden, G.; et al. Circulating Folate, Vitamin B12, Homocysteine, Vitamin B12, Transport Proteins, and Risk of Prostate Cancer: A Case-Control Study, Systematic Review, and Meta-analysis. *Cancer Epidemiol. Biomark. Prev.* **2010**, *19*, 1632. [CrossRef] [PubMed]
131. Chiche, L.; Jean, R.; Romain, F.; Roux, F.; Thomas, G.; Canavese, S.; Branger, S.; Harlé, J.R.; Durand, J.M. Implications cliniques de la découverte d'une hypervitaminémie B_{12} en médecine interne. *Rev. Med. Interne* **2008**, *29*, 187–194. [CrossRef]
132. Beard, M.F.; Pitney, W.R.; Sanneman, E.H. Serum concentrations of vitamin B_{12} in patients suffering from leukemia. *Blood* **1954**, *9*, 789–794. [CrossRef]
133. Mollin, D.; Ross, G. Serum vitamin B_{12} concentrations in leukaemia and in some other haematological conditions. *Br. J. Haematol.* **1955**, *1*, 155–172. [CrossRef]
134. Gilbert, H.S.; Krauss, S.; Pasternack, B.; Herbert, V.; Wasserman, L.R. Serum vitamin B_{12} content and unsaturated vitamin B_{12}-binding capacity in myeloproliferative disease: Value in differential diagnosis and as indicators of disease activity. *Ann. Intern. Med.* **1969**, *71*, 719–729. [CrossRef] [PubMed]
135. Gimsing, P. Cobalamin forms and analogues in plasma and myeloid cells during chronic myelogenous leukaemia related to clinical condition. *Br. J. Haematol.* **1995**, *89*, 812–819. [CrossRef] [PubMed]
136. Hall, C.A.; Finkler, A.E. Abnormal Transport of Vitamin B_{12} in Plasma in Chronic Myelogenous Leukemia. *Nature* **1964**, *204*, 1207. [CrossRef] [PubMed]
137. Gimsing, P.; Overballe-Petersen, C.; Hippe, E. Cobalamin and cobalamin-binding proteins in plasma related to the clinical condition in chronic myelogenous leukemia. *Leukemia* **1995**, *9*, 1604–1609. [PubMed]
138. Deneuville, T.; Mario, N.; Tiev, K.P.; Toledano, C.; Josselin-Mahr, L.; Gain, M.; Pateron, D.; Guidet, B.; Retbi, A.; Taright, N.; et al. Concentration plasmatique élevée de la vitamine B_{12}: Un indicateur des maladies hépatiques ou tumorales? *Rev. Med. Interne* **2009**, *30*. [CrossRef]
139. Carmel, R. Extreme elevation of serum transcobalamin I in patients with metastatic cancer. *N. Engl. J. Med.* **1975**, *292*, 282–284. [CrossRef]
140. Frémont, S.; Champigneulle, B.; Gérard, P.; Felden, F.; Lambert, D.; Guéant, J.L.; Nicolas, J.P. Blood transcobalamin levels in malignant hepatoma. *Tumour Biol.* **1991**, *12*, 353–359. [CrossRef]
141. Liu, G.; Wang, Y.; Yue, M.; Zhao, L.; Guo, Y.-D.; Liu, Y.; Yang, H.; Liu, F.; Zhang, X.; Zhi, L.; et al. High expression of TCN1 is a negative prognostic biomarker and can predict neoadjuvant chemosensitivity of colon cancer. *Sci. Rep. (Nat. Publ. Group)* **2020**, *10*. [CrossRef]
142. Lee, Y.Y.; Wei, Y.C.; Tian, Y.F.; Sun, D.P.; Sheu, M.J.; Yang, C.C.; Lin, L.C.; Lin, C.Y.; Hsing, C.H.; Li, W.S.; et al. Overexpression of Transcobalamin 1 is an Independent Negative Prognosticator in Rectal Cancers Receiving Concurrent Chemoradiotherapy. *J. Cancer* **2017**, *8*, 1330–1337. [CrossRef]
143. Brasky, T.M.; White, E.; Chen, C.-L. Long-Term, Supplemental, One-Carbon Metabolism-Related Vitamin B Use in Relation to Lung Cancer Risk in the Vitamins and Lifestyle (VITAL) Cohort. *J. Clin. Oncol.* **2017**, *35*, 3440–3448. [CrossRef]
144. Fanidi, A.; Carreras-Torres, R.; Larose, T.L.; Yuan, J.-M.; Stevens, V.L.; Weinstein, S.J.; Albanes, D.; Prentice, R.; Pettinger, M.; Cai, Q.; et al. Is high vitamin B_{12} status a cause of lung cancer? *Int. J. Cancer* **2019**, *145*, 1499–1503. [CrossRef] [PubMed]
145. Figueiredo, J.C.; Grau, M.V.; Haile, R.W.; Sandler, R.S.; Summers, R.W.; Bresalier, R.S.; Burke, C.A.; McKeown-Eyssen, G.E.; Baron, J.A. Folic acid and risk of prostate cancer: Results from a randomized clinical trial. *J. Natl. Cancer Inst.* **2009**, *101*, 432–435. [CrossRef]
146. Oliai Araghi, S.; Kiefte-de Jong, J.C.; van Dijk, S.C.; Swart, K.M.A.; van Laarhoven, H.W.; van Schoor, N.M.; de Groot, L.; Lemmens, V.; Stricker, B.H.; Uitterlinden, A.G.; et al. Folic Acid and Vitamin B12 Supplementation and the Risk of Cancer: Long-term Follow-up of the B Vitamins for the Prevention of Osteoporotic Fractures (B-PROOF) Trial. *Cancer Epidemiol. Biomark. Prev.* **2019**, *28*, 275–282. [CrossRef] [PubMed]

147. Naghshi, S.; Sadeghi, O.; Willett, W.C.; Esmaillzadeh, A. Dietary intake of total, animal, and plant proteins and risk of all cause, cardiovascular, and cancer mortality: Systematic review and dose-response meta-analysis of prospective cohort studies. *BMJ* **2020**, *370*, m2412. [CrossRef] [PubMed]
148. Troen, A.M.; Mitchell, B.; Sorensen, B.; Wener, M.H.; Johnston, A.; Wood, B.; Selhub, J.; McTiernan, A.; Yasui, Y.; Oral, E.; et al. Unmetabolized folic acid in plasma is associated with reduced natural killer cell cytotoxicity among postmenopausal women. *J. Nutr.* **2006**, *136*, 189–194. [CrossRef] [PubMed]
149. Henry, C.J.; Nemkov, T.; Casas-Selves, M.; Bilousova, G.; Zaberezhnyy, V.; Higa, K.C.; Serkova, N.J.; Hansen, K.C.; D'Alessandro, A.; DeGregori, J. Folate dietary insufficiency and folic acid supplementation similarly impair metabolism and compromise hematopoiesis. *Haematologica* **2017**, *102*, 1985–1994. [CrossRef] [PubMed]
150. Tsai, T.-Y.; Lee, T.-H.; Wang, H.-H.; Yang, T.-H.; Chang, I.J.; Huang, Y.-C. Serum Homocysteine, Folate, and Vitamin B12 Levels in Patients with Systemic Lupus Erythematosus: A Meta-Analysis and Meta-Regression. *J. Am. Coll. Nutr.* **2020**, 1–11. [CrossRef]
151. Ermens, A.A.; Vlasveld, L.T.; Lindemans, J. Significance of elevated cobalamin (vitamin B_{12}) levels in blood. *Clin. Biochem.* **2003**, *36*, 585–590. [CrossRef]
152. Baker, H.; Leevy, C.B.; DeAngelis, B.; Frank, O.; Baker, E.R. Cobalamin (Vitamin B_{12}) and Holotranscobalamin Changes in Plasma and Liver Tissue in Alcoholics with Liver Disease. *J. Am. Coll. Nutr.* **1998**, *17*, 235–238. [CrossRef]
153. McMahon, G.M.; Hwang, S.-J.; Tanner, R.M.; Jacques, P.F.; Selhub, J.; Muntner, P.; Fox, C.S. The association between vitamin B12, albuminuria and reduced kidney function: An observational cohort study. *BMC Nephrol.* **2015**, *16*, 7. [CrossRef]
154. Carmel, R.; Vasireddy, H.; Aurangzeb, I.; George, K. High serum cobalamin levels in the clinical setting–clinical associations and holo-transcobalamin changes. *Clin. Lab. Haematol.* **2001**, *23*, 365–371. [CrossRef] [PubMed]
155. Matthews, D.M.; Beckett, A.G. Serum vitamin B12 in renal failure. *J. Clin. Pathol.* **1962**, *15*, 456–458. [CrossRef]
156. Julian, T.; Syeed, R.; Glascow, N.; Angelopoulou, E.; Zis, P. B12 as a Treatment for Peripheral Neuropathic Pain: A Systematic Review. *Nutrients* **2020**, *12*, 2221. [CrossRef] [PubMed]
157. Xǔ, G.; Xu, S.; Tang, W.-Z.; Xú, G.; Cheng, C.; Xu, J. Local Injection of Methylcobalamin Combined with Lidocaine for Acute Herpetic Neuralgia. *Pain Med.* **2015**, *17*, 572–581. [CrossRef] [PubMed]
158. Xu, G.; Lv, Z.-W.; Feng, Y.; Tang, W.-Z.; Xu, G. A Single-Center Randomized Controlled Trial of Local Methylcobalamin Injection for Subacute Herpetic Neuralgia. *Pain Med.* **2013**, *14*, 884–894. [CrossRef] [PubMed]
159. Bowen, R.A.; Drake, S.K.; Vanjani, R.; Huey, E.D.; Grafman, J.; Horne, M.K., 3rd. Markedly increased vitamin B12 concentrations attributable to IgG-IgM-vitamin B12 immune complexes. *Clin. Chem.* **2006**, *52*, 2107–2114. [CrossRef]
160. Yadav, D.K.; Shrestha, S.; Lillycrop, K.A.; Joglekar, C.V.; Pan, H.; Holbrook, J.D.; Fall, C.H.D.; Yajnik, C.S.; Chandak, G.R. Vitamin B12 supplementation influences methylation of genes associated with Type 2 diabetes and its intermediate traits. *Epigenomics* **2017**, *10*, 71–90. [CrossRef]
161. Trautmann, C.; Bock, A.; Urbach, A.; Hübner, C.A.; Engmann, O. Acute vitamin B12 supplementation evokes antidepressant response and alters Ntrk-2. *Neuropharmacology* **2020**, *171*, 108112. [CrossRef]
162. de Queiroz, K.B.; Cavalcante-Silva, V.; Lopes, F.L.; Rocha, G.A.; D'Almeida, V.; Coimbra, R.S. Vitamin B_{12} is neuroprotective in experimental pneumococcal meningitis through modulation of hippocampal DNA methylation. *J. Neuroinflammation* **2020**, *17*, 96. [CrossRef]
163. Chang, S.E.; Littlefield, J.W. Elevated dihydrofolate reductase messenger RNA levels in methotrexate-resistant BHK cells. *Cell* **1976**, *7*, 391–396. [CrossRef]
164. Farber, S.; Diamond, L.K. Temporary remissions in acute leukemia in children produced by folic acid antagonist, 4-aminopteroyl-glutamic acid. *N. Engl. J. Med.* **1948**, *238*, 787–793. [CrossRef] [PubMed]
165. Wright, J.C.; Prigot, A.; Wright, B.; Weintraub, S.; Wright, L.T. An evaluation of folic acid antagonists in adults with neoplastic diseases: A study of 93 patients with incurable neoplasms. *J. Natl. Med. Assoc.* **1951**, *43*, 211–240. [PubMed]
166. Evans, W.E.; Crom, W.R.; Abromowitch, M.; Dodge, R.; Look, A.T.; Bowman, W.P.; George, S.L.; Pui, C.H. Clinical pharmacodynamics of high-dose methotrexate in acute lymphocytic leukemia. Identification of a relation between concentration and effect. *N. Engl. J. Med.* **1986**, *314*, 471–477. [CrossRef] [PubMed]

167. Vogler, W.R.; Huguley, C.M., Jr.; Kerr, W. Toxicity and Antitumor Effect of Divided Doses of Methotrexate. *Arch. Intern. Med.* **1965**, *115*, 285–293. [CrossRef] [PubMed]
168. Hersh, E.M.; Wong, V.G.; Henderson, E.S.; Freireich, E.J. Hepatotoxic effects of methotrexate. *Cancer* **1966**, *19*, 600–606. [CrossRef]
169. Levitt, M.; Mosher, M.B.; DeConti, R.C.; Farber, L.R.; Skeel, R.T.; Marsh, J.C.; Mitchell, M.S.; Papac, R.J.; Thomas, E.D.; Bertino, J.R. Improved therapeutic index of methotrexate with "leucovorin rescue". *Cancer Res.* **1973**, *33*, 1729–1734.
170. Longley, D.B.; Harkin, D.P.; Johnston, P.G. 5-fluorouracil: Mechanisms of action and clinical strategies. *Nat. Rev. Cancer* **2003**, *3*, 330–338. [CrossRef]
171. Vogler, W.R.; Jacobs, J. Toxic and therapeutic effects of methotrexate-folinic acid (Leucovorin) in advanced cancer and leukemia. *Cancer* **1971**, *28*, 894–901. [CrossRef]
172. Weinblatt, M.E.; Coblyn, J.S.; Fox, D.A.; Fraser, P.A.; Holdsworth, D.E.; Glass, D.N.; Trentham, D.E. Efficacy of low-dose methotrexate in rheumatoid arthritis. *N. Engl. J. Med.* **1985**, *312*, 818–822. [CrossRef]
173. Cronstein, B.N. Low-dose methotrexate: A mainstay in the treatment of rheumatoid arthritis. *Pharmacol. Rev.* **2005**, *57*, 163–172. [CrossRef]
174. Rossetti, M.; Spreafico, R.; Saidin, S.; Chua, C.; Moshref, M.; Leong, J.Y.; Tan, Y.K.; Thumboo, J.; van Loosdregt, J.; Albani, S. Ex vivo-expanded but not in vitro-induced human regulatory T cells are candidates for cell therapy in autoimmune diseases thanks to stable demethylation of the FOXP3 regulatory T cell-specific demethylated region. *J. Immunol.* **2015**, *194*, 113–124. [CrossRef] [PubMed]
175. Cribbs, A.P.; Kennedy, A.; Penn, H.; Amjadi, P.; Green, P.; Read, J.E.; Brennan, F.; Gregory, B.; Williams, R.O. Methotrexate Restores Regulatory T Cell Function Through Demethylation of the FoxP3 Upstream Enhancer in Patients With Rheumatoid Arthritis. *Arthritis Rheumatol.* **2015**, *67*, 1182–1192. [CrossRef]
176. Cheong, H.; Lu, C.; Lindsten, T.; Thompson, C.B. Therapeutic targets in cancer cell metabolism and autophagy. *Nat. Biotechnol.* **2012**, *30*, 671–678. [CrossRef] [PubMed]
177. Teicher, B.A.; Linehan, W.M.; Helman, L.J. Targeting cancer metabolism. *Clin. Cancer Res.* **2012**, *18*, 5537–5545. [CrossRef]
178. Chen, J.; Wang, Q.; Yin, F.-Q.; Zhang, W.; Yan, L.-H.; Li, L. MTRR silencing inhibits growth and cisplatin resistance of ovarian carcinoma via inducing apoptosis and reducing autophagy. *Am. J. Transl. Res.* **2015**, *7*, 1510–1527.
179. Richie, J.P., Jr.; Leutzinger, Y.; Parthasarathy, S.; Malloy, V.; Orentreich, N.; Zimmerman, J.A. Methionine restriction increases blood glutathione and longevity in F344 rats. *FASEB J.* **1994**, *8*, 1302–1307. [CrossRef] [PubMed]
180. Miller, R.A.; Buehner, G.; Chang, Y.; Harper, J.M.; Sigler, R.; Smith-Wheelock, M. Methionine-deficient diet extends mouse lifespan, slows immune and lens aging, alters glucose, T4, IGF-I and insulin levels, and increases hepatocyte MIF levels and stress resistance. *Aging Cell* **2005**, *4*, 119–125. [CrossRef]
181. Orentreich, N.; Matias, J.R.; DeFelice, A.; Zimmerman, J.A. Low methionine ingestion by rats extends life span. *J. Nutr.* **1993**, *123*, 269–274. [CrossRef]
182. Zimmerman, J.A.; Malloy, V.; Krajcik, R.; Orentreich, N. Nutritional control of aging. *Exp. Gerontol.* **2003**, *38*, 47–52. [CrossRef]
183. Ables, G.P.; Perrone, C.E.; Orentreich, D.; Orentreich, N. Methionine-restricted C57BL/6J mice are resistant to diet-induced obesity and insulin resistance but have low bone density. *PLoS ONE* **2012**, *7*, e51357. [CrossRef]
184. Malloy, V.L.; Krajcik, R.A.; Bailey, S.J.; Hristopoulos, G.; Plummer, J.D.; Orentreich, N. Methionine restriction decreases visceral fat mass and preserves insulin action in aging male Fischer 344 rats independent of energy restriction. *Aging Cell* **2006**, *5*, 305–314. [CrossRef] [PubMed]
185. Barcena, C.; Quiros, P.M.; Durand, S.; Mayoral, P.; Rodriguez, F.; Caravia, X.M.; Marino, G.; Garabaya, C.; Fernandez-Garcia, M.T.; Kroemer, G.; et al. Methionine Restriction Extends Lifespan in Progeroid Mice and Alters Lipid and Bile Acid Metabolism. *Cell Rep.* **2018**, *24*, 2392–2403. [CrossRef] [PubMed]
186. Grandison, R.C.; Piper, M.D.; Partridge, L. Amino-acid imbalance explains extension of lifespan by dietary restriction in Drosophila. *Nature* **2009**, *462*, 1061–1064. [CrossRef] [PubMed]
187. Liu, G.; Yu, L.; Fang, J.; Hu, C.A.; Yin, J.; Ni, H.; Ren, W.; Duraipandiyan, V.; Chen, S.; Al-Dhabi, N.A.; et al. Methionine restriction on oxidative stress and immune response in dss-induced colitis mice. *Oncotarget* **2017**, *8*, 44511–44520. [CrossRef] [PubMed]

188. Martinez, Y.; Li, X.; Liu, G.; Bin, P.; Yan, W.; Mas, D.; Valdivie, M.; Hu, C.A.; Ren, W.; Yin, Y. The role of methionine on metabolism, oxidative stress, and diseases. *Amino Acids* **2017**, *49*, 2091–2098. [CrossRef] [PubMed]
189. Sharma, S.; Dixon, T.; Jung, S.; Graff, E.C.; Forney, L.A.; Gettys, T.W.; Wanders, D. Dietary Methionine Restriction Reduces Inflammation Independent of FGF21 Action. *Obesity* **2019**, *27*, 1305–1313. [CrossRef] [PubMed]
190. Sun, L.; Sadighi Akha, A.A.; Miller, R.A.; Harper, J.M. Life-span extension in mice by preweaning food restriction and by methionine restriction in middle age. *J. Gerontol. Biol. Sci. Med. Sci.* **2009**, *64*, 711–722. [CrossRef]
191. Wanders, D.; Ghosh, S.; Stone, K.P.; Van, N.T.; Gettys, T.W. Transcriptional impact of dietary methionine restriction on systemic inflammation: Relevance to biomarkers of metabolic disease during aging. *Biofactors* **2014**, *40*, 13–26. [CrossRef]
192. Tsai, H.C.; Li, H.; Van Neste, L.; Cai, Y.; Robert, C.; Rassool, F.V.; Shin, J.J.; Harbom, K.M.; Beaty, R.; Pappou, E.; et al. Transient low doses of DNA-demethylating agents exert durable antitumor effects on hematological and epithelial tumor cells. *Cancer Cell* **2012**, *21*, 430–446. [CrossRef]
193. Herman, J.G.; Baylin, S.B. Gene silencing in cancer in association with promoter hypermethylation. *N. Engl. J. Med.* **2003**, *349*, 2042–2054. [CrossRef]
194. Kulis, M.; Esteller, M. DNA methylation and cancer. *Adv. Genet.* **2010**, *70*, 27–56. [CrossRef] [PubMed]
195. Paz, M.F.; Fraga, M.F.; Avila, S.; Guo, M.; Pollan, M.; Herman, J.G.; Esteller, M. A systematic profile of DNA methylation in human cancer cell lines. *Cancer Res.* **2003**, *63*, 1114–1121. [PubMed]
196. Ceol, C.J.; Houvras, Y.; Jane-Valbuena, J.; Bilodeau, S.; Orlando, D.A.; Battisti, V.; Fritsch, L.; Lin, W.M.; Hollmann, T.J.; Ferré, F.; et al. The histone methyltransferase SETDB1 is recurrently amplified in melanoma and accelerates its onset. *Nature* **2011**, *471*, 513–517. [CrossRef] [PubMed]
197. Dalgliesh, G.L.; Furge, K.; Greenman, C.; Chen, L.; Bignell, G.; Butler, A.; Davies, H.; Edkins, S.; Hardy, C.; Latimer, C.; et al. Systematic sequencing of renal carcinoma reveals inactivation of histone modifying genes. *Nature* **2010**, *463*, 360–363. [CrossRef]
198. Delhommeau, F.; Dupont, S.; Valle, V.D.; James, C.; Trannoy, S.; Massé, A.; Kosmider, O.; Le Couedic, J.-P.; Robert, F.; Alberdi, A.; et al. Mutation in TET2 in Myeloid Cancers. *N. Engl. J. Med.* **2009**, *360*, 2289–2301. [CrossRef]
199. Figueroa, M.E.; Abdel-Wahab, O.; Lu, C.; Ward, P.S.; Patel, J.; Shih, A.; Li, Y.; Bhagwat, N.; Vasanthakumar, A.; Fernandez, H.F.; et al. Leukemic IDH1 and IDH2 mutations result in a hypermethylation phenotype, disrupt TET2 function, and impair hematopoietic differentiation. *Cancer Cell* **2010**, *18*, 553–567. [CrossRef]
200. Jones, S.; Wang, T.L.; Shih Ie, M.; Mao, T.L.; Nakayama, K.; Roden, R.; Glas, R.; Slamon, D.; Diaz, L.A., Jr.; Vogelstein, B.; et al. Frequent mutations of chromatin remodeling gene ARID1A in ovarian clear cell carcinoma. *Science* **2010**, *330*, 228–231. [CrossRef]
201. Ley, T.J.; Ding, L.; Walter, M.J.; McLellan, M.D.; Lamprecht, T.; Larson, D.E.; Kandoth, C.; Payton, J.E.; Baty, J.; Welch, J.; et al. DNMT3A mutations in acute myeloid leukemia. *N. Engl. J. Med.* **2010**, *363*, 2424–2433. [CrossRef]
202. Cavuoto, P.; Fenech, M.F. A review of methionine dependency and the role of methionine restriction in cancer growth control and life-span extension. *Cancer Treat. Rev.* **2012**, *38*, 726–736. [CrossRef]
203. Cellarier, E.; Durando, X.; Vasson, M.P.; Farges, M.C.; Demiden, A.; Maurizis, J.C.; Madelmont, J.C.; Chollet, P. Methionine dependency and cancer treatment. *Cancer Treat. Rev.* **2003**, *29*, 489–499. [CrossRef]
204. Sugimura, T.; Birnbaum, S.M.; Winitz, M.; Greenstein, J.P. Quantitative nutritional studies with water-soluble, chemically defined diets. VIII. The forced feeding of diets each lacking in one essential amino acid. *Arch. Biochem. Biophys.* **1959**, *81*, 448–455. [CrossRef]
205. Guo, H.Y.; Herrera, H.; Groce, A.; Hoffman, R.M. Expression of the biochemical defect of methionine dependence in fresh patient tumors in primary histoculture. *Cancer Res.* **1993**, *53*, 2479–2483. [PubMed]
206. Halpern, B.C.; Clark, B.R.; Hardy, D.N.; Halpern, R.M.; Smith, R.A. The effect of replacement of methionine by homocystine on survival of malignant and normal adult mammalian cells in culture. *Proc. Natl. Acad. Sci. USA* **1974**, *71*, 1133–1136. [CrossRef] [PubMed]
207. Mecham, J.O.; Rowitch, D.; Wallace, C.D.; Stern, P.H.; Hoffman, R.M. The metabolic defect of methionine dependence occurs frequently in human tumor cell lines. *Biochem. Biophys. Res. Commun.* **1983**, *117*, 429–434. [CrossRef]

208. Hoshiya, Y.; Kubota, T.; Inada, T.; Kitajima, M.; Hoffman, R.M. Methionine-depletion modulates the efficacy of 5-fluorouracil in human gastric cancer in nude mice. *Anticancer Res.* **1997**, *17*, 4371–4375. [PubMed]
209. Sinha, R.; Cooper, T.K.; Rogers, C.J.; Sinha, I.; Turbitt, W.J.; Calcagnotto, A.; Perrone, C.E.; Richie, J.P., Jr. Dietary methionine restriction inhibits prostatic intraepithelial neoplasia in TRAMP mice. *Prostate* **2014**, *74*, 1663–1673. [CrossRef]
210. Hens, J.R.; Sinha, I.; Perodin, F.; Cooper, T.; Sinha, R.; Plummer, J.; Perrone, C.E.; Orentreich, D. Methionine-restricted diet inhibits growth of MCF10AT1-derived mammary tumors by increasing cell cycle inhibitors in athymic nude mice. *BMC Cancer* **2016**, *16*, 349. [CrossRef]
211. Jeon, H.; Kim, J.H.; Lee, E.; Jang, Y.J.; Son, J.E.; Kwon, J.Y.; Lim, T.-G.; Kim, S.; Park, J.H.Y.; Kim, J.-E.; et al. Methionine deprivation suppresses triple-negative breast cancer metastasis in vitro and in vivo. *Oncotarget* **2016**, *7*, 67223–67234. [CrossRef]
212. Miousse, I.R.; Tobacyk, J.; Quick, C.M.; Jamshidi-Parsian, A.; Skinner, C.M.; Kore, R.; Melnyk, S.B.; Kutanzi, K.R.; Xia, F.; Griffin, R.J.; et al. Modulation of dietary methionine intake elicits potent, yet distinct, anticancer effects on primary versus metastatic tumors. *Carcinogenesis* **2018**, *39*, 1117–1126. [CrossRef]
213. Goseki, N.; Yamazaki, S.; Shimojyu, K.; Kando, F.; Maruyama, M.; Endo, M.; Koike, M.; Takahashi, H. Synergistic effect of methionine-depleting total parenteral nutrition with 5-fluorouracil on human gastric cancer: A randomized, prospective clinical trial. *Jpn. J. Cancer Res.* **1995**, *86*, 484–489. [CrossRef]
214. Molina-Montes, E.; Salamanca-Fernández, E.; Garcia-Villanova, B.; Sánchez, M.J. The Impact of Plant-Based Dietary Patterns on Cancer-Related Outcomes: A Rapid Review and Meta-Analysis. *Nutrients* **2020**, *12*. [CrossRef] [PubMed]
215. Olteanu, H.; Munson, T.; Banerjee, R. Differences in the efficiency of reductive activation of methionine synthase and exogenous electron acceptors between the common polymorphic variants of human methionine synthase reductase. *Biochemistry* **2002**, *41*, 13378–13385. [CrossRef] [PubMed]
216. Gaughan, D.J.; Kluijtmans, L.A.; Barbaux, S.; McMaster, D.; Young, I.S.; Yarnell, J.W.; Evans, A.; Whitehead, A.S. The methionine synthase reductase (MTRR) A66G polymorphism is a novel genetic determinant of plasma homocysteine concentrations. *Atherosclerosis* **2001**, *157*, 451–456. [CrossRef]
217. Fang, D.H.; Ji, Q.; Fan, C.H.; An, Q.; Li, J. Methionine synthase reductase A66G polymorphism and leukemia risk: Evidence from published studies. *Leuk. Lymphoma* **2014**, *55*, 1910–1914. [CrossRef] [PubMed]
218. Wang, P.; Li, S.; Wang, M.; He, J.; Xi, S. Association of MTRR A66G polymorphism with cancer susceptibility: Evidence from 85 studies. *J. Cancer* **2017**, *8*, 266–277. [CrossRef] [PubMed]
219. Bose, S.; Allen, A.E.; Locasale, J.W. The Molecular Link from Diet to Cancer Cell Metabolism. *Mol. Cell* **2020**, *78*, 1034–1044. [CrossRef] [PubMed]

2

B Vitamins and their Role in Immune Regulation and Cancer

Christine Tara Peterson [1], **Dmitry A. Rodionov** [2,3], **Andrei L. Osterman** [4] and **Scott N. Peterson** [5,*]

1. Center of Excellence for Research and Training in Integrative Health, Department of Family Medicine and Public Health, UC San Diego, School of Medicine, La Jolla, CA 92093, USA; chpeterson@ucsd.edu
2. Bioinformatics and Structural Biology Program, Sanford Burnham Prebys Medical Discovery Institute, La Jolla, CA 92037, USA; rodionov@SBPdiscovery.org
3. A.A. Kharkevich Institute for Information Transmission Problems, Russian Academy of Sciences, 119991 Moscow, Russia
4. Immunity and Pathogenesis Program, Infectious and Inflammatory Diseases Center, Sanford Burnham Prebys Medical Discovery Institute, La Jolla, CA 92037, USA; osterman@SBPdiscovery.org
5. Tumor Microenvironment and Cancer Immunology Program, Sanford Burnham Prebys Medical Discovery Institute, La Jolla, CA 92037, USA

* Correspondence: speterson@SBPdiscovery.org

Abstract: B group vitamins represent essential micronutrients for myriad metabolic and regulatory processes required for human health, serving as cofactors used by hundreds of enzymes that carry out essential functions such as energy metabolism, DNA and protein synthesis and other critical functions. B vitamins and their corresponding vitamers are universally essential for all cellular life forms, from bacteria to humans. Humans are unable to synthesize most B vitamins and are therefore dependent on their diet for these essential micronutrients. More recently, another source of B vitamins has been identified which is derived from portions of the 10^{13} bacterial cells inhabiting the gastrointestinal tract. Here we review the expanding literature examining the relationship between B vitamins and the immune system and diverse cancers. Evidence of B vitamin's role in immune cell regulation has accumulated in recent years and may help to clarify the disparate findings of numerous studies attempting to link B vitamins to cancer development. Much work remains to be carried out to fully clarify these relationships as the complexity of B vitamins' essential functions complicates an unequivocal assessment of their beneficial or detrimental effects in inflammation and cancers.

Keywords: thiamine; riboflavin; niacin; pantothenic acid; pyridoxine; biotin; folate; cobalamin; gut microbiota; inflammation; oxidative stress; cancer

---

1. Introduction

B vitamins (B1, thiamine, B2, riboflavin, B3, niacin, B5, pantothenic acid B6, pyridoxine, B7, biotin B9, folate and B12, cobalamin) are essential micronutrients for all cellular life. The essentiality of B vitamins stems from the fact that B vitamins are key intermediates of pathways that generate essential cofactors such as: B1, Thiamine PyroPhosphate (TPP), B2, Flavin MonoNucleotide/Flavin Adenine Dinucleotide (FMN/FAD), B3, Nicotinamide Adenine Dinucleotide (NAD), B5, Coenzyme A (CoA), B6, PyroxidaL Phosphate (PLP), B7, Biotin-Adenine MonoPhosphate (biotin-AMP) and B9, TetraHydroFolate (THF) and B12, cobalamin that are required for hundreds of enzymes carrying out critical cellular functions. The pleiotropic nature of B vitamins emphasizes their importance to cell function and homeostasis but also complicates studies aimed at determining the contexts where B vitamins promote beneficial or detrimental effects on human health, when B vitamins are in insufficient or excessive supply. The World Health Organization (WHO) provides guidelines for the minimal daily consumption of B vitamins in the adult diet (B1: 1.1–1.2 mg, B2: 1.0–1.3 mg, B3: 11–12 mg, B5: 5 mg, B6: 1.3–1.7 mg, B7: 30 μg, B9: 400 μg and B12: 2.4 μg). The variation in B vitamin demands represents a complex relationship between the absorption, stability and number of enzymes requiring these cofactors.

Dietary B vitamins are supplied by plants and animal products in ample quantities, although a variety of conditions can increase the demand and cause deficiencies in B vitamins. Malnutrition, which remains a prevalent problem in developed and developing countries world-wide [1], exercise, stress, drug abuse, alcohol consumption and pregnancy also increase cellular demands for B vitamins [2]. Notably, vitamin B12 is not produced by plants, placing vegans and vegetarians solely reliant on microbial sources, thereby placing them at risk for B12 deficiency in the absence of supplementation. In the following sections, we describe a newly discovered source of B vitamins, as well as experimental and clinical findings that relate each B vitamin to its role in immune regulation and the related area of cancer.

2. Gut Microbes Generate B Vitamins.

Beyond acquisition of B vitamins from the diet, the gut microbiota is now recognized as a potential source of B vitamins. One useful distinction between dietary and microbial B vitamins is that dietary B vitamins are absorbed most prominently in the small intestine, whereas the majority of bacterial-generated B vitamins are produced and absorbed in the large intestine. It remains unclear whether these distinct sites of B vitamin absorption have any differential effects on the host. It is conceivable that gut immune cell populations that are differentially represented in the small and large intestine may be differentially activated/repressed in a site-specific manner, although direct evidence of this possibility remains unverified. Numerous species resident in gut microbiota synthesize B vitamins. Perhaps surprising, not all gut microbes are prototrophic for B vitamin biosynthesis, despite their essentiality for cellular life. Indeed, B vitamin auxotrophs for vitamins B1, B2, B3, B5 and B9 represent ~20–25% of bacterial communities, whereas B7 and B12 auxotrophy is more prevalent comprising 30 and >50% of the microbial community, respectively [3]. Given the universal essentiality of B vitamin-derived cofactors, the presence of auxotrophs led us to test the hypothesis that B vitamin prototrophs must share B vitamins with auxotrophs and presumably also with their host. Gnotobiotic mice colonized with human fecal material were provided diets lacking B vitamins or containing them in normal quantities or in 30-fold excess. Surprisingly, after 4 weeks on any of these diets, the percentage of auxotrophs for each B vitamin remained unchanged, suggesting that B vitamin sharing is able to sustain the relative fitness of B vitamin auxotrophs and that the quantities shared were not limiting [4]. It remains unclear whether the microbial provision of B vitamins is through active secretion or more trivially due to cell lysis or whether the supply of B vitamins is sufficient to sustain the health and fitness of their host in the absence of adequate dietary supplementation. The occurrence of B vitamin deficiencies in human populations, would suggest that microbial B vitamin provisions are insufficient in the long-term to sustain health.

Bacterial biosynthesis of thiamine is complex and may be initiated using a number of amino acid substrates such as tyrosine, glycine or cysteine (Figure 1). Biosynthesis of riboflavin uses ribose-5-phosphate and GTP as substrates. Riboflavin is then converted in a single-step to the active cofactors, FMN and FAD generated by riboflavin kinase and FAD synthase, respectively, that act as electron carriers for a number of critical redox reactions. Bacterial synthesis of niacin and its resulting cofactors utilizes aspartic acid or tryptophan to form quinolate. Nicotinate, nicotinamide or *N*-ribosyl nicotinamide that is converted to nicotinic acid mononucleotide is subsequently used to form NAD in a two-step reaction. Bacterial biosynthesis of pantothenic acid is initiated with aspartic acid that is converted to β-alanine, which is then linked to pantoate and subsequently converted to pantothenate. Pantothenate is then converted in a multistep reaction to CoA. Bacterial biosynthesis of pyridoxine is the simplest vitamin production pathway that uses either 4-hydroxyl-L-threonine-phosphate or through an alternative route, combines ribose 5-phosphate, glutamine and glyceraldehyde phosphate as substrates. Bacteria synthesize biotin through one of two primary pathways, in one malonyl-acyl carrier protein (ACP) is converted to malonyl-ACP methyl ester and subsequently converted to pimeloyl-ACP methyl ester which may also be used as substrate directly to produce pimeloyl-ACP. A third pathway uses pimelate as substrate that is converted to pimeloyl-CoA. These pathways then converge in a four-step reaction to form biotin. Folate is produced by bacteria from chorismate and GTP as precursors. Chorismate is converted to 4-aminobenzoic acid (PABA) in a two-step reaction where it combines the GTP arm of the pathway to form THF. Cobalamin biosynthesis is by far the most gene-intensive pathway used by bacteria for any B vitamin, requiring 23 separate genes. This may be the reason why B12 auxotrophs are significantly more prevalent compared to any other B vitamin produced by bacteria.

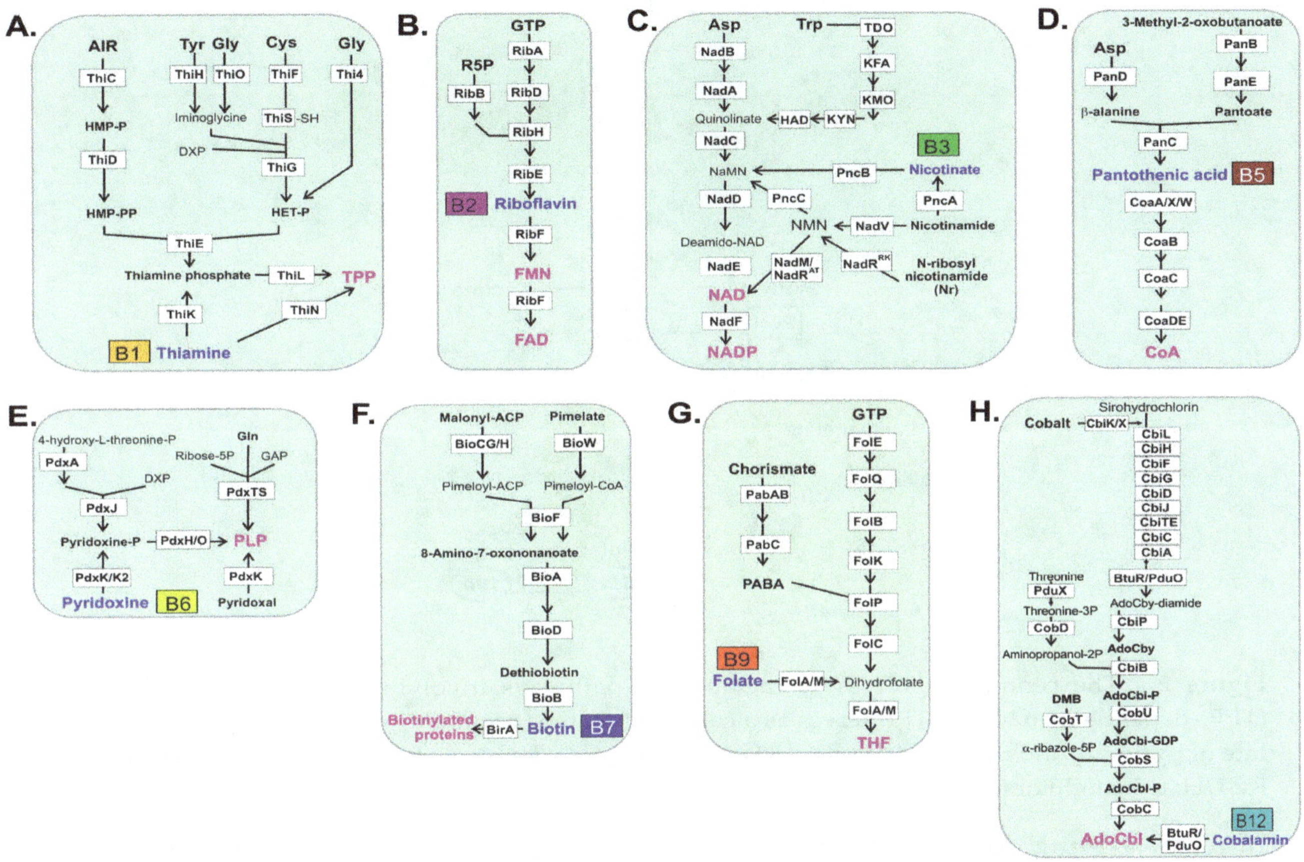

Figure 1. Biochemical pathways for vitamin/cofactor biosynthesis in human gut microbiome. (**A**) thiamine pyrophosphate (TPP); (**B**) Flavin MonoNucleotide/Flavin Adenine Dinucleotide FMN/FAD; (**C**) Nicotinamide Adenine Dinucleotide (Phosphate) NAD/NADP; (**D**) coenzyme A (CoA); (**E**) pyridoxal-phosphate (PLP); (**F**) biotin; (**G**) tetrahydrofolate (THF); (**H**) adenosylcobalamine (AdoCbl). Enzymes are shown in white boxes. B-vitamins/cofactors are in blue/magenta text.

3. Thiamine B1

In the human host, thiamine-derived molecules serve as an important cofactor for numerous enzymes, notably those involved in energy production via the tricarboxylic acid (TCA) cycle [5]. The active form of thiamine is thiamine pyrophosphate (TPP). Within mitochondria, pyruvate dehydrogenase and α-ketoglutarate dehydrogenase utilize TPP as a cofactor, whereas TPP is also important in converting amino acids and fatty acids to Acetyl CoA. TPP is a cofactor for transketolase that generates ribose-5-phosphate for RNA and DNA synthesis. A recent concept considers energy metabolism and the balance between glycolysis and TCA cycle activities as a determinant controlling immune cell function, referred to as immunometabolism [6]. Thiamine-derived cofactors play an important role in enzymes involved in these pathways (Figure 2). T-regulatory cells (Tregs), resting macrophage and naïve T cells generate energy mostly through the TCA cycle, whereas activated macrophage and Th1, Th2 and Th17 cells shift the balance toward aerobic glycolysis to complement energy derived from the TCA cycle [7]. This phenomenon has also been documented for B cells [8]. The relevance of B1 in immunometabolism was illustrated in mice fed a B1-deficient diet that curtailed the maintenance of naïve B cells but had little effect on differentiated IgA producing plasma cells [9]. This mirrors the behavior of malignant cell growth that reprograms its metabolism to favor glycolysis in the so-called Warburg effect.

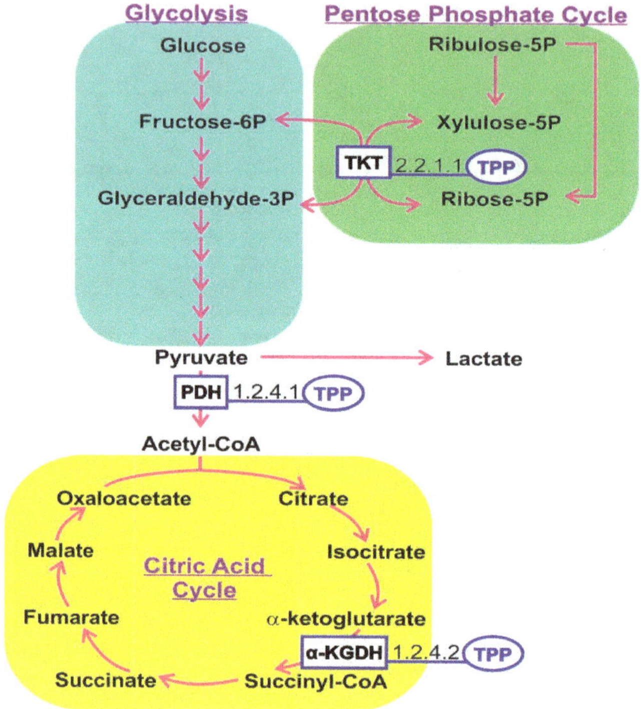

Figure 2. The central carbohydrate metabolism pathways involving thiamine pyrophosphate (TPP)-dependent enzymes. TPP serves as a cofactor for steps regulating the pentose phosphate cycle, fate of pyruvate and the tricarboxylic acid cycle. TKT; transketolase, PDH; pyruvate dehydrogenase, KGDH; α-ketoglutarate dehydrogenase.

In mice, varying doses of thiamine (50, 100 and 125 mg/kg) were injected intraperitoneally in the context of xylene-induced edema. All doses of thiamine were analgesic with higher doses displaying a more prolonged effect. Similarly, edema was curtailed by all doses of thiamine indicating an anti-inflammatory effect in that setting [10]. Thiamine deficiency is a well-established feature of neurodegenerative diseases such as Alzheimer's Disease (AD). Thiamine deficiency in this model shows congruent patterns of neuronal death occurring in brain regions displaying reduced thiamine-dependent enzyme activities [11]. Thiamine deficiency induced ferritin expression in activated microglia in vulnerable regions of the brain. Microglial cells are loaded with redox active iron that may directly contribute to oxidative stress and neuronal death in AD [12]. Thiamine–immune cell interactions are mediated by hemin-dependent oxygenases that impact the release of IntraCellular Adhesion Molecules (ICAMs) which serve to localize cells expressing various integrins [13]. Thiamine has antioxidative effects on neutrophils that protect sulfhydryl groups on the cell surface [14]. In macrophages, thiamine suppresses oxidative stress-induced activation of NF-κB and pro-inflammatory cytokine release [15].

Multiple reports have examined the effect of thiamine as part of a regimen to treat acute sepsis in conjunction with hydrocortisone and ascorbic acid [16]. Death due to sepsis is regarded as a consequence of the host response rather than the infection per se. Thiamine deficiency in septic patients is prevalent (20–70%) and thought to contribute to a variety of phenotypes associated with septic shock including decreased ATP production and increased Reactive Oxygen Species (ROS) [17]. A study of 88 patients with sepsis showed that the thiamine treatment group had significantly lower levels of lactate indicating a restoration of mitochondrial function and ATP production and corresponding reductions in mortality rates [17]. Additional studies are required to clarify the effects of thiamine on immune cell functions and inflammation.

The speculation of a role for thiamine in cancer stems from its role in mediating enzyme activities that are relevant to tumor cells' increased proliferation and accompanying energy demands. Further investigation regarding thiamine supplementation to support nutrition is warranted, given thiamine's unknown oncogenic potential. This consideration highlights an important unanswered question for all B vitamins that should strive to distinguish protective effects in healthy individuals distinctly from their role in cancer patients, where B vitamins may be therapeutic or contribute to oncogenesis.

An in vitro study using the breast cancer cell line MCF7, compared to the non-tumorigenic line MCF10A, treated with various doses of thiamine showed that high doses (1 mg and 2 mg/mL for 24 h) significantly reduced cell proliferation in MCF7 cells only. This reduction was associated with reduced glycolysis and activation of the pyruvate dehydrogenase (PDH) complex [18]. The hypoxia-inducible factor Hif-1α increases thiamine uptake in tumor cells under hypoxic conditions [19]. In a study involving seven tumor cell lines under hypoxic conditions, thiamine pyrophosphate kinase-1 (TPK1) that converts thiamine to TPP is upregulated. Despite the upregulation of TPK1, intracellular TPP was decreased. SiRNA knockdown of TPK1 reduced tumor cell proliferation, suggesting that increased TPP supports increased tumor growth [20]. A study motivated by the observation of poor thiamine bioavailability in tumors developed thiamine mimetics to improve delivery to cells. Administration of these mimetics increased intracellular TPP and reduced PDH phosphorylation by PDK while reducing tumor cell proliferation. PDK is over-expressed in tumor cells and phosphorylation of PDH drives aerobic glycolysis to complement TCA cycle energy generation. One of the mimetics tested (benfotiamine but not sulbutiamine) reduced growth of subcutaneous xenograft tumors in mice [21].

Using Erlich's ascites tumor model, administration of 25-fold excess compared to FDA guidelines for thiamine increased tumor growth; however, at 2500 times the recommended daily allowance, modest tumor growth inhibition was observed. This attenuation of tumor growth was enhanced when high-dose thiamine was administered 7 days prior to tumor inoculation [22]. Taken together, these results suggest that thiamine may promote or inhibit tumorigenesis depending on the cancer type analyzed or the effective dose or amount of intracellular TPP.

Thiamine supplementation has been investigated with respect to cancer risk and its effect on tumorgenicity. The results of studies are mixed, some studies showing protective effects and others no significant differences. A study of an Italian ORDET cohort including 391 breast cancer cases and B vitamin intake indicated that, overall, thiamine was protective and particularly protective in estrogen- and progesterone receptor-negative HER2-positive cases [23]. By contrast, a similar study examining a broad set of cancers in Canadian women failed to show a significant correlation between thiamine intake and cancer risk [24]. A study conducted in rats examined the effect of a reduced thiamine diet and found that thiamine deficiency was associated with increased frequency of aberrant crypt foci in the colon [25].

Both in vitro and in vivo studies generate disparate findings with respect to thiamine's role in cancer and may be nuanced and dependent on cancer subtypes. Taken together, current knowledge suggests that additional work should be undertaken to resolve apparent disagreements between studies and analyze thiamine's impact on cancer at a higher resolution involving cancer subtypes.

4. Riboflavin B2

In humans, several FAD-dependent enzymes, such as glutathione reductase, that facilitate the redox cycle of glutathione point to riboflavin's role as a regulator of oxidative stress. Indeed, riboflavin deficiency, clinically referred to as ariboflavinosis, leads to elevated oxidative stress [26]. Riboflavin protects against oxidant-mediated inflammatory injury in lungs [27]. Detailed biochemical analyses have shown that riboflavin or FAD plays a central role in regulating the activity of phagocytic NADPH oxidase that generates superoxide anions in response to infection [28]. Riboflavin activates phagocytosis and proliferation of macrophages and neutrophils [29]. Interestingly, riboflavin inhibited neutrophil migration and infiltration and accumulation of activated granulocytes at peripheral sites that may decrease inflammatory responses [30]. Riboflavin inhibits the lipopolysaccharide (LPS)-induced ROS that leads to activation of NF-kB, thereby downregulating TNF-α and NO in a variety of experimental models [31]. A study involving undifferentiated pro-monocytic lymphoma cells demonstrated that riboflavin did not impact cell proliferation or apoptosis. Riboflavin did significantly decrease cell migration in a trans-well assay and also downregulated the expression of the checkpoint protein PD-L1 that downregulates cytotoxic $CD8^+$ T cell effector functions [32].

Among a variety of immune modulatory effects hypothesized for riboflavin, the most intensively studied is its role in activation of Mucosal-Associated Invariant T (MAIT) cells. MAIT cells are abundant innate-like lymphocytes that predominantly reside in barrier tissues, where microbes coexist. Indeed, it is likely that MAIT cells' primary function may be to protect the host from bacterial infection. Germ-free mice have very low MAIT cell abundance compared to conventional mice [33]. MAIT cell ligands include riboflavin-derived molecules that are presented by MR1, a non-polymorphic major histocompatibility complex class I-like molecule [34]. A study examining a panel of *S. pneumoniae* serotype 19A isolates assessed the activation of MAIT cells and effector functions [35]. Human monocyte-derived dendritic cells (DCs) infected with *S. pneumoniae* isolates displayed high variability in MAIT cell activation. Attempts to analyze metabolites tracked with MAIT cell activation efficiency were carried out. Among the known MAIT cell ligands are precursors of riboflavin 6,7-dimethyl-8-ribityllumazine (DMRL) and the downstream gene product, 5-amino-6-ribityluracil (5-A-RU). 5-A-RU is the most potent MAIT cell ligand [34,36]. 5-A-RU can be linked to either glyoxal or methylglyoxal to form additional ligands. ribD encodes a pyrimidine deaminase/reductase which generates 5-A-RU. Indeed, *S. pneumoniae* ribD knockout strains were unable to activate MAIT cells.

A number of studies indicate that riboflavin reduces mortality in LPS-induced septic shock by reducing a number of inflammatory cytokines, such as IL-1, IL-1β, IL-6, IFN-γ and NO, in mice [37]. In addition, riboflavin is involved with reduced oxidative stress via increased expression of inducible nitric oxide synthase (iNOS) and catalase [38]. The optimization of ROS in combatting bacterial infections by *Listeria monocytogenes* and *S. aureus* is dependent on riboflavin [39].

Riboflavin reversed liver cancer progression in animal models using carcinogenic inducers. The mechanism proposed for this effect was due to increased expression of apoptotic genes and decreases in antiapoptotic factors [40]. Studies in riboflavin-deficient rats treated with *N*-nitrosomethylbenzene to induce esophageal tumors showed increased chronic inflammation-associated genomic instability, which was elevated compared to control animals provided a normal riboflavin diet [41]. Riboflavin inhibited melanoma metastasis to the lung in animal models [42].

Riboflavin deficiency has been defined as a risk factor for cancer in general, although some data are conflicting in this regard [43]. A meta-analysis of 27 studies involving nearly 50,000 cases and over 1.2 million individuals analyzing riboflavin and other B vitamins concluded that B2 might decrease the risk of breast cancer, although significance was borderline [44]. Another meta-analysis examining components of one-carbon metabolism and the risk of renal carcinoma found no significant correlations with any B vitamins and cancer risk [45]. Riboflavin concentrations in the blood of patients with esophageal squamous cell carcinoma is reduced compared to healthy subjects [46]. Similar reports suggest that riboflavin may decrease the risk of colorectal cancer in women, potentially through FAD-dependent methylenetetrahydrofolate reductase (MTHFR) [47]. Analysis of riboflavin and the risk of ovarian cancer failed to identify any association [24]. In non-smoking women, increased riboflavin intake was associated with a decrease in the risk of lung cancer [48].

While results are mixed, the role of FAD as a regulator of redox, TCA and ROS in the cell appears to influence cancer risk, which is supported by some findings indicating negative correlations between riboflavin and cancer. The present lack of clarity and mechanisms through which riboflavin may alter cancer risk suggest that additional studies on riboflavin are required to determine potential protective effects in additional cancer types and contexts. Further studies focused on the role of MAIT cells as potential mediators of antitumor responses represent another important area of exploration.

5. Niacin B3

Niacin (nicotinic acid) is a precursor of NAD and NADP, a cofactor utilized by multiple enzymes throughout the body. Unlike other B vitamin-derived cofactors, human cells can synthesize NAD through a number of salvage pathways that are independent of niacin. NAD is involved in numerous redox reactions where NAD (oxidizing agent) and NADH (reducing agent) are interconverted. A second role of NAD is to act as a substrate for sirtuins (see below), which mediate deacetylation reactions and also facilitate the activity of a number of ADP-ribosylation enzymes. NAD is also involved in the maintenance of genomic stability and regulation of enzymes involved in epigenetic regulation [49]. NAD-dependent enzymes are involved in base excision repair [50]. High NAD levels (NAD/NADH) inhibit ROS production [51].

The conversion of NAD to NADP by NAD kinase yields a form of the cofactor for enzymes predominantly involved in anabolic biosynthetic reactions such as fatty acid synthesis, whereas NAD is more characteristic of catabolic reactions generating energy from the TCA cycle. Niacin deficiency can result in Pellagra, a rare disease in developed countries resulting in inflamed skin, diarrhea and/or dementia. Tryptophan metabolism is a source of NAD. Diets deficient in tryptophan can also lead to pellagra or an inability to utilize niacin. Carcinoid syndrome involves gastrointestinal neuroendocrine tumors that use tryptophan as an energy source, producing large quantities of serotonin that limit availability of both niacin and tryptophan.

Obesity, long considered a condition of metabolic imbalance, is now viewed as an inflammatory disease. A key component of obesity is the LPS activation of infiltrating macrophages in adipose tissue. In high-fat diet-fed mice, niacin increased adiponectin (hormone regulating fatty acid catabolism) gene and protein expression and decreased MCP-1, IL-1β and the frequency of activated M1 macrophage [52]. Niacin is touted for its drug-like efficacy in increasing low-density lipoprotein (LDL) and reducing serum triglyceride levels. These effects include anti-inflammatory action as shown in humans with non-ST elevated acute coronary syndrome, where hs-CRP is significantly reduced following niacin treatment [53]. In ApoE$^{-/-}$ mice, which manifests elevated cholesterol levels, niacin inhibited the progression of atherosclerosis while suppressing inflammatory cytokines and adhesion molecules, NF-κB and apoptosis of vascular smooth muscle [54]. In a high fat diet (HFD) model of liver steatosis, niacin decreased liver fat content and oxidative products in rats. These effects were also noted in mice with pre-existing steatosis prior to niacin treatment. Niacin treatment resulted in reduced diacylglycerol acyltransferase, an enzyme in triglyceride synthesis [55]. These results have been recapitulated in humans [56]. In another study, niacin was shown to reduce liver cholesteryl ester transfer protein (CETP) expression via its effects on reducing hepatic macrophage [57]. Niacin inhibited carrageenan-activated neutrophil migration in mice further suggesting its anti-inflammatory role through mechanisms involving alterations in chemoattraction [58]. Niacin signals through GPR109A, the same receptor as the short chain fatty acid (SCFA), butyrate. Monocytes and macrophages express GPR109A. When treated with LPS (a TLR4 agonist), niacin reduced inflammatory cytokine secretion of TNF-α, IL-6 and MCP-1; these results were also observed following monocyte stimulation with heat-killed *L. monocytogenes*, TLR2 agonists. Niacin reduced the amount of NF-κB nuclear localization, chemotaxis and adhesion to human umbilical vein endothelial cell (HUVEC) and vascular cell adhesion molecule (VCAM) via integrin very late antigen 4 [59]. In rats treated with LPS to induce endotoxemia, high-dose niacin inhibited NF-κB activation and inflammatory cytokine gene expression in lungs and tissue damage, thereby increasing survival. Niacin treatment increased glutathione levels and decreased malondialdehyde levels (a marker of oxidative stress) [60]. In nephretomized rats used to model chronic kidney disease, niacin administration reduced MCP-1, plasminogen activator inhibitor (PAI-1), TGF-β, p47(phox), p22(phox), COX-1 and NF-κB activation, concomitant with reduced hypertension, proteinuria, glomerulosclerosis and tubulointerstitial injury [61].

Mice fed a diet enriched in saturated fatty acids to induce blood-brain barrier (BBB) defects and neuroinflammation, were completely protected by treatment with either niacin or nicotinamide [62]. Parkinson's Disease patients provided low-dose niacin showed an increased M2 macrophage at the expense of the M1 macrophage, which was associated with an improved quality of life [63]. Immune activation by treatment of mice with LPS, TNF-α or IL-1 led to an increase in GPR109A expression in adipose tissue and LPS increased receptor expression in the spleen, as did lipoteichoic acid, poly dI:dC and macrophage-produced TNF-α and IL-1 [64]. GPR109A influences physiology in a tissue-dependent manner; in colonocytes, its activation is anti-inflammatory and induces apoptosis, whereas in keratinocytes niacin induces flushing via COX-2 inflammatory pathways [65]. GPR109A is expressed in normal mammary tissue but is shut off in human primary breast tumors. Furthermore, GPR109A deletion triggers earlier onset of tumors and lung metastases in an mouse mammary tumor virus (MMTV)-Neu mouse model of breast cancer [65].

Nicotinamide is a B3 vitamer that also has therapeutic activity. NAD is a substrate of the enzyme sirtuin 1 (SIRT1) involved in deacetylation reactions and poly ADP-ribose polymerase (PARP1), involved in poly ADP-ribosylation [66]. Many non-redox enzymes convert NAD to nicotinamide, including SIRT1 and PARP1 [67]. SIRT1 is an NAD-dependent enzyme that deacetylates histones and transcription factors thereby regulating gene expression, impacting DNA repair, apoptosis, cell proliferation, hormone responses and metabolism [68]. PARP1 is activated by DNA damage and DNA breaks [69]. Extreme DNA damage over-activates PARP1 thereby depleting NAD and ATP levels resulting in cell necrosis [69,70]. Interestingly, nicotinamide and NADH represses the activities of SIRT1 and PARP1 [67]. Therefore, the activity of these enzymes represent an important "sensing" mechanism of NAD/NADH ratios in the cell.

Nicotinamide is anti-inflammatory and downregulates NF-κB via SIRT1 deacetylation [67]. A number of in vitro, ex vivo and animal studies have examined the effect of nicotinamide showing the efficacy of nicotinamide in reducing immunosuppression following UV irradiation, enhanced DNA repair in keratinocytes and melanocytes, suppression of inflammatory cytokines in keratinocytes and suppression of tumor formation in animals, reviewed in [70]. In human clinical trials, oral nicotinamide reduced the incidence of actinic keratosis, squamous cell carcinoma and basal cell carcinoma. Additional animal studies show that nicotinamide suppressed chemically induced lung tumors, liver tumors, non-lymphocytic leukemia and kidney tumors [70]. Finally, clinical trials involving Accelerated Radiotherapy with CarbOgen and Nicotinamide (ARCON) showed efficacy in treating head and neck cancers, larynx and bladder cancers, reduction in tumor hypoxia in primary colon tumors and metastasis to the liver in animal models. Nicotinamide did not show significant effects in clinical trials attempting to treat glioblastoma or non-small cell lung carcinoma [70]. However, in a 16-year follow up study, consisting of nearly 650 hepatocellular carcinoma (HCC) cases, higher niacin intake was associated with a lower risk of HCC, which displayed an inverse dose response association [71].

While evidence for a beneficial role of niacin in certain cancer types appear solid, interpretation of the mechanisms through which niacin acts is complicated as they may be attributed to NAD/P as redox cofactors, or the products generated via sirtuin degradation. It is noteworthy that an active field of research, beyond the scope of this review, involves efforts to develop inhibitors of nicotinamide phosphoribosyl transferase (NAMPT) which mediates the rate-limiting step of an NAD salvage pathway (reviewed in [72]).

6. Pantothenic Acid B5

Pantothenic acid is an essential vitamin as it is required for the synthesis of CoA, a key cofactor in the TCA cycle and fatty acid metabolism. CoA is also required for acylation reactions. Deficiency in B5 is very rare as it is available in a variety of plants and animal products and therefore has not been studied in great detail. Uptake of pantothenic acid occurs via the sodium-dependent multivitamin transporter (SMVT), which also transports biotin (B7). Intestinal deletion of SMVT results in stunted growth, spontaneous and severe inflammation, increased gut permeability and early death. Surprisingly, supplementation of these mice with pantothenic acid and biotin curtailed these phenotypes [73]. These results suggest an alternative mechanism for these B vitamins' absorption other than through SMVT. In a follow-up study, confirmation that biotin levels in SMVT-deficient mice were decreased but not eliminated supports this conjecture [74]. Given that the transporter facilitates the transport of both B5 and B7, the attribution of phenotypes to biotin vs. pantothenic acid remains obscured but suggests that one or both of these vitamins plays a role in maintaining gut homeostasis.

Greater insights as to the role of pantothenic acid have come from the study of a family of proteins encoded by vanin genes. CoA catabolism generates pantetheine that is acted upon by vanins, otherwise known as pantetheinases, which generate pantothenate and cysteamine, the latter of which potentiates inflammation [75]. Mice deficient in vanin-1 are resistant to apoptotic oxidative tissue injury caused by γ-irradiation or paraquot [76]. These mice also attenuated chemically induced inflammation in models of colitis [77]. PPARγ inhibitors blocked the anti-inflammatory phenotypes of vanin-1-deficient mice, suggesting that the activity of vanin-1 antagonizes PPARγ [77]. Exposure of human mononuclear cells to oxidative stress inducers led to an increase in vanin-1 expression and a decrease in PPARγ [78]. Studies of vanin-1-deficient mice show a reduced ability to control *Shistosoma manosoni* and *Coxiella burnetii* infections suggesting that the role of vanin-1 induces inflammatory responses to infections [77,79]. Vanin-1-deficient mice display elevated levels of reduced glutathione in multiple tissues. Cysteamine breaks disulfide bonds that inactivate proteins and directly inhibits γ-glutamylcysteine synthase, the rate-limiting step in glutathione synthesis [76]. These findings point to cysteamine as the source of oxidative stress (ROS) generated during inflammation in vanin-1-deficient mice rather than pantothenate. Cysteamine administration to vanin-1 mice restores the inflammation observed to levels comparable to wild-type mice [76,80].

Compared to other B vitamins, the direct effects of vitamin B5 supplementation are scant. Therefore, the impact of B5 must be gathered through its known metabolism that has thus far highlighted cysteamine's pro-inflammatory properties. Given the importance of CoA, additional studies appear warranted to determine their effect on inflammatory processes and cancer. Analysis of pantothenate in the absence of pantetheinase activities, while challenging, may shed light on the more subtle roles of pantetheine in human health.

7. Pyridoxine B6

Despite the simplicity of pyridoxine synthesis (Figure 1), conversion of pyridoxin to its associated vitamers in human cells is complex. Pyridoxin (PN) and its vitamers pyridoxal (PL) and pyridoxamine are phosphorylated by pyridoxal kinase (PDXK) to generate pyridoxin-5′-phosphate (PNP), pyridoxol-5′-phosphate (PLP) and pyridoxamine-5′-phosphate (PMP). Each form of B6 are present in various foods; however, before absorption, they must be dephosphorylated by intestinal alkaline phosphatase [81]. Among these forms of vitamin B6, PN and PLP have received the greatest amount of attention, due to their more significant impact on human processes.

Vitamin B6-derived metabolites (PLP and PMP) serve as interconverting cofactors (transaminase) for >140 enzymatic reactions and have been estimated to be essential for 4% of all enzyme activities in the human genome. These reactions are important for amino acid, carbohydrate and fatty acid metabolism, and neurotransmitter production. PLP is a cofactor of decarboxylases and racemases, where PLP is not converted to PMP. PLP acts as a cosubstrate (phosphate donor) for glycogen phosphorylase.

Several studies have demonstrated the bioactivity of B6 and its vitamers in cancer models in vitro as inhibitors of cell proliferation, enhancement of chemotherapy cytotoxicity and alterations in gene expression. PN inhibits the growth of both murine and human melanoma cell lines and in this context PL displayed substantially greater effects than PN [82]. These observations have been extended to additional cell lines including hepatoma HepG2 and gastric cancer MKN45 cells [83], MCF-7 breast cancer and PANC-1 human pancreatic cancer cells [84]. The inhibition of cell proliferation in these models was assumed or verified as being correlated with elevated PLP.

Studies of PN and PLP in animal models of cancer have yielded mixed results. Some studies have reported an inverse correlation between PLP and different cancers [85]. In an examination of bile acids that are a risk factor for developing colorectal cancer (CRC), B6 supplementation increased fecal mucin levels and reduced the ratio of lithocholic acid to deoxycholic acid in a dose-dependent manner [86]. A study of rats exposed to 1,2-dimethylhydrazine to induce intestinal damage observed that vitamin B6 supplementation reduced the expression of alkaline phosphatase, a marker of intestinal damage and reduced cell proliferation [87]. Vitamin B6 was shown to stimulate proliferation of blood and splenic lymphocytes [88]. Using BALB/c mice fed varying doses of B6, very high doses of B6 (7.7 and 74.3 mg/day) exhibited the greatest impact on tumor volume reduction. Strong negative correlations were noted for PLP and tumor volume in these mice that also exhibited increased lymphocyte proliferation [88]. These results do not allow clear discrimination between whether the tumor inhibition following B6 feeding is due to an intrinsic effect on tumor growth or, alternatively, a greater stimulation of the antitumor immune response.

Treatment of A549 human non-small lung carcinoma (NSCLC) cells with a combination of PN and cisplatin potentiated the cytotoxicity of cisplatin by increasing the intracellular accumulation of cisplatin [85,89]. These studies concluded that PDXK activity was important for the observed enhancement of cisplatin. This is consistent with a report indicating that PDXK expression was positively correlated with overall survival of NSCLC patients treated with cisplatin. Treatment of human colon cancer and HEPG2 cells with 0.5-mM PL increased the expression of the cyclin inhibitor p21 as the result of p53 repression [90]. Similarly, PL treatment of HT29 colon cancer and HEPG2 cells increased the expression of insulin growth factor binding protein 1, a tumor suppressor [84]; the same finding was reported in MCF-7 breast cancer cells [84].

Reduced dietary intake of vitamin B6 has been documented as a risk factor for developing cancer [85,91]. Other studies have noted an inverse correlation between some cancers and vitamin B6 and/or serum PLP levels [85,92]. These include pancreatic, gastric adenocarcinoma, prostate, oral/pharyngeal, lung and colon cancers. It has been shown that B6 deficiency decreases the activity of serine hydroxymethyltransferase (SHMT) and betaine-homocysteine methyltransferase (BHMT), which reduce the pool of methylene groups for 5,10-methylene-THF resulting in an increase in the frequency of uracil incorporation during DNA synthesis that may be associated with mutation, and the DNA strand breaks [93]. The extent that this promotes carcinogenesis remains only partially characterized. In patients with non-small cell lung carcinoma, elevated levels of PDXK was identified as a good prognostic marker [92]. A meta-analysis of studies examining vitamin B6 in renal cell carcinoma patients concluded that B6 was protective and a useful biomarker; however, variability across studies made these conclusions tentative [45]. In a similar analysis of breast cancer risk involving nearly 50,000 cases, vitamin B6 levels were borderline significant in estrogen/progesterone receptor-negative tumors but not ER/PR + tumors [44]. Finally, an assessment of esophageal cancer found that an increase of 1 mg/day of vitamin B6 corresponded to a 16% reduction in cancer risk [94]. Hand–foot syndrome (HFS) is a dermatological reaction to toxicities generated by some cancer chemotherapies. Pyridoxine has been used to prevent HFS, although a meta-analysis of studies examining the efficacy of pyridoxine to prevent HFS found no significant differences in prevention of low-grade HFS compared to placebo controls; however, higher doses of B6 (400 mg daily) were statistically preventative [95].

8. Biotin B7

While biotin is available in many foods that are part of a standard diet, it is usually presented as a protein-bound form of biotin that is not readily available to cell metabolism. Peptide- or lysine-bound (biotinyl-lysine) biotin is released by the action of the pancreatic enzyme biotinidase and transported into cells by a number of different transporters [96]. Once inside the cell, biotin is covalently bound to biotin carboxyl carrier protein (BCCP) which serves as a prosthetic group for a number of carboxylases/decarboxylases regulating gluconeogenesis, lipogenesis, fatty acid synthesis and catabolism of branched-chain amino acids as well as valine and isovalerate. Biotinyl-AMP represents the activated form of biotin that is formed in the course of BCCP biotinylation. Biotin plays an indirect role in regulating gene expression as it has been reported that deprivation alters gene expression of multiple genes in the liver [97], including NO-like functions that increase cGMP via increased guanylate cyclase [98]. Biotin deficiency stems primarily from genetic changes in biotinidase which is required for cleavage from BCCP and recycling, resulting in alopecia, delays in development, seizures, aciduria and others neurological conditions. Biotin deficiency is also associated with elevated inflammation [99].

Neurodegenerative diseases are associated with mitochondrial dysfunction and oxidative stress and cell death. Myelin producing oligodendrocytes treated with biotin partially restored mitochondrial function, reduced oxygen free radicals and apoptosis [100]. Monocyte-derived DCs cultured in biotin-deficient medium produced elevated inflammatory cytokines in response to an LPS challenge [99]. In a study of monozygotic twins discordant for body mass index (BMI), BMI was anticorrelated with serum biotin levels and inflammation and hypertriglyceridemia [101].

Biotin deficiency impacts the expression of transcription factors such as NF-κB and SP1/3 highlighting the role of biotin in regulation of immunological phenomenon in a manner outside of its carboxylation/decarboxylation function [102]. While the molecular targets of biotin have been studied in some detail, there is much still to learn about the role of biotin in immune regulation and cancer and at present remain highly understudied.

9. Folate B9

Folate is transported into human cells as a monoglutamate form of the vitamin. Once inside the cell, tetrahydrofolate polyglutamates are formed, representing the active form of the vitamin. Concerns over meeting the daily minimum requirements for folate has led to the fortification of a variety of foods—e.g., cereals. This practice has led to an appreciable decrease in developmental problems associated with neural tube defects where folate plays an important role [103]. While the literature clearly illustrates the detrimental effects of folate deficiency, the metabolism of rapidly dividing malignant cells generate additional requirements for folate, thereby drawing into question whether folate supplementation may do more harm than good in this context.

There is a general lack of literature examining the role of folate in the regulation of the immune system; however, its role as a key regulator of one-carbon metabolism is well-studied and described in a subsequent section. Both folate and vitamin B12 deficiency are associated with the reduction in glutathione, a major antioxidant protein in the cell. Azoxymethane (AOM) is used in many models to induce tumors and to induce oxidative stress. AOM-treated rats display oxidative stress, glutathione depletion, oxidation of proteins and oxidative damage of DNA. Folate and B12 reduced oxidative stress and the cytotoxic effects of AOM in mice [104]. Folate deficiency has been shown to have negative consequences for some immune functions. Treatment of $CD8^+$ T cells and phytohaemaggutinin and IL-2 promotes cell proliferation but stimulation was inhibited when folic acid was absent. This activity did not affect $CD4^+$ T cells [105]. Folate deficiency in primary human lymphocytes reduced cell proliferation and resulted in increased DNA strand breaks, apoptosis and cell cycle arrest [106]. Folate deficiency has also been linked to reduced DC maturation and effector functions including: reduced IL-2, TNF-α, IL-6 and IL1-β in response to LPS stimulation. These changes were coupled to reduced $CD4^+$ T cell differentiation with reduced Th1 and Treg cell populations [107]. Anti-inflammatory Treg cells express the folate receptor constitutively and at high levels. Blockade of this receptor leads to reductions in Treg cell populations [108]. Finally, high oral doses of folic acid reduced the inflammatory response of mice with allergic dermatitis through inhibition of T cell cytokine secretion [109].

In mice implanted with tumor cells derived from various MMTV-Wnt breast tumors, differential effects of folic acid withdrawal were observed in a comparison of non-metastatic epithelial, non-metastatic mesenchymal, or metastatic mesenchymal cell lines. After 72-h growth in the absence of folic acid, the non-metastatic mesenchymal cell line displayed the largest change in its transcriptome. The type I interferon signaling pathway was activated under folic acid insufficiency. This pathway is downregulated in aggressive triple-negative breast cancers [110]. This differential response is consistent with other data indicating that folic acid supplementation impacts cell migration and metastasis. In a similar study using nasopharyngeal epidermoid carcinoma cell growth in folate-deficient medium, hypermethylation of H-cadherin promoter sequences were observed, which corresponded to reduced expression [111].

A number of in vitro and animal studies have shown that folate deficiency may drive oncogenic events, whereas high folate intake promotes the growth and progression of established tumors [112]. Low folate intake has been associated with increased expression of immune-related genes, urokinase and iNOS, and the downregulation of genes encoding adhesion proteins—protocadherin-4, nidogen and integrin αV. Gene expression changes in the intestine were pronounced in aged rats fed a folate-deficient diet including reduced expression of urokinase, p53, insulin-like growth factor binding protein-3 and the vav-1 oncogene [113]. Using three normal colonic cell lines with varying doses of folate, gene expression was altered including the upregulation of folate receptor-1 which was inversely proportional with folate levels. Oncogenes p53, p21, p16 and β-catenin followed a similar pattern. DNA strand breaks were increased with decreased folate. Other changes included the Wnt/APC pathway and genes involved in cell adhesion, migration and invasion [114]. Folate antagonists, methotrexate and trimetrexate treatment of glioma cell lines reduced cell migration but had no impact on invasion potential [115].

A study of a small number of women at high risk for developing breast cancer (BRCA1/2) found that high plasma levels of folate were associated with high risk [116]. Other studies come to an opposing conclusion indicating a protective effect of folic acid supplementation in women with BRCA1 mutation [117]. No such association was attributed to B6 or B12 [116]. Epidemiological and clinical studies indicate that folate intake and blood levels are both inversely correlated with colorectal cancer risk. The risk reduction for CRC is substantial when comparing the upper and lower quartiles of folate intake, corresponding to a 40% reduction [118]. High serum folate in men with prostate cancer was associated with elevated cell proliferation [119]. Similarly, folate intake was positively associated with risk of recurrence in patients with non-muscle-invasive bladder cancer [120]. Despite these findings, reports of serum folate in hepatocellular carcinoma patients were found to be inversely associated with tumor size, tumor multiplicity and metastasis [121]. Interestingly, serum folate levels were reduced with HCC stage progression. Using an HCC xenograft mouse model, folate-deficient feeding promoted tumorigenesis and metastasis [122]. Similarly, folate deprivation of cultured epithelial colon cancer cells enhanced cell migration and invasion resembling an epithelial–mesencymal transition, associated with snail gene expression and E-cadherin repression with increased expression of β1 integrin and proteolysis activity of MMP2. These patterns were abolished by the inhibition of sonic hedgehog due to the hypomethylation of its promoter or NFκB [123]. High folate intake is inversely associated with ovarian cancer risk [124]. Carcinomas have been reported to over-express folate receptor α. Ovarian tumors over-express folate receptor α but display a decreased expression of another transporter, reduced folate carrier. These outcomes were associated with folate receptor α gene amplification and hypermethylation of the reduced folate carrier. Folate promoted proliferation, migration and invasion in vitro. Knock down of folate receptor α or over-expression of the reduced folate carrier negated these effects. In summary, folate deficiency is negatively correlated with cancer risk for a number of malignancies; however, there is increasing concern that folate supplementation in individuals with an already developed cancer may further drive cancer progression. The major role of folate relates to one-carbon metabolism which is discussed below.

10. One-Carbon Metabolism

One-carbon metabolism refers to a complex network of biochemical pathways involving homocysteine, methionine and B vitamins (B2, B6, B9 and B12). The folate cycle and methionine cycle are coordinated and mediate diverse cellular processes including: DNA synthesis (purines and thymidine), energy (ATP), redox potential (NADPH) and lipid, polyamine, amino acids and phospholipid biosynthesis (Figure 3). Importantly one-carbon metabolism generates *S*-adenosylmethionine (SAM) which is a universal methyl donor for methylation of DNA and RNA and histones, thereby regulating transcription and translation.

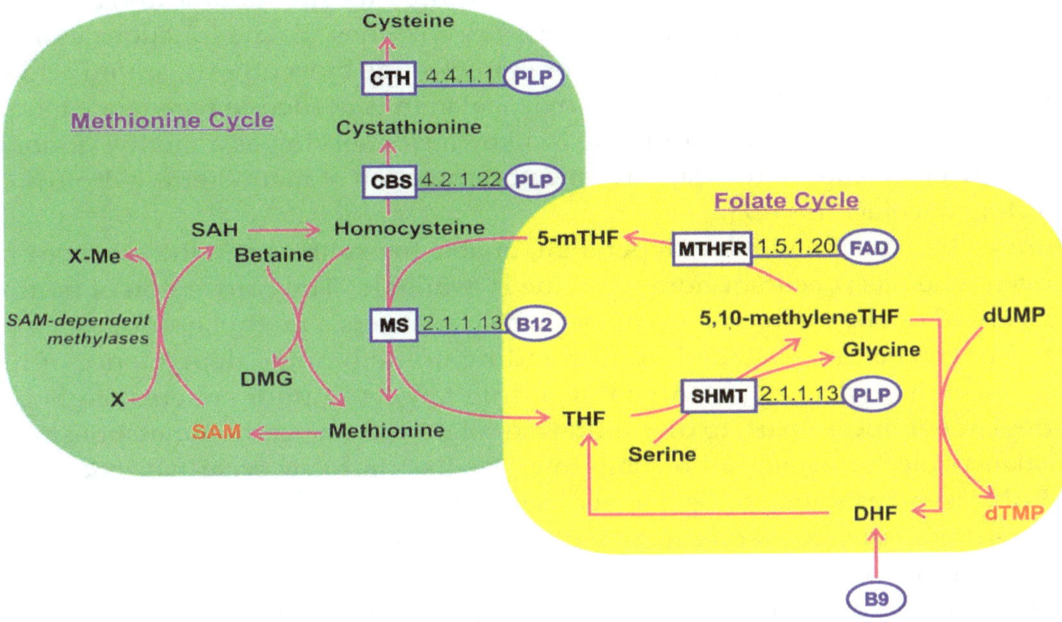

Figure 3. The methionine and folate cycle pathways involving PLP-, FAD- and B12-dependent enzymes. The folate cycle begins with the conversion of dietary folate (B9) into dihydrofolate (DHF), which is then reduced to tetrahydrofolate (THF) by the enzyme dihydrofolate reductase (DHFR). THF is next converted to 5,10-methyleneTHF by serine hydroxymethyltransferase (SHMT), a reaction that is coupled with the hydroxylation of serine (Ser) to glycine (Gly) and requires PLP as a cofactor. Thymidylate synthase (TS) uses 5,10-methyleneTHF as a methyl donor to methylate deoxyuridine monophosphate (dUMP), creating deoxythymidine monophosphate (dTMP). This step regenerates DHF for continued cycling. Alternatively, 5,10-methyleneTHF can be reduced by methylenetetrahydrofolate reductase (MTHFR) to 5-methytetrahydrofolate (5-mTHF) using FAD as a cofactor. As part of the methionine cycle, 5-mTHF donates a methyl group to regenerate methionine from homocysteine (Hcy), which is catalyzed by methionine synthase (MS) that requires B12, in the form of methylcobalamin, as a cofactor. To generate the methyl donor *S*-adenosylmethionine (SAM) for use by multiple methyltransferases. SAM is demethylated during the methyltransferase reactions to form *S*-adenosylhomocysteine (SAH) which is then hydrolysed by *S*-adenosylhomocysteine hydrolase (AHCY) to form Hcy. Hcy can also enter the trans-sulfuration pathway catalyzed by cystathionine beta synthase (CBS) and cystathionine gamma lyase (CTH), both requiring PLP as a cofactor, to create cysteine.

Inputs for the folate cycle include serine and glycine. The folate cycle is segregated in the cytoplasm and the reactions occurring in the mitochondria. The methionine cycle requires methionine to generate cysteine, a key component of a third pathway referred to as trans-sulfuration, which generates glutathione—a mediator of redox balance, inhibitor of ROS-induced oxidative stress and which generates SAM. An exciting research area considers that maternal intake of B vitamins involved in one-carbon metabolism may impact the long-term cancer risks of offspring through modulation of epigenetic imprinting. While several studies have reported evidence in this direction, the field is fraught with contradictory findings at this stage and is therefore considered too premature for detailed description here [125]. Folate and cobalamin deficiency can alter the balance of one-carbon metabolism pathways. PLP, derived from vitamin B6, plays an essential role as a cofactor for enzymes in homocysteine metabolism, encompassing both folate-mediated one-carbon metabolism and the trans-sulfuration pathway. As such, vitamin B6 is involved in purine, thymidylate and methionine synthesis. These activities have highlighted vitamin B6's potential role in genome stability and epigenetic regulation [126]. Glutamylated folate is involved in the carriage and transfer of one-carbon units (formate) in the form of 10-formyltetrahydrofolate, required for purine biosynthesis, (formaldehyde) in the form of methylenetetrahydrofolate required for thymidylate biosynthesis or (methanol) in the form of 5-methyltetrahydrofolate, required for methionine and SAM biosynthesis. Each of these forms serves as a cofactor for one or more enzymes. Folate functions as a coenzyme in numerous reactions involving one-carbon transfer in nucleotide biosynthesis, amino acid metabolism. The action of folate and B12 are linked since methylcobalamin is needed to regenerate tetrahydrofolate from methyltetrahydrofolate. Tetrahydrofolate is a key factor serving as a methyl donor in multiple pathways. B12 deficiency leads to the trapping and accumulation of methyltetrahydrofolate disrupting the normal cycling of cofactors [127].

Many tumors become methionine-dependent, unable to proliferate in the absence of exogenous methionine even when its precursor homocysteine is available. The conversion of homocysteine to methionine is carried out by methionine synthase which transfers a methyl group from 5-methyl THF in the presence of cobalamin. Detailed understanding of methionine dependence of tumors is an area of active research to identify potential novel drug targets. Tumor spheres of glioblastoma are methionine-dependent due, in part, to disruptions in folate and one-carbon metabolism. One-carbon metabolism balances the flux of one-carbon units toward either the folate cycle that generates nucleotides for DNA and RNA synthesis and energy metabolism or alternatively, toward the methionine cycle for methionine generation where it serves as precursor of SAM, which is required for the methylation of DNA, RNA, histones and proteins impacting gene expression (reviewed in [128]). Vitamin B12 deprivation results in a decrease in SAM concentrations and strong reductions in cancer cell growth [129]. Hyperhomocysteinemia is a risk factor for cardiovascular disease. Using apoE-null mice provided a diet rich in methionine but depleted in vitamins B6, B9 and B12, increased cardiovascular signatures were found to develop in said mice, including elevated expression of the receptor for advanced glycation products, VCAM-1 and MMP-9 in the vasculature; provision of the B vitamins alleviated these effects [130]. By contrast, a human clinical trial where patients who experienced ischemic attack or stroke were provided vitamins B6, B9 and B12 to lower homocysteine levels; while such treatments indeed lowered homocysteine levels, markers of vascular inflammation were unaffected [131].

A meta-analysis of one-carbon metabolism-related vitamins (B6, B9 and B12) concluded that there was no association between B12 and breast cancer risk [44]. In another meta-analysis study examining methylenetetrahydrofolate reductase polymorphisms (MTHFR C677T) and B9 and B12 intake concluded that low intake of folate was associated with increased risk of breast cancer, whereas no association were found for B12 [132]. A study seeking to find genetic associations between vitamins and five cancers also concluded that B12 was not relevant to colorectal, breast, prostate, malignant melanoma or squamous cell carcinoma [133]. A study of B vitamins involved in one-carbon metabolism in the setting of esophageal cancer found that vitamin B2 and B12 were positively correlated with cancer risk, whereas vitamin B6 and B9 were inversely correlated [94]. From an analysis of nearly 4000 incident lung cancer cases, B6 intake was deemed protective, whereas B9 and B12 intake were not associated with lung cancer risk [134]. In a large meta-analysis of patients (757,185 subjects) for all cancers, elevated B12 was identified as a risk factor for cancer; this was particularly evident in liver, pancreatic and myeloid malignancies [135]. Finally, a meta-analysis of prostate cancer risk found that both vitamin B9 and B12 were positively associated [136].

11. Cobalamin B12

B12 absorption requires release of the vitamin from dietary proteins. Once released it may bind to gastric intrinsic factor which is absorbed in the gastrointestinal tract (ileum) through a receptor-mediated process. Individuals that do not produce adequate quantities of intrinsic factor suffer from pernicious anemia due to the low bioavailability of cobalamin. Additionally, certain medicines can interfere with B12 absorption including chloramphenicol, metformin, proton pump inhibitors and histamine. B12 absorption is saturable and relatively inefficient as ~1% of dietary B12 is absorbed and the remainder is excreted in urine.

Vitamin B12 is important in the regulation of select immune cell types, including NK cells and $CD8^+$ T cells through an upregulation of their expansion [137]. In aged rats, B12 deficiency was associated with a decline in NK cell activity and a reduction in a subset of B lymphocytes [138]. Interestingly, this study also highlighted the importance of maintaining normal levels of folate and B12, since the age-induced B12 reductions were most evident when folate was supplemented. NK cell activity was compromised in association with free unmetabolized folic acid illustrating the importance of achieving a proper balance between folate and B12 levels.

High serum cobalamin levels were associated with poor survival in patients with HCC [139]. A study of non-small cell lung carcinoma examined plasma levels of cobalamin and cobalamin carrier proteins—transcobalamin, holotranscobalamin and haptocorrin. Among the analytes examined, significant associations were determined only for haptocorrin that was significantly elevated in patients with NSCLC, suggesting that this may be a useful biomarker for diagnostic purposes [140]. Similarly, in a case-control study of prostate cancer, B12 and holo-haptocorrin levels were positively associated with cancer risk [141]. In a nested case-control study, blood B12 levels were positively associated with overall lung cancer risk [142].

12. Conclusions

The accumulated knowledge of B vitamins and their vitamers as cofactors to a large number of essential enzymes and cellular activities is impressive. Overall, evidence for some B vitamins having a protective role in various cancers remains elusive, begging the question, why? The answers are likely to be complex, owing to the number of variables associated with any B vitamin such as absorption, bioactivity and variability of vitamer generation to name a few. B vitamins influence the function of such a wide spectrum of cell functions, so it should perhaps not be surprising that studies aimed at assessing their role as regulators of immune function and cancer are variable. It may not be adequate to simply interogate B vitamin intake or even blood concentrations of B vitamins. Animal studies allow a more direct assessment of individual B vitamers and in some cases give greater clarity of the beneficial and detrimental effects of B vitamin consumption. Ultimately, these results are very challenging to translate to humans in the form of intervention studies since the design of cancer prevention studies would require compliance for many years in very large cohorts. Alternatively, human studies in the future may require more comprehensive molecular analyses of B vitamins and their corresponding vitamers to be coupled with a high-resolution analysis of a variety of immune functions and tumor subtypes that may allow stronger and more convincing associations to be uncovered. As appears to be the case for folate (B9), B vitamins may provide protection from developing cancer but play a detrimental role in patients diagnosed with cancer. This single example suggests that a more detailed and sophisticated analysis of B vitamins will be of high potential importance.

Acknowledgments: The authors wish to thank Lisa Hamilton for assistance with references and manuscript preparation.

References

1. Whatham, A.; Bartlett, H.; Eperjesi, F.; Blumenthal, C.; Allen, J.; Suttle, C.; Gaskin, K. Vitamin and mineral deficiencies in the developed world and their effect on the eye and vision. *Ophthalmic Physiol. Opt.* **2008**, *28*, 1–12. [CrossRef] [PubMed]
2. Revuelta, J.L.; Buey, R.M.; Ledesma-Amaro, R.; Vandamme, E.J. Microbial biotechnology for the synthesis of (pro)vitamins, biopigments and antioxidants: Challenges and opportunities. *Microb. Biotechnol.* **2016**, *9*, 564–567. [CrossRef]
3. Rodionov, D.A.; Arzamasov, A.A.; Khoroshkin, M.S.; Iablokov, S.N.; Leyn, S.A.; Peterson, S.N.; Novichkov, P.S.; Osterman, A.L. Micronutrient requirements and sharing capabilities of the human gut microbiome. *Front. Microbiol.* **2019**, *10*, 1316. [CrossRef]
4. Sharma, V.; Rodionov, D.A.; Leyn, S.A.; Tran, D.; Iablokov, S.N.; Ding, H.; Peterson, D.A.; Osterman, A.L.; Peterson, S.N. B-vitamin sharing promotes stability of gut microbial communities. *Front. Microbiol.* **2019**, *10*, 1485. [CrossRef]
5. Frank, R.A.; Leeper, F.J.; Luisi, B.F. Structure, mechanism and catalytic duality of thiamine-dependent enzymes. *Cell Mol. Life Sci.* **2007**, *64*, 892–905. [CrossRef]
6. Mathis, D.; Shoelson, S.E. Immunometabolism: An emerging frontier. *Nat. Rev. Immunol.* **2011**, *11*, 81. [CrossRef]
7. Buck, M.D.; Sowell, R.T.; Kaech, S.M.; Pearce, E.L. Metabolic instruction of immunity. *Cell* **2017**, *169*, 570–586. [CrossRef]
8. Shikina, T.; Hiroi, T.; Iwatani, K.; Jang, M.H.; Fukuyama, S.; Tamura, M.; Kubo, T.; Ishikawa, H.; Kiyono, H. IgA class switch occurs in the organized nasopharynx- and gut-associated lymphoid tissue, but not in the diffuse lamina propria of airways and gut. *J. Immunol.* **2004**, *172*, 6259–6264. [CrossRef]
9. Kunisawa, J.; Sugiura, Y.; Wake, T.; Nagatake, T.; Suzuki, H.; Nagasawa, R.; Shikata, S.; Honda, K.; Hashimoto, E.; Suzuki, Y.; et al. Mode of bioenergetic metabolism during B cell differentiation in the intestine determines the distinct requirement for vitamin B1. *Cell Rep.* **2015**, *13*, 122–131. [CrossRef]
10. Moallem, S.A.; Hosseinzadeh, H.; Farahi, S. A study of acute and chronic anti-nociceptive and anti-inflammatory effects of thiamine in mice. *Iran. Biomed. J.* **2008**, *12*, 173–178. [PubMed]
11. Gibson, G.E.; Ksiezak-Reding, H.; Sheu, K.F.; Mykytyn, V.; Blass, J.P. Correlation of enzymatic, metabolic, and behavioral deficits in thiamin deficiency and its reversal. *Neurochem. Res.* **1984**, *9*, 803–814. [CrossRef]
12. Calingasan, N.Y.; Chun, W.J.; Park, L.C.; Uchida, K.; Gibson, G.E. Oxidative stress is associated with region-specific neuronal death during thiamine deficiency. *J. Neuropathol. Exp. Neurol.* **1999**, *58*, 946–958. [CrossRef]
13. Wegner, C.D.; Gundel, R.H.; Reilly, P.; Haynes, N.; Letts, L.G.; Rothlein, R. Intercellular adhesion molecule-1 (ICAM-1) in the pathogenesis of asthma. *Science* **1990**, *247*, 456–459. [CrossRef]
14. Jones, P.T.; Anderson, R. Oxidative inhibition of polymorphonuclear leukocyte motility mediated by the peroxidase/H_2O_2/halide system: Studies on the reversible nature of the inhibition and mechanism of protection of migratory responsiveness by ascorbate, levamisole, thiamine and cysteine. *Int. J. Immunopharmacol.* **1983**, *5*, 377–389. [CrossRef]
15. Yadav, U.C.; Kalariya, N.M.; Srivastava, S.K.; Ramana, K.V. Protective role of benfotiamine, a fat-soluble vitamin B1 analogue, in lipopolysaccharide-induced cytotoxic signals in murine macrophages. *Free Radic. Biol. Med.* **2010**, *48*, 1423–1434. [CrossRef] [PubMed]
16. Marik, P.E. Hydrocortisone, Ascorbic Acid and Thiamine (HAT Therapy) for the treatment of sepsis. Focus on ascorbic acid. *Nutrients* **2018**, *10*, 1762. [CrossRef] [PubMed]
17. Cruickshank, A.M.; Telfer, A.B.; Shenkin, A. Thiamine deficiency in the critically ill. *Intensive Care Med.* **1988**, *14*, 384–387. [CrossRef]
18. Liu, X.; Montissol, S.; Uber, A.; Ganley, S.; Grossestreuer, A.V.; Berg, K.; Heydrick, S.; Donnino, M.W. The effects of thiamine on breast cancer cells. *Molecules* **2018**, *23*, 1464. [CrossRef]
19. Sweet, R.; Paul, A.; Zastre, J. Hypoxia induced upregulation and function of the thiamine transporter, SLC19A3 in a breast cancer cell line. *Cancer Biol. Ther.* **2010**, *10*, 1101–1111. [CrossRef]
20. Jonus, H.C.; Hanberry, B.S.; Khatu, S.; Kim, J.; Luesch, H.; Dang, L.H.; Bartlett, M.G.; Zastre, J.A. The adaptive regulation of thiamine pyrophosphokinase-1 facilitates malignant growth during supplemental thiamine conditions. *Oncotarget* **2018**, *9*, 35422–35438. [CrossRef]

21. Jonus, H.C.; Byrnes, C.C.; Kim, J.; Valle, M.L.; Bartlett, M.G.; Said, H.M.; Zastre, J.A. Thiamine mimetics sulbutiamine and benfotiamine as a nutraceutical approach to anticancer therapy. *Biomed. Pharmacother.* **2020**, *121*, 109648. [CrossRef]
22. Comin-Anduix, B.; Boren, J.; Martinez, S.; Moro, C.; Centelles, J.J.; Trebukhina, R.; Petushok, N.; Lee, W.N.; Boros, L.G.; Cascante, M. The effect of thiamine supplementation on tumour proliferation. A metabolic control analysis study. *Eur. J. Biochem.* **2001**, *268*, 4177–4182. [CrossRef]
23. Cancarini, I.; Krogh, V.; Agnoli, C.; Grioni, S.; Matullo, G.; Pala, V.; Pedraglio, S.; Contiero, P.; Riva, C.; Muti, P.; et al. Micronutrients involved in one-carbon metabolism and risk of breast cancer subtypes. *PLoS ONE* **2015**, *10*, e0138318. [CrossRef]
24. Kabat, G.C.; Miller, A.B.; Jain, M.; Rohan, T.E. Dietary intake of selected B vitamins in relation to risk of major cancers in women. *Br. J. Cancer* **2008**, *99*, 816–821. [CrossRef]
25. Bruce, W.R.; Furrer, R.; Shangari, N.; O'Brien, P.J.; Medline, A.; Wang, Y. Marginal dietary thiamin deficiency induces the formation of colonic aberrant crypt foci (ACF) in rats. *Cancer Lett.* **2003**, *202*, 125–129. [CrossRef]
26. Powers, H.J. Current knowledge concerning optimum nutritional status of riboflavin, niacin and pyridoxine. *Proc. Nutr. Soc.* **1999**, *58*, 435–440. [CrossRef]
27. Seekamp, A.; Hultquist, D.E.; Till, G.O. Protection by vitamin B2 against oxidant-mediated acute lung injury. *Inflammation* **1999**, *23*, 449–460. [CrossRef]
28. Hashida, S.; Yuzawa, S.; Suzuki, N.N.; Fujioka, Y.; Takikawa, T.; Sumimoto, H.; Inagaki, F.; Fujii, H. Binding of FAD to cytochrome b558 is facilitated during activation of the phagocyte NADPH oxidase, leading to superoxide production. *J. Biol. Chem.* **2004**, *279*, 26378–26386. [CrossRef]
29. Araki, S.; Suzuki, M.; Fujimoto, M.; Kimura, M. Enhancement of resistance to bacterial infection in mice by vitamin B2. *J. Vet. Med. Sci.* **1995**, *57*, 599–602. [CrossRef]
30. Verdrengh, M.; Tarkowski, A. Riboflavin in innate and acquired immune responses. *Inflamm. Res.* **2005**, *54*, 390–393. [CrossRef]
31. Qureshi, A.A.; Tan, X.; Reis, J.C.; Badr, M.Z.; Papasian, C.J.; Morrison, D.C.; Qureshi, N. Suppression of nitric oxide induction and pro-inflammatory cytokines by novel proteasome inhibitors in various experimental models. *Lipids Health Dis.* **2011**, *10*, 177. [CrossRef] [PubMed]
32. Mikkelsen, K.; Prakash, M.D.; Kuol, N.; Nurgali, K.; Stojanovska, L.; Apostolopoulos, V. Anti-tumor effects of vitamin B2, B6 and B9 in promonocytic lymphoma cells. *Int. J. Mol. Sci.* **2019**, *20*, 3763. [CrossRef]
33. Koay, H.F.; Gherardin, N.A.; Enders, A.; Loh, L.; Mackay, L.K.; Almeida, C.F.; Russ, B.E.; Nold-Petry, C.A.; Nold, M.F.; Bedoui, S.; et al. A three-stage intrathymic development pathway for the mucosal-associated invariant T cell lineage. *Nat. Immunol.* **2016**, *17*, 1300–1311. [CrossRef]
34. Corbett, A.J.; Eckle, S.B.; Birkinshaw, R.W.; Liu, L.; Patel, O.; Mahony, J.; Chen, Z.; Reantragoon, R.; Meehan, B.; Cao, H.; et al. T-cell activation by transitory neo-antigens derived from distinct microbial pathways. *Nature* **2014**, *509*, 361–365. [CrossRef]
35. Hartmann, N.; McMurtrey, C.; Sorensen, M.L.; Huber, M.E.; Kurapova, R.; Coleman, F.T.; Mizgerd, J.P.; Hildebrand, W.; Kronenberg, M.; Lewinsohn, D.M.; et al. Riboflavin metabolism variation among clinical isolates of streptococcus pneumoniae results in differential activation of mucosal-associated invariant T cells. *Am. J. Respir. Cell Mol. Biol.* **2018**, *58*, 767–776. [CrossRef] [PubMed]
36. Patel, O.; Kjer-Nielsen, L.; Le Nours, J.; Eckle, S.B.; Birkinshaw, R.; Beddoe, T.; Corbett, A.J.; Liu, L.; Miles, J.J.; Meehan, B.; et al. Recognition of vitamin B metabolites by mucosal-associated invariant T cells. *Nat. Commun.* **2013**, *4*, 2142. [CrossRef]
37. Toyosawa, T.; Suzuki, M.; Kodama, K.; Araki, S. Effects of intravenous infusion of highly purified vitamin B2 on lipopolysaccharide-induced shock and bacterial infection in mice. *Eur. J. Pharmacol.* **2004**, *492*, 273–280. [CrossRef]
38. Al-Harbi, N.O.; Imam, F.; Nadeem, A.; Al-Harbi, M.M.; Korashy, H.M.; Sayed-Ahmed, M.M.; Hafez, M.M.; Al-Shabanah, O.A.; Nagi, M.N.; Bahashwan, S. Riboflavin attenuates lipopolysaccharide-induced lung injury in rats. *Toxicol. Mech. Methods* **2015**, *25*, 417–423. [CrossRef]
39. Schramm, M.; Wiegmann, K.; Schramm, S.; Gluschko, A.; Herb, M.; Utermohlen, O.; Kronke, M. Riboflavin (vitamin B2) deficiency impairs NADPH oxidase 2 (Nox2) priming and defense against Listeria monocytogenes. *Eur. J. Immunol.* **2014**, *44*, 728–741. [CrossRef]
40. Gupta, T.K.; Vishnuvajjala, B.R.; Witiak, D.T.; Gerald, M.C. Antagonism of amphetamine stereotyped behavior by diastereoisomeric dihydrodibenzothiepin neuroleptics. *Experientia* **1977**, *33*, 65. [CrossRef]

41. Pan, F.; Chen, Y.; He, J.Z.; Long, L.; Chen, Y.; Luo, H.J.; Xu, Y.W.; Pang, X.X.; Yang, Q.; Wang, J.J.; et al. Dietary riboflavin deficiency promotes N-nitrosomethylbenzylamine-induced esophageal tumorigenesis in rats by inducing chronic inflammation. *Am. J. Cancer Res.* **2019**, *9*, 2469–2481.
42. Machado, D.; Shishido, S.M.; Queiroz, K.C.; Oliveira, D.N.; Faria, A.L.; Catharino, R.R.; Spek, C.A.; Ferreira, C.V. Irradiated riboflavin diminishes the aggressiveness of melanoma in vitro and in vivo. *PLoS ONE* **2013**, *8*, e54269. [CrossRef]
43. Powers, H.J. Riboflavin (vitamin B-2) and health. *Am. J. Clin. Nutr.* **2003**, *77*, 1352–1360. [CrossRef]
44. Zeng, J.; Gu, Y.; Fu, H.; Liu, C.; Zou, Y.; Chang, H. Association between one-carbon metabolism-related vitamins and risk of breast cancer: A systematic review and meta-analysis of prospective studies. *Clin. Breast Cancer* **2020**, *20*, e469–e480. [CrossRef] [PubMed]
45. Clasen, J.L.; Heath, A.K.; Scelo, G.; Muller, D.C. Components of one-carbon metabolism and renal cell carcinoma: A systematic review and meta-analysis. *Eur. J. Nutr.* **2020**. [CrossRef]
46. Li, S.S.; Tan, H.Z.; Xu, Y.W.; Wu, Z.Y.; Wu, J.Y.; Zhao, X.K.; Wang, L.D.; Long, L.; Li, E.M.; Xu, L.Y.; et al. [The association between the whole blood riboflavin level and the occurrence, development and prognosis of esophageal squamous cell carcinoma]. *Zhonghua Yu Fang Yi Xue Za Zhi* **2019**, *53*, 1124–1129. [CrossRef]
47. de Vogel, S.; Dindore, V.; van Engeland, M.; Goldbohm, R.A.; van den Brandt, P.A.; Weijenberg, M.P. Dietary folate, methionine, riboflavin, and vitamin B-6 and risk of sporadic colorectal cancer. *J. Nutr.* **2008**, *138*, 2372–2378. [CrossRef]
48. Takata, Y.; Cai, Q.; Beeghly-Fadiel, A.; Li, H.; Shrubsole, M.J.; Ji, B.T.; Yang, G.; Chow, W.H.; Gao, Y.T.; Zheng, W.; et al. Dietary B vitamin and methionine intakes and lung cancer risk among female never smokers in China. *Cancer Causes Control.* **2012**, *23*, 1965–1975. [CrossRef]
49. Kirkland, J.B.; Meyer-Ficca, M.L. Niacin. *Adv. Food Nutr. Res.* **2018**, *83*, 83–149. [CrossRef] [PubMed]
50. Lohani, M.; Dhasmana, A.; Haque, S.; Dar, S.A.; Jawed, A.; Wahid, M.; Mandal, R.K.; Akhter, N.; Farasani, A.; Hobani, Y.H.; et al. Niacin deficiency modulates genes involved in cancer: Are smokers at higher risk? *J. Cell Biochem.* **2019**, *120*, 232–242. [CrossRef]
51. Choi, H.J.; Jang, S.Y.; Hwang, E.S. High-dose nicotinamide suppresses ros generation and augments population expansion during CD8(+) T cell activation. *Mol. Cells* **2015**, *38*, 918–924. [CrossRef] [PubMed]
52. Wanders, D.; Graff, E.C.; White, B.D.; Judd, R.L. Niacin increases adiponectin and decreases adipose tissue inflammation in high fat diet-fed mice. *PLoS ONE* **2013**, *8*, e71285. [CrossRef]
53. Karacaglar, E.; Atar, I.; Altin, C.; Yetis, B.; Cakmak, A.; Bayraktar, N.; Coner, A.; Ozin, B.; Muderrisoglu, H. The effects of niacin on inflammation in patients with non-ST elevated acute coronary syndrome. *Acta Cardiol. Sin.* **2015**, *31*, 120–126. [CrossRef]
54. Su, G.; Sun, G.; Liu, H.; Shu, L.; Zhang, J.; Guo, L.; Huang, C.; Xu, J. Niacin suppresses progression of atherosclerosis by inhibiting vascular inflammation and apoptosis of vascular smooth muscle cells. *Med. Sci. Monit.* **2015**, *21*, 4081–4089. [CrossRef]
55. Ganji, S.H.; Kukes, G.D.; Lambrecht, N.; Kashyap, M.L.; Kamanna, V.S. Therapeutic role of niacin in the prevention and regression of hepatic steatosis in rat model of nonalcoholic fatty liver disease. *Am. J. Physiol. Gastrointest. Liver Physiol.* **2014**, *306*, G320–G327. [CrossRef]
56. Kashyap, M.L.; Ganji, S.; Nakra, N.K.; Kamanna, V.S. Niacin for treatment of nonalcoholic fatty liver disease (NAFLD): Novel use for an old drug? *J. Clin. Lipidol.* **2019**, *13*, 873–879. [CrossRef] [PubMed]
57. Li, Z.; Wang, Y.; van der Sluis, R.J.; van der Hoorn, J.W.; Princen, H.M.; Van Eck, M.; Van Berkel, T.J.; Rensen, P.C.; Hoekstra, M. Niacin reduces plasma CETP levels by diminishing liver macrophage content in CETP transgenic mice. *Biochem. Pharmacol.* **2012**, *84*, 821–829. [CrossRef]
58. Ferreira, R.G.; Matsui, T.C.; Gomides, L.F.; Godin, A.M.; Menezes, G.B.; de Matos Coelho, M.; Klein, A. Niacin inhibits carrageenan-induced neutrophil migration in mice. *Naunyn Schmiedebergs Arch. Pharmacol.* **2013**, *386*, 533–540. [CrossRef]
59. Digby, J.E.; Martinez, F.; Jefferson, A.; Ruparelia, N.; Chai, J.; Wamil, M.; Greaves, D.R.; Choudhury, R.P. Anti-inflammatory effects of nicotinic acid in human monocytes are mediated by GPR109A dependent mechanisms. *Arterioscler. Thromb. Vasc. Biol.* **2012**, *32*, 669–676. [CrossRef] [PubMed]
60. Kwon, W.Y.; Suh, G.J.; Kim, K.S.; Kwak, Y.H. Niacin attenuates lung inflammation and improves survival during sepsis by downregulating the nuclear factor-kappaB pathway. *Crit. Care Med.* **2011**, *39*, 328–334. [CrossRef]

61. Cho, K.H.; Kim, H.J.; Rodriguez-Iturbe, B.; Vaziri, N.D. Niacin ameliorates oxidative stress, inflammation, proteinuria, and hypertension in rats with chronic renal failure. *Am. J. Physiol. Renal. Physiol.* **2009**, *297*, F106–F113. [CrossRef] [PubMed]
62. Takechi, R.; Pallebage-Gamarallage, M.M.; Lam, V.; Giles, C.; Mamo, J.C. Nutraceutical agents with anti-inflammatory properties prevent dietary saturated-fat induced disturbances in blood-brain barrier function in wild-type mice. *J. Neuroinflamm.* **2013**, *10*, 73. [CrossRef]
63. Wakade, C.; Giri, B.; Malik, A.; Khodadadi, H.; Morgan, J.C.; Chong, R.K.; Baban, B. Niacin modulates macrophage polarization in Parkinson's disease. *J. NeuroImmunol.* **2018**, *320*, 76–79. [CrossRef]
64. Feingold, K.R.; Moser, A.; Shigenaga, J.K.; Grunfeld, C. Inflammation stimulates niacin receptor (GPR109A/HCA2) expression in adipose tissue and macrophages. *J. Lipid Res.* **2014**, *55*, 2501–2508. [CrossRef]
65. Elangovan, S.; Pathania, R.; Ramachandran, S.; Ananth, S.; Padia, R.N.; Lan, L.; Singh, N.; Martin, P.M.; Hawthorn, L.; Prasad, P.D.; et al. The niacin/butyrate receptor GPR109A suppresses mammary tumorigenesis by inhibiting cell survival. *Cancer Res.* **2014**, *74*, 1166–1178. [CrossRef]
66. Nikas, I.P.; Paschou, S.A.; Ryu, H.S. The role of nicotinamide in cancer chemoprevention and therapy. *Biomolecules* **2020**, *10*, 477. [CrossRef]
67. Hwang, E.S.; Song, S.B. Nicotinamide is an inhibitor of SIRT1 in vitro, but can be a stimulator in cells. *Cell Mol. Life Sci.* **2017**, *74*, 3347–3362. [CrossRef]
68. Alves-Fernandes, D.K.; Jasiulionis, M.G. The role of SIRT1 on DNA damage response and epigenetic alterations in cancer. *Int. J. Mol. Sci.* **2019**, *20*, 3153. [CrossRef]
69. Surjana, D.; Halliday, G.M.; Damian, D.L. Role of nicotinamide in DNA damage, mutagenesis, and DNA repair. *J. Nucleic Acids* **2010**, *2010*, 157591. [CrossRef]
70. Fania, L.; Mazzanti, C.; Campione, E.; Candi, E.; Abeni, D.; Dellambra, E. Role of nicotinamide in genomic stability and skin cancer chemoprevention. *Int. J. Mol. Sci.* **2019**, *20*, 5946. [CrossRef]
71. Antwi, S.O.; Petrick, J.L.; Campbell, P.T.; Norez, D.A.; Stevens, V.L.; Liao, L.M.; Roberts, L.R.; Patel, T.; McGlynn, K.A. One-carbon metabolism-related micronutrients intake and risk for hepatocellular carcinoma: A prospective cohort study. *Int. J. Cancer* **2020**, *147*, 2075–2090. [CrossRef]
72. Galli, U.; Colombo, G.; Travelli, C.; Tron, G.C.; Genazzani, A.A.; Grolla, A.A. Recent advances in NAMPT inhibitors: A novel immunotherapic strategy. *Front. Pharmacol.* **2020**, *11*, 656. [CrossRef] [PubMed]
73. Sabui, S.; Kapadia, R.; Ghosal, A.; Schneider, M.; Lambrecht, N.W.G.; Said, H.M. Biotin and pantothenic acid oversupplementation to conditional SLC5A6 KO mice prevents the development of intestinal mucosal abnormalities and growth defects. *Am. J. Physiol. Cell Physiol.* **2018**, *315*, C73–C79. [CrossRef]
74. Ghosal, A.; Lambrecht, N.; Subramanya, S.B.; Kapadia, R.; Said, H.M. Conditional knockout of the Slc5a6 gene in mouse intestine impairs biotin absorption. *Am. J. Physiol. Gastrointest. Liver Physiol.* **2013**, *304*, G64–G71. [CrossRef]
75. Nitto, T.; Onodera, K. Linkage between coenzyme a metabolism and inflammation: Roles of pantetheinase. *J. Pharmacol. Sci.* **2013**, *123*, 1–8. [CrossRef]
76. Berruyer, C.; Martin, F.M.; Castellano, R.; Macone, A.; Malergue, F.; Garrido-Urbani, S.; Millet, V.; Imbert, J.; Duprè, S.; Pitari, G.; et al. Vanin-1-/- mice exhibit a glutathione-mediated tissue resistance to oxidative stress. *Mol. Cell Biol.* **2004**, *24*, 7214–7224. [CrossRef]
77. Berruyer, C.; Pouyet, L.; Millet, V.; Martin, F.M.; LeGoffic, A.; Canonici, A.; Garcia, S.; Bagnis, C.; Naquet, P.; Galland, F. Vanin-1 licenses inflammatory mediator production by gut epithelial cells and controls colitis by antagonizing peroxisome proliferator-activated receptor gamma activity. *J. Exp. Med.* **2006**, *203*, 2817–2827. [CrossRef]
78. Zhang, B.; Lo, C.; Shen, L.; Sood, R.; Jones, C.; Cusmano-Ozog, K.; Park-Snyder, S.; Wong, W.; Jeng, M.; Cowan, T.; et al. The role of vanin-1 and oxidative stress-related pathways in distinguishing acute and chronic pediatric ITP. *Blood* **2011**, *117*, 4569–4579. [CrossRef]
79. Meghari, S.; Berruyer, C.; Lepidi, H.; Galland, F.; Naquet, P.; Mege, J.L. Vanin-1 controls granuloma formation and macrophage polarization in Coxiella burnetii infection. *Eur. J. Immunol.* **2007**, *37*, 24–32. [CrossRef]
80. Pouyet, L.; Roisin-Bouffay, C.; Clément, A.; Millet, V.; Garcia, S.; Chasson, L.; Issaly, N.; Rostan, A.; Hofman, P.; Naquet, P.; et al. Epithelial vanin-1 controls inflammation-driven carcinogenesis in the colitis-associated colon cancer model. *Inflamm. Bowel Dis.* **2010**, *16*, 96–104. [CrossRef]

81. Fedde, K.N.; Whyte, M.P. Alkaline phosphatase (tissue-nonspecific isoenzyme) is a phosphoethanolamine and pyridoxal-5′-phosphate ectophosphatase: Normal and hypophosphatasia fibroblast study. *Am. J. Hum. Genet.* **1990**, *47*, 767–775.
82. DiSorbo, D.M.; Wagner, R., Jr.; Nathanson, L. In vivo and in vitro inhibition of B16 melanoma growth by vitamin B6. *Nutr. Cancer* **1985**, *7*, 43–52. [CrossRef]
83. Matsuo, T.; Fujiwara, A.; Nakamura, K.; Sadzuka, Y. The effects of vitamin B(6) compounds on cell proliferation and melanogenesis in B16F10 melanoma cells. *Oncol. Lett.* **2018**, *15*, 5181–5184. [CrossRef]
84. Zhang, P.; Suidasari, S.; Hasegawa, T.; Yanaka, N.; Kato, N. High concentrations of pyridoxal stimulate the expression of IGFBP1 in HepG2 cells through upregulation of the ERK/c-Jun pathway. *Mol. Med. Rep.* **2013**, *8*, 973–978. [CrossRef]
85. Hartman, T.J.; Woodson, K.; Stolzenberg-Solomon, R.; Virtamo, J.; Selhub, J.; Barrett, M.J.; Albanes, D. Association of the B-vitamins pyridoxal 5′-phosphate (B(6)), B(12), and folate with lung cancer risk in older men. *Am. J. Epidemiol.* **2001**, *153*, 688–694. [CrossRef]
86. Okazaki, Y.; Utama, Z.; Suidasari, S.; Zhang, P.; Yanaka, N.; Tomotake, H.; Sakaguchi, E.; Kato, N. Consumption of vitamin B(6) reduces fecal ratio of lithocholic acid to deoxycholic acid, a risk factor for colon cancer, in rats fed a high-fat diet. *J. Nutr. Sci. Vitaminol.* **2012**, *58*, 366–370. [CrossRef]
87. Kayashima, T.; Tanaka, K.; Okazaki, Y.; Matsubara, K.; Yanaka, N.; Kato, N. Consumption of vitamin B6 reduces colonic damage and protein expression of HSP70 and HO-1, the anti-tumor targets, in rats exposed to 1,2-dimethylhydrazine. *Oncol. Lett.* **2011**, *2*, 1243–1246. [CrossRef]
88. Gebhard, K.J.; Gridley, D.S.; Stickney, D.R.; Shulz, T.D. Enhancement of immune status by high levels of dietary vitamin B-6 without growth inhibition of human malignant melanoma in athymic nude mice. *Nutr. Cancer* **1990**, *14*, 15–26. [CrossRef] [PubMed]
89. Galluzzi, L.; Marsili, S.; Vitale, I.; Senovilla, L.; Michels, J.; Garcia, P.; Vacchelli, E.; Chatelut, E.; Castedo, M.; Kroemer, G. Vitamin B6 metabolism influences the intracellular accumulation of cisplatin. *Cell Cycle* **2013**, *12*, 417–421. [CrossRef]
90. Zhang, P.; Suidasari, S.; Hasegawa, T.; Yanaka, N.; Kato, N. Vitamin B_6 activates p53 and elevates p21 gene expression in cancer cells and the mouse colon. *Oncol. Rep.* **2014**, *31*, 2371–2376. [CrossRef]
91. Sujol, G.; Docquier, A.; Boulahtouf, A.; Castet-Nicolas, A.; Cavaillès, V. Vitamin B6 and cancer: From clinical data to molecularly mechanisms. *Bull. Cancer* **2011**, *98*, 1201–1208. [CrossRef] [PubMed]
92. Galluzzi, L.; Vacchelli, E.; Michels, J.; Garcia, P.; Kepp, O.; Senovilla, L.; Vitale, I.; Kroemer, G. Effects of vitamin B6 metabolism on oncogenesis, tumor progression and therapeutic responses. *Oncogene* **2013**, *32*, 4995–5004. [CrossRef]
93. Bourquin, F.; Capitani, G.; Grütter, M.G. PLP-dependent enzymes as entry and exit gates of sphingolipid metabolism. *Protein Sci.* **2011**, *20*, 1492–1508. [CrossRef] [PubMed]
94. Qiang, Y.; Li, Q.; Xin, Y.; Fang, X.; Tian, Y.; Ma, J.; Wang, J.; Wang, Q.; Zhang, R.; Wang, J.; et al. Intake of dietary one-carbon metabolism-related B vitamins and the risk of esophageal cancer: A dose-response meta-analysis. *Nutrients* **2018**, *10*, 835. [CrossRef]
95. Chen, M.; Zhang, L.; Wang, Q.; Shen, J. Pyridoxine for prevention of hand-foot syndrome caused by chemotherapy: A systematic review. *PLoS ONE* **2013**, *8*, e72245. [CrossRef]
96. Hymes, J.; Wolf, B. Biotinidase and its roles in biotin metabolism. *Clin. Chim. Acta* **1996**, *255*, 1–11. [CrossRef]
97. Chauhan, J.; Dakshinamurti, K. Transcriptional regulation of the glucokinase gene by biotin in starved rats. *J. Biol. Chem.* **1991**, *266*, 10035–10038.
98. Spence, J.T.; Koudelka, A.P. Effects of biotin upon the intracellular level of cGMP and the activity of glucokinase in cultured rat hepatocytes. *J. Biol. Chem.* **1984**, *259*, 6393–6396.
99. Agrawal, S.; Agrawal, A.; Said, H.M. Biotin deficiency enhances the inflammatory response of human dendritic cells. *Am. J. Physiol. Cell Physiol.* **2016**, *311*, C386–C391. [CrossRef] [PubMed]
100. Sghaier, R.; Zarrouk, A.; Nury, T.; Badreddine, I.; O'Brien, N.; Mackrill, J.J.; Vejux, A.; Samadi, M.; Nasser, B.; Caccia, C.; et al. Biotin attenuation of oxidative stress, mitochondrial dysfunction, lipid metabolism alteration and 7beta-hydroxycholesterol-induced cell death in 158N murine oligodendrocytes. *Free Radic. Res.* **2019**, *53*, 535–561. [CrossRef]
101. Järvinen, E.; Ismail, K.; Muniandy, M.; Bogl, L.H.; Heinonen, S.; Tummers, M.; Miettinen, S.; Kaprio, J.; Rissanen, A.; Ollikainen, M.; et al. Biotin-dependent functions in adiposity: A study of monozygotic twin pairs. *Int. J. Obes.* **2016**, *40*, 788–795. [CrossRef]

102. Kuroishi, T. Regulation of Immunological and inflammatory functions by biotin. *Can. J. Physiol. Pharmacol.* **2015**, *93*, 1091–1096. [CrossRef]
103. Honein, M.A.; Paulozzi, L.J.; Mathews, T.J.; Erickson, J.D.; Wong, L.Y. Impact of folic acid fortification of the US food supply on the occurrence of neural tube defects. *JAMA* **2001**, *285*, 2981–2986. [CrossRef]
104. Padmanabhan, S.; Waly, M.I.; Taranikanti, V.; Guizani, N.; Ali, A.; Rahman, M.S.; Al-Attabi, Z.; Al-Malky, R.N.; Al-Maskari, S.N.M.; Al-Ruqaishi, B.R.S.; et al. Folate/Vitamin B12 supplementation combats oxidative stress-associated carcinogenesis in a rat model of colon cancer. *Nutr. Cancer* **2019**, *71*, 100–110. [CrossRef]
105. Courtemanche, C.; Elson-Schwab, I.; Mashiyama, S.T.; Kerry, N.; Ames, B.N. Folate deficiency inhibits the proliferation of primary human CD8+ T lymphocytes in vitro. *J. Immunol.* **2004**, *173*, 3186–3192. [CrossRef]
106. Courtemanche, C.; Huang, A.C.; Elson-Schwab, I.; Kerry, N.; Ng, B.Y.; Ames, B.N. Folate deficiency and ionizing radiation cause DNA breaks in primary human lymphocytes: A comparison. *FASEB J.* **2004**, *18*, 209–211. [CrossRef]
107. Yamaguchi, T.; Hirota, K.; Nagahama, K.; Ohkawa, K.; Takahashi, T.; Nomura, T.; Sakaguchi, S. Control of immune responses by antigen-specific regulatory T cells expressing the folate receptor. *Immunity* **2007**, *27*, 145–159. [CrossRef]
108. Wu, C.H.; Huang, T.C.; Lin, B.F. Folate deficiency affects dendritic cell function and subsequent T helper cell differentiation. *J. Nutr. Biochem.* **2017**, *41*, 65–72. [CrossRef]
109. Makino, E.; Fukuyama, T.; Watanabe, Y.; Tajiki-Nishino, R.; Tajima, H.; Ohnuma-Koyama, A.; Takahashi, N.; Ohtsuka, R.; Okazaki, Y. Subacute oral administration of folic acid elicits anti-inflammatory response in a mouse model of allergic dermatitis. *J. Nutr. Biochem.* **2019**, *67*, 14–19. [CrossRef]
110. Kok, D.E.; O'Flanagan, C.H.; Coleman, M.F.; Ashkavand, Z.; Hursting, S.D.; Krupenko, S.A. Effects of folic acid withdrawal on transcriptomic profiles in murine triple-negative breast cancer cell lines. *Biochimie* **2020**, *173*, 114–122. [CrossRef]
111. Jhaveri, M.S.; Wagner, C.; Trepel, J.B. Impact of extracellular folate levels on global gene expression. *Mol. Pharmacol.* **2001**, *60*, 1288–1295. [CrossRef]
112. Hansen, M.F.; Jensen, S.; Füchtbauer, E.M.; Martensen, P.M. High folic acid diet enhances tumour growth in PyMT-induced breast cancer. *Br. J. Cancer* **2017**, *116*, 752–761. [CrossRef] [PubMed]
113. Crott, J.W.; Choi, S.W.; Ordovas, J.M.; Ditelberg, J.S.; Mason, J.B. Effects of dietary folate and aging on gene expression in the colonic mucosa of rats: Implications for carcinogenesis. *Carcinogenesis* **2004**, *25*, 69–76. [CrossRef] [PubMed]
114. Crott, J.W.; Liu, Z.; Keyes, M.K.; Choi, S.W.; Jang, H.; Moyer, M.P.; Mason, J.B. Moderate folate depletion modulates the expression of selected genes involved in cell cycle, intracellular signaling and folate uptake in human colonic epithelial cell lines. *J. Nutr. Biochem.* **2008**, *19*, 328–335. [CrossRef]
115. Terzis, A.J.; Fiskerstrand, T.; Refsum, H.; Ueland, P.M.; Arnold, H.; Bjerkvig, R. Proliferation, migration and invasion of human glioma cells exposed to antifolate drugs. *Int. J. Cancer* **1993**, *54*, 112–118. [CrossRef]
116. Kim, S.J.; Zuchniak, A.; Sohn, K.J.; Lubinski, J.; Demsky, R.; Eisen, A.; Akbari, M.R.; Kim, Y.I.; Narod, S.A.; Kotsopoulos, J. Plasma folate, vitamin B-6, and vitamin B-12 and breast cancer risk in BRCA1- and BRCA2-mutation carriers: A prospective study. *Am. J. Clin. Nutr.* **2016**, *104*, 671–677. [CrossRef]
117. Kim, S.J.; Zhang, C.X.W.; Demsky, R.; Armel, S.; Kim, Y.I.; Narod, S.A.; Kotsopoulos, J. Folic acid supplement use and breast cancer risk in BRCA1 and BRCA2 mutation carriers: A case-control study. *Breast Cancer Res. Treat.* **2019**, *174*, 741–748. [CrossRef]
118. Kim, Y.I. Folate, colorectal carcinogenesis, and DNA methylation: Lessons from animal studies. *Environ. Mol. Mutagen.* **2004**, *44*, 10–25. [CrossRef]
119. Tomaszewski, J.J.; Cummings, J.L.; Parwani, A.V.; Dhir, R.; Mason, J.B.; Nelson, J.B.; Bacich, D.J.; O'Keefe, D.S. Increased cancer cell proliferation in prostate cancer patients with high levels of serum folate. *Prostate* **2011**, *71*, 1287–1293. [CrossRef] [PubMed]
120. Tu, H.; Dinney, C.P.; Ye, Y.; Grossman, H.B.; Lerner, S.P.; Wu, X. Is folic acid safe for non-muscle-invasive bladder cancer patients? An evidence-based cohort study. *Am. J. Clin. Nutr.* **2018**, *107*, 208–216. [CrossRef]
121. Kuo, C.S.; Lin, C.Y.; Wu, M.Y.; Lu, C.L.; Huang, R.F. Relationship between folate status and tumour progression in patients with hepatocellular carcinoma. *Br. J. Nutr.* **2008**, *100*, 596–602. [CrossRef]
122. Su, Y.H.; Huang, W.C.; Huang, T.H.; Huang, Y.J.; Sue, Y.K.; Huynh, T.T.; Hsiao, M.; Liu, T.Z.; Wu, A.T.; Lin, C.M. Folate deficient tumor microenvironment promotes epithelial-to-mesenchymal transition and cancer stem-like phenotypes. *Oncotarget* **2016**, *7*, 33246–33256. [CrossRef]

123. Wang, T.P.; Hsu, S.H.; Feng, H.C.; Huang, R.F. Folate deprivation enhances invasiveness of human colon cancer cells mediated by activation of sonic hedgehog signaling through promoter hypomethylation and cross action with transcription nuclear factor-kappa B pathway. *Carcinogenesis* **2012**, *33*, 1158–1168. [CrossRef]
124. Larsson, S.C.; Giovannucci, E.; Wolk, A. Dietary folate intake and incidence of ovarian cancer: The Swedish Mammography Cohort. *J. Natl. Cancer Inst.* **2004**, *96*, 396–402. [CrossRef]
125. Dugué, P.A.; Chamberlain, J.A.; Bassett, J.K.; Hodge, A.M.; Brinkman, M.T.; Joo, J.E.; Jung, C.H.; Wong, E.M.; Makalic, E.; Schmidt, D.F.; et al. Overall lack of replication of associations between dietary intake of folate and vitamin B-12 and DNA methylation in peripheral blood. *Am. J. Clin. Nutr.* **2020**, *111*, 228–230. [CrossRef]
126. Wu, X.Y.; Lu, L. Vitamin B6 deficiency, genome instability and cancer. *Asian Pac. J. Cancer Prev.* **2012**, *13*, 5333–5338. [CrossRef]
127. Paul, L.; Selhub, J. Interaction between excess folate and low vitamin B12 status. *Mol. Asp. Med.* **2017**, *53*, 43–47. [CrossRef] [PubMed]
128. Guéant, J.L.; Oussalah, A.; Zgheib, R.; Siblini, Y.; Hsu, S.B.; Namour, F. Genetic, epigenetic and genomic mechanisms of methionine dependency of cancer and tumor-initiating cells: What could we learn from folate and methionine cycles. *Biochimie* **2020**, *173*, 123–128. [CrossRef]
129. Guéant, J.L.; Caillerez-Fofou, M.; Battaglia-Hsu, S.; Alberto, J.M.; Freund, J.N.; Dulluc, I.; Adjalla, C.; Maury, F.; Merle, C.; Nicolas, J.P.; et al. Molecular and cellular effects of vitamin B12 in brain, myocardium and liver through its role as co-factor of methionine synthase. *Biochimie* **2013**, *95*, 1033–1040. [CrossRef]
130. Hofmann, M.A.; Lalla, E.; Lu, Y.; Gleason, M.R.; Wolf, B.M.; Tanji, N.; Ferran, L.J., Jr.; Kohl, B.; Rao, V.; Kisiel, W.; et al. Hyperhomocysteinemia enhances vascular inflammation and accelerates atherosclerosis in a murine model. *J. Clin. Investig.* **2001**, *107*, 675–683. [CrossRef]
131. Dusitanond, P.; Eikelboom, J.W.; Hankey, G.J.; Thom, J.; Gilmore, G.; Loh, K.; Yi, Q.; Klijn, C.J.; Langton, P.; van Bockxmeer, F.M.; et al. Homocysteine-lowering treatment with folic acid, cobalamin, and pyridoxine does not reduce blood markers of inflammation, endothelial dysfunction, or hypercoagulability in patients with previous transient ischemic attack or stroke: A randomized substudy of the VITATOPS trial. *Stroke* **2005**, *36*, 144–146. [CrossRef]
132. Chen, X.; Ahamada, H.; Zhang, T.; Bai, Z.; Wang, C. Association of intake folate and related gene polymorphisms with breast cancer. *J. Nutr. Sci. Vitaminol.* **2019**, *65*, 459–469. [CrossRef]
133. Cheng, W.W.; Wang, Z.K.; Shangguan, H.F.; Zhu, Q.; Zhang, H.Y. Are vitamins relevant to cancer risks? A Mendelian randomization investigation. *Nutrition* **2020**, *78*, 110870. [CrossRef]
134. Brasky, T.M.; Ray, R.M.; Navarro, S.L.; Schenk, J.M.; Newton, A.M.; Neuhouser, M.L. Supplemental one-carbon metabolism related B vitamins and lung cancer risk in the Women's Health Initiative. *Int. J. Cancer* **2020**, *147*, 1374–1384. [CrossRef]
135. Arendt, J.F.H.; Sørensen, H.T.; Horsfall, L.J.; Petersen, I. Elevated vitamin B12 levels and cancer risk in UK primary care: A THIN database cohort study. *Cancer Epidemiol. Biomark. Prev.* **2019**, *28*, 814–821. [CrossRef] [PubMed]
136. Collin, S.M. Folate and B12 in prostate cancer. *Adv. Clin. Chem.* **2013**, *60*, 1–63. [CrossRef] [PubMed]
137. Tamura, J.; Kubota, K.; Murakami, H.; Sawamura, M.; Matsushima, T.; Tamura, T.; Saitoh, T.; Kurabayshi, H.; Naruse, T. Immunomodulation by vitamin B12: Augmentation of CD8+ T lymphocytes and natural killer (NK) cell activity in vitamin B12-deficient patients by methyl-B12 treatment. *Clin. Exp. Immunol.* **1999**, *116*, 28–32. [CrossRef]
138. Partearroyo, T.; Úbeda, N.; Montero, A.; Achón, M.; Varela-Moreiras, G. Vitamin B(12) and folic acid imbalance modifies NK cytotoxicity, lymphocytes B and lymphoprolipheration in aged rats. *Nutrients* **2013**, *5*, 4836–4848. [CrossRef]
139. Lin, C.Y.; Kuo, C.S.; Lu, C.L.; Wu, M.Y.; Huang, R.F. Elevated serum vitamin B(12) levels in association with tumor markers as the prognostic factors predictive for poor survival in patients with hepatocellular carcinoma. *Nutr. Cancer* **2010**, *62*, 190–197. [CrossRef]
140. Lo-Bisgaard, T.; Espelund, U.; Frystyk, J.; Rasmussen, T.R.; Nexo, E.; Arendt, J.F.H. Vitamin B12 and its binding proteins in patients with non-small cell lung cancer referred to fast-track diagnostic work-up for lung cancer. *Scand. J. Clin. Lab. Investig.* **2020**, *80*, 14–19. [CrossRef]

141. Collin, S.M.; Metcalfe, C.; Refsum, H.; Lewis, S.J.; Zuccolo, L.; Smith, G.D.; Chen, L.; Harris, R.; Davis, M.; Marsden, G.; et al. Circulating folate, vitamin B12, homocysteine, vitamin B12 transport proteins, and risk of prostate cancer: A case-control study, systematic review, and meta-analysis. *Cancer Epidemiol. Biomark. Prev.* **2010**, *19*, 1632–1642. [CrossRef]
142. Fanidi, A.; Carreras-Torres, R.; Larose, T.L.; Yuan, J.M.; Stevens, V.L.; Weinstein, S.J.; Albanes, D.; Prentice, R.; Pettinger, M.; Cai, Q.; et al. Is high vitamin B12 status a cause of lung cancer? *Int. J. Cancer* **2019**, *145*, 1499–1503. [CrossRef] [PubMed]

3

Effects of Two-Year Vitamin B12 and Folic Acid Supplementation on Depressive Symptoms and Quality of Life in Older Adults with Elevated Homocysteine Concentrations: Additional Results from the B-PROOF Study, an RCT

Elisa J. de Koning [1,2,*,†], Nikita L. van der Zwaluw [3,†], Janneke P. van Wijngaarden [3], Evelien Sohl [1,2], Elske M. Brouwer-Brolsma [3], Harm W. J. van Marwijk [1,4,5], Anke W. Enneman [6], Karin M. A. Swart [1,2], Suzanne C. van Dijk [6], Annelies C. Ham [6], Nathalie van der Velde [6], André G. Uitterlinden [6], Brenda W. J. H. Penninx [1,7], Petra J. M. Elders [4], Paul Lips [1,8], Rosalie A. M. Dhonukshe-Rutten [3], Natasja M. van Schoor [1,2] and Lisette C. P. G. M. de Groot [3]

1. EMGO Institute for Health and Care Research, VU University Medical Center, P.O. Box 7057, 1007 MB Amsterdam, The Netherlands; e.sohl@vumc.nl (E.S.); harm.vanmarwijk@manchester.ac.uk (H.W.J.v.M.); k.swart@vumc.nl (K.M.A.S.); b.penninx@vumc.nl (B.W.J.H.P.); p.lips@vumc.nl (P.L.); nm.vanschoor@vumc.nl (N.M.v.S.)
2. Department of Epidemiology and Biostatistics, VU University Medical Center, P.O. Box 7057, 1007 MB Amsterdam, The Netherlands
3. Division of Human Nutrition, Wageningen University, P.O. Box 8129, 6700 EV Wageningen, The Netherlands; nikitavanderzwaluw@gmail.com (N.L.v.d.Z.); janneke.vanwijngaarden@gmail.com (J.P.v.W.); elkse.brouwer-brolsma@wur.nl (E.M.B.-B.); rosalie-dhonukshe-rutten@wur.nl (R.A.M.D.-R.); lisette.degroot@wur.nl (L.C.P.G.M.d.G.)
4. Department of General Practice and Elderly Care Medicine, VU University Medical Center, P.O. Box 7057, 1007 MB Amsterdam, The Netherlands; p.elders@vumc.nl
5. Primary Care Research Center, Institute of Population Health, University of Manchester, Oxford Road, M13 9PL Manchester, UK
6. Department of Internal Medicine, Erasmus University Medical Center, P.O. Box 2040, 3000 CA Rotterdam, The Netherlands; a.enneman@erasmusmc.nl (A.W.E.); s.c.vandijk@erasmusmc.nl (S.C.v.D.); a.ham@erasmusmc.nl (A.C.H.); n.vandervelde@erasmusmc.nl (N.v.d.V.); a.g.uitterlinden@erasmusmc.nl (A.G.U.)
7. Department of Psychiatry, VU University Medical Center/GGZ inGeest, P.O. Box 7057, 1007 MB Amsterdam, The Netherlands
8. Department of Internal Medicine/Endocrinology, VU University Medical Center, P.O. Box 7057, 1007 MB Amsterdam, The Netherlands

* Correspondence: ej.dekoning@vumc.nl

† These authors contributed equally to this work.

Abstract: Lowering elevated plasma homocysteine (Hcy) concentrations by supplementing vitamin B_{12} and folic acid may reduce depressive symptoms and improve health-related quality of life (HR-QoL) in older adults. This study aimed to test this hypothesis in a randomized controlled trial. Participants (N = 2919, ≥65 years, Hcy concentrations ≥12 μmol/L) received either 500 μg vitamin B_{12} and 400 μg folic acid daily or placebo for two years. Both tablets contained 15 μg vitamin D_3. Depressive symptoms were measured with the Geriatric Depression Scale-15 (GDS-15). HR-QoL was assessed with the SF-12 Mental and Physical component summary scores and the EQ-5D Index score and Visual Analogue Scale. Differences in two-year change scores were analyzed with Analysis of Covariance (ANCOVA). Hcy concentrations decreased more in the intervention group, but two-year change scores of the GDS-15 and three of four HR-QoL measures did not differ between groups. The EQ-5D Index score declined less in the intervention group than in the placebo group (mean change 0.00 vs. −0.02, $p = 0.004$). In conclusion, two-year supplementation with vitamin B_{12} and folic acid in older adults with hyperhomocysteinemia showed that lowering Hcy concentrations does not reduce depressive symptoms, but it may have a small positive effect on HR-QoL.

Keywords: homocysteine; hyperhomocysteinemia; depressive symptoms; quality of life; vitamin B_{12}; folic acid; older adults; randomized controlled trial

---

1. Introduction

Depression is a leading cause of disability worldwide and induces substantial individual and societal burden [1]. In addition, health-related quality of life (HR-QoL) can be compromised by both mental disorders and reduced physical functioning [2,3]. Depression and low HR-QoL increase the risk of institutionalization and mortality [4]. Especially in older adults, management of depression is often suboptimal, for instance due to side-effects of antidepressant medication or interactions with other drugs [5]. Such complexities emphasize the need for simple and safe interventions for both the prevention and treatment of depression.

Elevated plasma homocysteine (Hcy) concentrations are common in older adults [6,7]. Hyperhomocysteinemia has been associated with various adverse health conditions, including cardiovascular disease [6], fractures [7], dementia [8], decreased physical functioning [9], and mortality [10]. In addition, observational studies suggest a link between elevated Hcy concentrations and depressive symptoms [11–14] and lower HR-QoL [15,16]. A meta-analysis of nine observational studies showed that persons with Hcy ≥12.5 μmol/L had a 70% higher risk of prevalent depression than persons with Hcy concentrations <12.5 μmol/L [17]. Supplementation with vitamin B_{12} and folic acid decreases Hcy concentrations [18] and may thereby reduce depressive symptoms and improve HR-QoL. However, trials investigating these effects are scarce and show inconsistent results [16,19–24]. Heterogeneity in study duration, study samples, and supplement dose may explain the observed differences.

Insufficient amounts of folate and vitamin B_{12} limit the conversion of Hcy into methionine. Methionine is a direct precursor of *S*-adenosylmethionine (SAM). SAM plays an important role in the methylation of neurotransmitters involved in depression, such as serotonin, dopamine, and noradrenalin [25,26]. In accordance with this, lower concentrations of SAM and monoamine neurotransmitter metabolites were observed in the cerebrospinal fluid of severely depressed patients who had high Hcy concentrations, compared to similar patients who did not have elevated Hcy concentrations [27].

The current amount of evidence regarding the role of Hcy, vitamin B_{12}, and folic acid in depression and HR-QoL is limited. To gain more insight into these complex relationships, we investigated a large sample of older adults with mildly elevated homocysteine concentrations both cross-sectionally and after two years of supplementation with vitamin B_{12} and folic acid. It was hypothesized that Hcy is positively associated with depressive symptoms, and inversely associated with HR-QoL at baseline, and that supplementation with vitamin B_{12} and folic acid decreases Hcy concentrations, thereby reducing depressive symptoms and improving HR-QoL.

2. Materials and Methods

2.1. Study Design and Participants

Data from the B-vitamins for the PRevention Of Osteoporotic Fractures (B-PROOF) study were used for the present study. The B-PROOF study is a multi-center, randomized, parallel-group, double-blind, placebo-controlled intervention trial investigating the effect of two-year daily vitamin B_{12} (500 μg) and folic acid (400 μg) supplementation versus placebo on fracture incidence in a large sample of older adults [28,29]. Depressive symptoms and HR-QoL were predefined secondary outcome measures of the B-PROOF study.

The B-PROOF study included 2919 older adults (≥65 years) from the general population. Participants were recruited from three regions in The Netherlands: Wageningen, Amsterdam, and Rotterdam. Participants were included if they had elevated Hcy concentrations (12–50 μmol/L). Exclusion criteria included cancer diagnosis within the last 5 years (except for non-melanoma skin cancer), being bedridden, serum creatinine concentration of >150 μmol/L, current or recent (<4 months) intramuscular injections of vitamin B_{12}, use of high-dose folic acid supplements (>300 μg per day), and participation in other intervention studies. Detailed information concerning recruitment, participants, and study procedures has been extensively reported elsewhere [28].

This study was conducted according to the guidelines laid down in the Declaration of Helsinki and all procedures involving human subjects were approved by the Medical Ethics Committee of Wageningen University. Local feasibility was approved by the Medical Ethics Committees of Erasmus Medical Center Rotterdam and VU University Medical Center Amsterdam. Written informed consent was obtained from all participants prior to the start of the intervention. The B-PROOF trial is registered with clinicaltrials.gov as NCT00696514 and with the Netherlands Trial Register as NTR1333.

2.2. *Intervention*

Participants were randomized in a 1:1 ratio to either the intervention group or the placebo group. Randomization was performed by an independent person by means of computer-generated numbers in stratified permuted blocks of size 4, stratified by sex, age (65–80 years, ≥80 years), study center, and Hcy concentrations (12–18 μmol/L, ≥18 μmol/L). Both groups received a daily oral tablet for a duration of two years. The tablets of the intervention group contained 500 μg vitamin B_{12}, 400 μg folic acid, and 15 μg vitamin D_3 (cholecalciferol). The placebo tablets contained 15 μg vitamin D_3. Tablets were similar in appearance, smell, and taste. Vitamin D_3 was added to both types of tablets to ensure adequate vitamin D concentrations, which was of importance for the primary outcome measure of the B-PROOF study: fracture incidence. At baseline and at the end of the trial, a structured interview took place, including questionnaires and physical measurements.

2.3. *Outcomes*

2.3.1. Depressive Symptoms

The Geriatric Depression Scale-15 (GDS-15) was used to assess depressive symptoms at baseline and after two years of supplementation. The GDS-15 is a short version of the original 30-item GDS [30] and is a widely used instrument that displays good psychometric properties in various elderly populations [31,32]. Scores range from 0 to 15, with higher scores indicating more symptoms. A score of 5 or higher indicates the presence of clinically relevant depressive symptoms [31].

2.3.2. Health-Related Quality of Life

HR-QoL is a multidimensional construct. We therefore used both the 12-item Short Form Health Survey (SF-12) [3] and the EuroQol 5 Dimensions (EQ-5D) [33] to take into account different aspects of HR-QoL (mental, physical, and general HR-QoL). Both questionnaires are self-rated, widely used, have been validated in various populations, have good test-retest reliability [3,33], and they complement each other [34].

The SF-12 is derived from the SF-36 questionnaire [35] and assesses eight health aspects: physical functioning, bodily pain, role limitations due to physical problems, general health, vitality, social functioning, role limitations due to emotional problems, and mental health. Mental (MCS) and physical (PCS) component summary scores were calculated. These scores were standardized to US general population norms [36], as Dutch norms are currently not available. Scores range from 0 to 100, with 0 representing lowest HR-QoL and 100 indicating best possible HR-QoL, with a normalized mean around 50 and a standard deviation (SD) of 10.

The EQ-5D covers five dimensions of HR-QoL: mobility, self-care, usual activities, pain/discomfort, and anxiety/depression [33]. A standardized index score (EQ-5D Index) was calculated based on Dutch norm data, ranging from −0.33 to 1, with higher scores indicating better HR-QoL [36]. Finally, the visual analogue scale of the EQ-5D (EQ-5D VAS) was used to indicate current health status on a visual scale ranging from 0 to 100, with higher scores representing better HR-QoL.

2.4. Baseline Characteristics

Information about marital status, highest level of completed education, alcohol intake (light, moderate, excessive/very excessive) [37], smoking habits (never, former, current), and physical activity [38] was obtained through structured questionnaires. Weight was measured using a calibrated scale. Height was measured with a stadiometer. Subsequently, body mass index (BMI) was calculated as weight/height^2 (kg/m^2). The Mini-Mental State Examination (MMSE) was used to assess global cognitive function (score range: 0–30) [39].

2.5. Biochemical Analyses

Venous blood samples were obtained from participants in a fasted state or after a restricted light breakfast. Samples were stored at −80 °C until analysis. Plasma Hcy concentrations were measured at baseline and after two years using either the Architect i2000 RS analyzer (VU University Medical Center; Abbott Diagnostics, Wiesbaden, Germany, intra-assay CV: 2%, inter-assay CV: 4%), HPLC method (Wageningen University, intra assay CV: 3.1%, inter assay CV: 5.9%), or liquid chromatography tandem mass spectrometry (LC-MS/MS) method (Erasmus Medical Center Rotterdam; CV: 3.1%). Cross-calibration showed that the outcomes of the three centers did not differ significantly. Serum folate and three markers of vitamin B_{12} status, i.e., serum vitamin B_{12}, serum holotranscobalamin (HoloTC), and serum methylmalonic acid (MMA), were measured at the Erasmus Medical Center at baseline. Folate and serum vitamin B_{12} were assessed with an electrochemiluminescence immunoassay (Elecsys 2010, Roche GmbH, Mannheim, Germany) (CV folate: 5.9% at 5.7 nmol/L and 2.8% at 23.4 nmol/L; CV vitamin B_{12}: 5.1% at 125 pmol/L and 2.9% at 753 pmol/L). Serum HoloTC was assessed with the AxSYM analyser (Abbott Diagnostics, Wiesbaden, Germany) (CV: <8%) and serum MMA was measured by LC-MS/MS.

2.6. Statistical Analyses

Data were analyzed using SPSS version 22 (SPSS Inc., Chicago, IL, USA). A two-sided p-value of <0.05 was regarded as statistically significant. Data are reported as N (%), or as median (interquartile range (IQR)). Baseline characteristics were compared between treatment groups using non-parametric Mann-Whitney tests or Pearson Chi-square tests. Participants who dropped out during the study were compared to participants who completed the study with respect to age, sex, baseline Hcy concentration, depressive symptoms, and HR-QoL.

2.6.1. Cross-Sectional Analyses

The GDS-15 and HR-QoL scores were non-normally distributed, even after transformation. Therefore, baseline associations of Hcy concentrations with depressive symptoms and HR-QoL were examined using Cox regression analyses with fixed time points. In this analysis, a constant risk period was assigned (time was fixed to 1). This technique was chosen because the obtained hazard ratio from this analysis can be interpreted as a risk ratio (RR) [40]. In case of a high prevalence of the condition of interest, this is a more conservative estimate of the true effect than an odds ratio (OR). Participants with a GDS-15 score of ≥ 5, indicating clinically relevant depressive symptoms [31], and participants who scored in the lowest quartile of the HR-QoL measures were considered 'cases'. It was examined whether higher Hcy concentrations were associated with a higher risk of having depressive symptoms or low HR-QoL. Analyses were performed without adjustments (crude model), adjusted for age, sex, and study center (Model 1), and additional adjustments for education level, smoking behavior, alcohol consumption, creatinine concentrations, BMI, and MMSE (Model 2). These covariates were added because of their possible influence on both the determinant (Hcy) and the outcomes (depressive symptoms, HR-QoL) [2,41,42].

2.6.2. Effect Study

We performed both intention-to-treat analyses, including all participants who completed baseline and follow-up measurements, and per-protocol analyses, including all participants who were compliant with the study protocol (≥80% of tablet intake in two years). The score distributions of the outcome variables violated normality assumptions.

Depressive symptoms—total sample: Due to the high number of null scores on the GDS-15 in the study sample, no change scores were calculated as this would lead to interpretation difficulties. Instead, to examine whether the treatment groups differed in number of persons with depressive symptoms after two years, logistic regression analyses were performed. The dichotomized follow-up GDS-15 score (0–4: no depressive symptoms; ≥5: depressive symptoms) [31] was taken as the outcome measure and treatment group as the independent variable. The dichotomized baseline GDS-15 score was added as a covariate to control for baseline values. Age, sex, study center, and baseline Hcy were added as covariates in a second, adjusted model as randomization was stratified based on these variables.

Depressive symptoms—subsample: To further examine the participants with depressive symptoms, a subgroup analysis was performed. Two-year change scores were calculated for participants who scored GDS-15 ≥5 at baseline and differences in change scores between treatment groups were analyzed using Analysis of Covariance (ANCOVA), with the GDS-15 change scores as the outcome measure, treatment as the fixed between-subjects factor, and baseline GDS-15 scores as a covariate. Age, sex, study center, and baseline Hcy were added as covariates in a second, adjusted model.

HR-QoL: For the HR-QoL analyses, two-year change scores were calculated for the four measures of HR-QoL (SF-12 MCS, SF-12 PCS, EQ-5D Index, and EQ-5D VAS). Subsequently, ANCOVA analyses were performed, similar to the GDS-15 subgroup analyses.

For all outcome measures, predefined interaction terms of treatment with sex, dichotomous age (65–80 and ≥80 years), and dichotomous Hcy concentration (<18 and ≥18 μmol/L) were examined in the adjusted models. The Hcy cutoff value of 18 μmol/L was chosen because stratification of the participants was also performed according to this value. If interaction terms had a *p*-value of <0.10, stratified subgroup analyses were performed. In explorative post-hoc analyses, interactions of the treatment group with plasma concentrations of vitamin B_{12}, HoloTC, and MMA (all indicators of vitamin B_{12} status) and folate were tested to investigate whether these baseline plasma concentrations influenced treatment effects. These variables were dichotomized at the median value (results shown in Table A1 in Appendix A).

As a final check of the effect, it was investigated whether change in Hcy concentration was associated with depressive symptoms and/or HR-QoL over time, irrespective of the treatment group. For this purpose, linear regression analyses were performed with two-year change in Hcy as the predictor and two-year change in the GDS-15 (≥5 subgroup) and HR-QoL measures as the outcome. These analyses were adjusted for baseline values of Hcy and GDS-15/HR-QoL (crude model), additionally adjusted for age, sex, and study center (Model 1), and additionally adjusted for education level, smoking behavior, alcohol consumption, creatinine concentrations, BMI, and MMSE (Model 2).

3. Results

3.1. Sample Characteristics

The baseline characteristics per treatment group are shown in Table 1. Median age of the total group was 73 years (IQR: 69–78 years) and was similar in both treatment groups. A similar number of women was included in the two groups (50%). Only HoloTC differed significantly between the groups, with the intervention group having slightly higher baseline HoloTC concentrations (median: 65, IQR: 48–86) than the placebo group (median: 63, IQR: 45–84; $p = 0.03$). The median GDS-15 score was 1 (IQR: 0–2), and 7% of the participants had a GDS score $\geq$5 at baseline ($N = 200$), indicating clinically relevant depressive symptoms (similar numbers in both groups). At follow-up, slightly more participants reported depressive symptoms (9%, $N = 223$, also similar in both groups). At baseline, 210 participants (7.3%) had a vitamin B_{12} deficiency (serum vitamin B_{12} < 150 pmol/L [43]) and 89 participants (3.1%) had a folate deficiency (serum folate <10 nmol/L [34]).

Compliance to the treatment was high; mean tablet intake was 90.1% in two years and 83.8% of participants had a tablet intake of $\geq$80% (similar in both treatment groups). The dropout percentage was 15.2% ($N = 222$) in the B-vitamin group and 13.7% ($N = 200$) in the placebo group. This group difference was not statistically significant ($p = 0.27$). Persons who dropped out were significantly older ($p < 0.001$), were more often female ($p = 0.01$), had higher baseline Hcy concentrations ($p < 0.001$), more depressive symptoms ($p < 0.001$), and lower scores on all four HR-QoL measures (SF-12 MCS: $p = 0.03$; SF-12 PCS: $p < 0.001$; EQ-5D Index: $p = 0.02$; EQ-5D VAS: $p < 0.001$) compared to persons who completed the study. Detailed information regarding dropout has been extensively reported elsewhere [29].

Table 1. Baseline characteristics of the two treatment groups (total $N = 2919$).

	Intervention ($N = 1461$)	Placebo ($N = 1458$)	p
Descriptive variables:			
Women	736 (50)	724 (50)	0.70
Age (years)	73 (69–78)	73 (69–78)	0.38
Education (years)	9 (6–15)	9 (6–15)	0.59
Study location:			0.91
WU (Wageningen)	426 (29)	431 (30)	
Erasmus MC (Rotterdam)	649 (44)	636 (44)	
VUmc (Amsterdam)	386 (26)	391 (27)	
Smoking			0.97
Current	139 (10)	142 (10)	
Former	828 (57)	821 (56)	
Never	494 (34)	495 (34)	
Alcohol use:			0.31
Light	994 (68)	972 (67)	
Moderate	417 (29)	422 (29)	
Excessive/very excessive	50 (3)	62 (4)	
Body mass index, kg/m^2	26.7 (24.6–29.2)	26.6 (24.6–29.4)	0.65
Physical activity (kcal/day)	546 (335–823)	556 (347–831)	0.32
MMSE (score 0–30)	28 (27–29)	28 (27–29)	0.10
Depressive symptoms/quality of life measures:			
GDS-15	1 (0–2)	1 (0–2)	0.45
SF12 MCS	57.1 (52.3–59.8)	56.6 (51.6–59.8)	0.29
SF12 PCS	51.3 (43.8–54.2)	50.8 (42.4–54.4)	0.32
EQ-5D Index	0.86 (0.81–1.00)	0.86 (0.81–1.00)	0.84
EQ-5D VAS	80 (75–90)	80 (75–90)	0.50
Biochemical analyses:			
Serum folate (nmol/L)	18.8 (14.9–24.7)	18.9 (14.8–24.5)	0.53
Serum vitamin B_{12} (pmol/L)	267 (213–341)	266 (204–343)	0.27
Serum holoTC (pmol/L)	65 (48–86)	63 (45–84)	0.03
Serum MMA (μmol/L)	0.22 (0.18–0.30)	0.23 (0.18–0.31)	0.26
Plasma Hcy (μmol/L)	14.3 (13.0–16.5)	14.5 (13.0–16.7)	0.46
Serum creatinine (mmol/L)	82.0 (71.0–94.0)	82.0 (71.0–94.0)	0.59

Values are displayed as N (%) or median (IQR); $p < 0.05$; N varies slightly between variables. MMSE: Mini-Mental State Examination; GDS-15: Geriatric Depression Scale 15-item version; SF-12: 12-item Short-Form Health Survey; MCS: Mental Component Summary score; PCS: Physical Component Summary score; EQ-5D: EuroQol 5 Dimensions; VAS: Visual Analogue Scale; holoTC: holotranscobalamin; MMA: methylmalonic acid; Hcy: homocysteine.

3.2. *Cross-Sectional Analyses*

Table 2 shows the results of the Cox regression analyses with fixed time points for the baseline association between Hcy concentrations and the GDS-15 and HR-QoL measures. The crude model showed a weak positive association between Hcy and the GDS-15, however, this association disappeared in the fully adjusted model (RR = 1.00; 95% CI: 0.96, 1.03; $p = 0.85$). For the HR-QoL measures, a similar pattern was observed, with significant crude associations between Hcy and the SF12-PCS, EQ-5D Index, and EQ-5D VAS, but after adjustment for covariates, the significance disappeared.

Table 2. Baseline associations (risk ratios) between Hcy concentrations and the risk of having depressive symptoms (GDS-15 $\geq$ 5) or being in the lowest HR-QoL quartile (intention-to-treat).

	Crude Model		Model 1 [a]		Model 2 (Fully Adjusted) [b]	
	RR (95% CI)	***p***	**RR (95% CI)**	***p***	**RR(95% CI)**	***p***
GDS-15	1.03 (1.00, 1.07)	0.04	1.02 (0.99, 1.06)	0.26	1.00 (0.96, 1.03)	0.85
SF-12 PCS	1.04 (1.02, 1.05)	<0.001	1.02 (1.00, 1.04)	0.04	1.01 (0.99, 1.03)	0.51
SF-12 MCS	1.02 (1.00, 1.04)	0.06	1.02 (1.00, 1.03)	0.13	1.01 (0.99, 1.03)	0.33
EQ-5D Index	1.03 (1.01, 1.05)	<0.001	1.02 (1.00, 1.04)	0.02	1.02 (1.00, 1.04)	0.11
EQ-5D VAS	1.04 (1.02, 1.05)	<0.001	1.03 (1.01, 1.04)	0.01	1.02 (1.00, 1.04)	0.15

[a] adjusted for age and sex; [b] additionally adjusted for study center, education level, smoking, alcohol use, creatinine, body mass index (BMI), and Mini-Mental State Examination (MMSE). *N* varies slightly between the models and variables. Hcy: homocysteine; GDS-15: Geriatric Depression Scale, 15-item version; HR-QoL: health-related quality of life; RR: Risk ratio; SF-12: 12-item Short-Form Health Survey; PCS: Physical Component Summary score; MCS: Mental Component Summary score; EQ-5D: EuroQol 5 Dimensions; VAS: Visual Analogue Scale.

3.3. *Effect Study*

As expected, Hcy concentrations decreased significantly more ($p < 0.001$) in the B-vitamin group (mean two-year change: −4.4 μmol/L, SD: 3.3) compared to the placebo group (mean two-year change: −0.2 μmol/L, SD: 4.1).

3.3.1. Depressive Symptoms

Total sample: Logistic regression analyses showed that the number of participants with depressive symptoms did not differ between the two treatment groups after two years, when controlled for baseline depressive symptoms (OR = 1.13. 95% CI: 0.83, 1.53, $p = 0.45$ in the fully adjusted model; see Table 3).

Subsample (GDS-15 $\geq$ 5): Table 3 also presents the results of the ANCOVA analyses for the subgroup of participants with depressive symptoms at baseline ($N = 161$). The fully adjusted model did not show significant differences in two-year GDS-15 change scores between the intervention group (mean change: 1.46, 95% CI: 0.71, 2.21) and placebo group (mean change: 1.76, 95% CI: 1.05, 2.47) ($p = 0.55$). Interaction terms of treatment with age, sex, and Hcy were not significant. Explorative post-hoc interaction analyses with vitamin B_{12} and folate status predictors revealed significant interaction terms for vitamin B_{12}, MMA, and folate, but stratified analyses did not show relevant differences between the intervention and placebo group (Appendix A: Table A1).

Table 3. Effect of the treatment on depressive symptoms, analyzed with logistic regression (total sample) and ANCOVA (subsample with symptoms) (intention-to-treat).

	Baseline	Two-Year Follow-up	Model 1 [a]			Model 2 (Fully Adjusted) [b]		
Logistic regression (total sample, N = 2588)	N with GDS-15 $\geq$ 5 (%)	N with GDS-15 $\geq$ 5 (%)	OR [c] (95% CI)	p		OR [c] (95% CI)	p	
			1.1 (0.8, 1.5)	0.56		1.1 (0.8, 1.5)	0.45	
B-vitamins	101 (7.0)	112 (8.6)						
Placebo	99 (6.8)	111 (8.5)						
ANCOVA (subsample GDS-15 $\geq$ 5, N = 161)	Median GDS-15 score (IQR)	Median GDS-15 score (IQR)	Mean change (95% CI)	F	p	Mean change (95% CI)	F	p
				0.57	0.45		0.36	0.55
B-vitamins	6 (5–8)	5 (3–7)	1.4 (0.7, 2.2)			1.5 (0.7, 2.2)		
Placebo	6 (5–8)	4 (3–6)	1.8 (1.1, 2.5)			1.8 (1.1, 2.5)		

[a] Adjusted for baseline values of the respective outcome variable; [b] additionally adjusted for age, sex, homocysteine, and study center; [c] odds ratio of having clinically relevant depressive symptoms (GDS-15 $\geq$ 5) after two years. GDS-15: Geriatric Depression Scale, 15-item version.

To further examine whether Hcy concentration is associated with depressive symptoms over time, linear regression analyses in the subsample with GDS-15 ≥ 5 (irrespective of treatment group) were conducted, with two-year change in Hcy as the predictor and two-year change in GDS-15 as the outcome. The crude and adjusted analyses did not reveal a significant association between the two change scores (Table 4). All per-protocol analyses yielded similar results (data not shown but available on request from the author).

Table 4. Linear regression analyses of the association of the two-year change in Hcy with the two-year change in depressive symptoms and HR-QoL (intention-to-treat).

	Crude Model [a]		Model 1 [b]		Model 2 (Fully Adjusted) [c]	
	β (SE)	*p*	β (SE)	*p*	β (SE)	*p*
GDS-15 (subgroup of ≥5)	0.07 (0.06)	0.27	0.05 (0.06)	0.38	0.05 (0.06)	0.43
SF-12 PCS	−0.14 (0.03)	<0.001	−0.10 (0.03)	0.003	−0.09 (0.03)	0.01
SF-12 MCS	−0.05 (0.04)	0.18	−0.05 (0.04)	0.15	−0.05 (0.04)	0.13
EQ-5D Index	−0.003 (0.001)	<0.001	−0.003 (0.001)	<0.001	−0.002 (0.001)	0.004
EQ-5D VAS	−0.15 (0.06)	0.02	−0.09 (0.06)	0.16	−0.09 0.06)	0.16

[a] Adjusted for baseline values of homocysteine and the respective outcome variable; [b] additionally adjusted for age, sex, and study center; [c] additionally adjusted for education level, smoking, alcohol use, creatinine, BMI, and MMSE. GDS-15: Geriatric Depression Scale, 15-item version; SF-12: 12-item Short-Form Health Survey; PCS: Physical Component Summary score; MCS: Mental Component Summary score; EQ-5D: EuroQol 5 Dimensions; VAS: Visual Analogue Scale.

3.3.2. Health-Related Quality of Life

Two-year change in the mental and physical component summary scales of the SF-12 and in the EQ-5D VAS did not differ significantly between treatment groups (Table 5). The EQ-5D Index score, however, remained stable over time in the intervention group (mean change: 0.00, 95% CI: −0.01, 0.00), whereas this score slightly decreased in the placebo group (mean change: −0.02, 95% CI: −0.03, −0.01) ($p = 0.004$).

For the EQ-5D VAS, the interaction of treatment with sex was significant ($p = 0.05$). Stratified analyses, however, did not show significant differences between treatment groups in men or women (Appendix A: Table A1). Exploratory post-hoc interaction analyses with vitamin B_{12} and folate predictors did not reveal significant interaction terms.

Linear regression analyses to investigate associations over time demonstrated that change in Hcy concentration was significantly associated with change in the EQ-5D Index score ($\beta = -0.002$; SE = 0.001; $p = 0.004$) and the SF-12 PCS score ($\beta = -0.09$; SE = 0.03; $p = 0.01$) over time (Table 4). This result indicates that these physical and general aspects of HR-QoL decreased as Hcy concentrations increased over time. Results of the per-protocol analyses were similar to the intention-to-treat analyses.

Table 5. Comparison of the two-year change scores of HR-QoL between the two treatment groups with Analysis of Covariance (ANCOVA, intention-to-treat).

			Model 1 [a]			Model 2 (Fully Adjusted) [b]		
	Baseline	Two-Year Follow-up	Change Scores			Change Scores		
	Median (IQR)	Median (IQR)	Mean Change (95% CI)	F	p	Mean Change (95% CI)	F	p
SF-12 PCS (N = 2594)				0.14	0.71		0.09	0.76
B-vitamins	51.6 (44.5–54.3)	51.1 (42.9–54.4)	−0.59 (−0.95, −0.23)			−0.60 (−0.95, −0.25)		
Placebo	51.5 (43.5–54.6)	50.8 (41.8–54.7)	−0.69 (−1.05, −0.32)			−0.68 (−1.03, −0.33)		
SF-12 MCS (N = 2594)				0.14	0.71		0.18	0.67
B-vitamins	57.2 (52.3–59.8)	56.8 (51.8–59.8)	−0.52 (−0.89, −0.15)			−0.53 (−0.90, −0.16)		
Placebo	56.8 (52.0–59.8)	56.6 (51.2–59.8)	−0.42 (−0.79, −0.05)			−0.42 (−0.79, −0.04)		
EQ-5D Index (N = 2617)				8.89	0.003		8.29	0.004
B-vitamins	0.86 (0.81–1.00)	0.89 (0.81–1.00)	0.00 (−0.01, 0.01)			0.00 (−0.01, 0.00)		
Placebo	0.8 (0.81–1.00)	0.84 (0.81–1.00)	−0.02 (−0.03, −0.01)			−0.02 (−0.03, −0.01)		
EQ-5D VAS (N = 2612)				0.20	0.65		0.17	0.68
B-vitamins	80 (75–90)	80 (70–90)	−1.06 (−1.73, −0.39)			−1.07 (−1.73, −0.41)		
Placebo	80 (75–90)	80 (70–90)	−1.28 (−1.95, −0.61)			−1.27 (−1.93, −0.61)		

[a] Adjusted for baseline values of the respective outcome variable; [b] additionally adjusted for age, sex, homocysteine, and study center. HR-QoL: health-related quality of life; SF-12: 12-item Short-Form Health Survey, PCS: Physical Component Summary score; MCS: Mental Component Summary score; EQ-5D: EuroQol 5 Dimensions; VAS: Visual Analogue Scale.

4. Discussion

This study investigated the role of Hcy concentrations and two years of supplementation with vitamin B_{12} and folic acid on depressive symptoms and HR-QoL in a large sample of Dutch older adults with elevated Hcy concentrations. Contrary to our hypotheses, no significant cross-sectional associations between Hcy concentrations and depressive symptoms or HR-QoL were observed, when controlling for confounding variables. Furthermore, supplementation with vitamin B_{12} and folic acid did not reveal significant differences between the two treatment groups (intervention vs. placebo) on depressive symptoms and three out of four HR-QoL measures after two years. The EQ-5D Index (measuring general HR-QoL), however, remained stable over time in the intervention group and decreased slightly but significantly in the placebo group, suggesting that B-vitamin supplementation did have a small positive effect on HR-QoL. Furthermore, the two-year change in Hcy (independent of group assignment) was associated with the two-year change in the EQ-5D Index and the physical component of the SF-12. This implies that a reduction of Hcy concentrations may lead to more stable—as opposed to declining—general and possibly also physical HR-QoL over time.

The results of the present study do not suggest a role of Hcy or vitamin B_{12} and folic acid supplementation in depressive symptoms in persons with mild hyperhomocysteinemia. Several observational studies have shown associations between Hcy and depressive symptoms [44–48], but some studies only found significant results in persons with low folate and/or vitamin B_{12} status [45,47]. Although Hcy concentrations were elevated in all B-PROOF participants, the number of persons with a vitamin B_{12} or folate deficiency was low (7.3% and 3.1%, respectively). Nevertheless, Hintakka et al. observed an association between vitamin B_{12} and depression in persons with vitamin B_{12} concentrations within the normal range [49].

In contrast to the present results, a prospective cohort study with 521 Korean persons (over 65 years old) from the general population observed a significant association of Hcy, vitamin B_{12}, and folate with incident depressive disorder over a follow-up period of 2–3 years [48]. In accordance with our results, previous trials did not observe a beneficial effect of B-vitamin supplementation on depressive symptoms either [50,51]. Supplementation dose and method, however, differed between the trials. The present study did account for some limitations of these previous studies, by including both men and women, as opposed to only men [50], and by using a long follow-up period of two years, in contrast to only four months [51].

Regarding HR-QoL, we observed a beneficial effect of B-vitamin supplementation on the EQ-5D Index score, whereas no effects were observed on the other three HR-QoL measures. The effect, however, was very small (the difference between groups was 0.02, on a scale of -0.33 to 1) and did not reach clinical relevance [52]. Comparison of the present HR-QoL results with other intervention studies is difficult due to the heterogeneity of study designs and samples. A Danish trial studied 140 adults with elevated MMA concentrations and found no effect on the SF-36 mental and physical summary scores after four weeks of vitamin B_{12} injections, but they did observe a positive effect on the general health subscale of this instrument [23]. Although these participants were not selected on the basis of their Hcy concentrations, most participants had mildly elevated Hcy concentrations. Another trial used a drink containing vitamin B_2, B_6, B_{12}, and folic acid that significantly lowered Hcy concentrations and improved HR-QoL (assessed with the General Health Survey) already after six weeks [16]. Other trials, however, did not observe effects on HR-QoL after study periods ranging from one to three years [20–22,24].

The observed significant treatment effect on the EQ-5D Index score, in contrast to the SF-12, was unexpected. In relatively healthy populations such as the B-PROOF sample, the SF-12 is usually a more sensitive instrument than the EQ-5D, as the EQ-5D may display ceiling effects [34,53]. For the scoring of the EQ-5D, Dutch norms were used, whereas the scoring system of the SF-12 was based on the US population because a Dutch sample is not currently available. The EQ-5D scoring system may have been better tailored for the B-PROOF sample, which could partly explain the observed discrepancy.

To the best of our knowledge, this study with almost 3000 participants is one of the largest studies investigating the effects of vitamin B_{12} and folic acid supplementation on mental health and well-being in older persons. The randomized placebo-controlled trial design, the large study sample, and the long follow-up period are major strengths of the B-PROOF study. In this way, relationships between Hcy, depressive symptoms, and HR-QoL could be studied both cross-sectionally and after supplementation. In addition, we were able to adequately control for possible covariates. The instruments that were used for assessing depressive symptoms and HR-QoL are widely used and have satisfactory psychometric properties. Compliance to the treatment was high, which was also reflected by the significantly decreased Hcy concentrations in the intervention group compared to the placebo group.

As depressive symptoms and HR-QoL were secondary outcome measures of the B-PROOF study, relatively few participants had clinically relevant depressive symptoms (7%) and participants generally perceived a high HR-QoL. This may have reduced the power of our analyses, especially in the subgroup of participants with depressive symptoms (N = 161). Furthermore, it should be mentioned that vitamin D_3 was added to both the B-vitamin and placebo tablets. Several observational and experimental studies have suggested that vitamin D supplementation reduces depressive symptoms and improves HR-QoL [54,55], which may have had an attenuating effect on our results.

By including persons with elevated Hcy concentrations, we aimed to include a sensitive sample for the effects of vitamin B_{12} and folic acid treatment. However, although elevated Hcy concentrations are common in the general older population [28], this selection may limit generalizability to the total elderly population. In addition, the restricted range of Hcy concentrations and the absence of participants with normal Hcy concentrations may have attenuated the results of the cross-sectional analyses.

Although the two-year supplementation in this study significantly lowered Hcy concentrations, our vitamin B_{12} dose of 500 μg/day may have been too low to observe an effect on depressive symptoms. A supplementation dose of at least 1000 μg/day may have been more effective [56,57]. Insufficient vitamin B_{12} status by itself has been associated with various neuropsychiatric symptoms, including depression [57]. Although we had only a low number of vitamin B_{12} deficient participants, a Finnish study showed that adult outpatients with clinical depression had a better treatment outcome when their B_{12} status was higher, even though all participants had normal or high vitamin B_{12} concentrations [49].

To further investigate the role of homocysteine in depression and HR-QoL, future research could focus on persons with hyperhomocysteinemia, low vitamin B_{12} or folate status, and on individuals with clinically relevant depressive symptoms and/or lower HR-QoL. These persons may possibly benefit more from B-vitamin supplementation. However, it should be mentioned that participants in the intervention group reported a higher incidence of cancer compared to the placebo group. This adverse effect of the B-vitamin supplementation has been reported previously [29]. Therefore, special caution is warranted in future studies with vitamin B_{12} and folic acid.

5. Conclusions

In conclusion, the results of the present study indicate that reducing Hcy concentrations by supplementation with vitamin B_{12} and folic acid in a generally healthy sample of older adults with mild hyperhomocysteinemia does not reduce depressive symptoms and may have a small positive effect on general HR-QoL.

Acknowledgments: We gratefully acknowledge all participants of the B-PROOF study. Furthermore, we would like to thank our colleagues and all students involved in the B-PROOF study for their valued help and dedication to the project. This study was supported and funded by The Netherlands Organization for Health Research and Development (ZonMw, Grant 6130.0031), the Hague; an unrestricted grant from the Dutch Dairy Association (NZO), Zoetermeer; MCO Health, Almere; the Netherlands Consortium Healthy Ageing (NCHA), Leiden/Rotterdam; Ministry of Economic Affairs, Agriculture and Innovation (project KB-15-004-003), the Hague; Wageningen University, Wageningen; VU University Medical Center, Amsterdam; and Erasmus Medical Center, Rotterdam. All organizations are based in the Netherlands. The funders had no role in the design, analysis or writing of this article.

Author Contributions: R.A.M.D.R., N.M.v.S., P.L., and L.C.P.G.M.d.G. conceived and designed the B-PROOF study; E.J.d.K., N.L.v.d.Z., J.P.v.W., E.M.B.-B., E.S., A.W.E., S.C.v.D., A.C.H., K.M.A.S. conducted the research and collected the data; E.J.d.K. and N.L.v.d.Z. analyzed and interpreted the data; E.J.d.K., N.L.v.d.Z., and N.M.v.S. drafted the manuscript; E.J.d.K., N.L.v.d.Z., J.P.v.W., N.M.v.S., and R.A.M.D.-R. had primary responsibility for the final content. All authors provided critical revision of the manuscript.

Appendix A

Table A1. Stratified analyses for significant interaction terms (stratified at the median, intention-to-treat analyses).

	N	Two-Year Change Scores in the Fully Adjusted Models Mean (95% CI)	*F* [a]	*p*
GDS-15: Stratified analyses for folate:				
Low Folate: (≤18.86 nmol/L)			1.63	0.21
B-vitamins	38	1.87 (0.76, 2.98)		
Placebo	41	0.86 (−0.21, 1.92)		
High Folate: (>18.86 nmol/L)			3.47	0.07
B-vitamins	38	1.19 (0.17, 2.20)		
Placebo	41	2.53 (1.56, 3.51)		
GDS-15: Stratified analyses for MMA:				
Low MMA: (≤0.23 µmol/L)			2.70	0.10
B-vitamins	38	0.63 (−0.50, 1.76)		
Placebo	41	1.95 (0.87, 3.04)		
High MMA: (>0.23 µmol/L)			1.12	0.29
B-vitamins	38	2.28 (1.34, 3.22)		
Placebo	41	1.57 (0.67, 2.48)		
GDS-15: Stratified analyses for Vitamin B_{12}:				
Low Vitamin B_{12}: (≤266.4 pmol/L)			1.07	0.30
B-vitamins	41	2.14 (1.13, 3.16)		
Placebo	39	1.36 (0.32, 2.41)		
High Vitamin B_{12}: (>266.4 pmol/L)			4.52	0.04
B-vitamins	41	0.55 (−0.60, 1.69)		
Placebo	39	2.21 (1.18, 3.24)		
EQ-5D VAS: Stratified analyses for sex:				
Men:			2.75	0.10
B-vitamins	657	−0.86 (−1.73, 0.02)		
Placebo	667	−1.90 (−2.76, −1.03)		
Women:			1.07	0.30
B-vitamins	645	−1.33 (−2.32, −0.33)		
Placebo	643	−0.58 (−1.58, 0.42)		

[a] Differences between the two treatment groups over time were tested with ANCOVA, adjusted for baseline values of the respective outcome variable, age, sex, homocysteine, and study center. GDS-15: Geriatric Depression Scale 15-item version; MMA: methylmalonic acid; EQ-5D VAS: EuroQol 5 Dimensions—Visual Analogue Scale.

References

1. World Health Organization: The Global Burden of Disease 2004 Update. Available online: http://www.who.int/healthinfo/global_burden_disease/GBD_report_2004update_full.pdf (accessed on 1 May 2014).
2. Blazer, D.G. Depression in late life: Review and commentary. *J. Gerontol. A Biol. Sci. Med. Sci.* **2003**, *58*, 249–265. [CrossRef] [PubMed]
3. Ware, J.; Kosinski, M.; Keller, S.D. A 12-Item Short-Form Health Survey: Construction of scales and preliminary tests of reliability and validity. *Med. Care* **1996**, *34*, 220–233. [CrossRef] [PubMed]
4. Idler, E.L.; Benyamini, Y. Self-rated health and mortality: A review of twenty-seven community studies. *J. Health Soc. Behav.* **1997**, *38*, 21–37. [CrossRef] [PubMed]
5. Prins, M.A.; Verhaak, P.F.; Hilbink-Smolders, M.; Spreeuwenberg, P.; Laurant, M.G.H.; van der Meer, K.; van Marwijk, H.W.J.; Penninx, B.W.J.H.; Bensing, J.M. Outcomes for depression and anxiety in primary

care and details of treatment: A naturalistic longitudinal study. *BMC Psychiatry* **2011**, *11*, 180. [CrossRef] [PubMed]

6. Wald, D.S.; Law, M.; Morris, J.K. Homocysteine and cardiovascular disease: Evidence on causality from a meta-analysis. *BMJ* **2002**, *325*, 1202. [CrossRef] [PubMed]
7. Van Wijngaarden, J.P.; Doets, E.L.; Szczecinska, A.; Souverein, O.W.; Duffy, M.E.; Dullemeijer, C.; Cavelaars, A.E.J.M.; Pietruszka, B.; van't Veer, P.; Brzozowska, A.; et al. Vitamin B_{12}, folate, homocysteine, and bone health in adults and elderly people: A systematic review with meta-analyses. *J. Nutr. Metab.* **2013**, *2013*, 486186. [CrossRef] [PubMed]
8. Malouf, R.; Grimley, E.J. Folic acid with or without vitamin B_{12} for the prevention and treatment of healthy elderly and demented people. *Cochrane Database Syst. Rev.* **2008**. [CrossRef]
9. Ng, T.P.; Aung, K.C.; Feng, L.; Scherer, S.C.; Yap, K.B. Homocysteine, folate, vitamin B-12, and physical function in older adults: Cross-sectional findings from the Singapore Longitudinal Ageing Study. *Am. J. Clin. Nutr.* **2012**, *96*, 1362–1368. [CrossRef] [PubMed]
10. Bates, C.J.; Mansoor, M.A.; Kristina, D.; Pentieva, K.D.; Hamer, M.; Mishra, G.D. Biochemical risk indices, including plasma homocysteine, that prospectively predict mortality in older British people: The National Diet and Nutrition Survey of People Aged 65 Years and Over. *Br. J. Nutr.* **2010**, *104*, 893–899. [CrossRef] [PubMed]
11. Sachdev, P.S.; Parslow, R.A.; Lux, O.; Salonikas, C.; Wen, W.; Naidoo, D.; Christensen, H.; Jorm, A.F. Relationship of homocysteine, folic acid and vitamin B_{12} with depression in a middle-aged community sample. *Psychol. Med.* **2005**, *35*, 529–538. [CrossRef] [PubMed]
12. Gariballa, S. Testing homocysteine-induced neurotransmitter deficiency, and depression of mood hypothesis in clinical practice. *Age Ageing* **2011**, *40*, 702–705. [CrossRef] [PubMed]
13. Bjelland, I.; Tell, G.S.; Vollset, S.E.; Refsum, H.; Ueland, P.M. Folate, vitamin B_{12}, homocysteine, and the MTHFR 677C->T polymorphism in anxiety and depression: The Hordaland Homocysteine Study. *Arch. Gen. Psychiatry* **2003**, *60*, 618–626. [CrossRef] [PubMed]
14. Almeida, O.P.; Lautenschlager, N.; Flicker, L.; Leedman, P.; Vasikaran, S.; Gelavis, A.; Ludlow, J. Association between homocysteine, depression, and cognitive function in community-dwelling older women from Australia. *J. Am. Geriatr. Soc.* **2004**, *52*, 327–328. [CrossRef] [PubMed]
15. Wong, Y.Y.; Almeida, O.P.; McCaul, K.A.; Yeap, B.B.; Hankey, G.J.; van Bockxmeer, F.M.; Flicker, L. Elevated homocysteine is associated with poorer self-perceived physical health in older men: The Health in Men Study. *Maturitas* **2012**, *73*, 158–163. [CrossRef] [PubMed]
16. Gariballa, S. Extending the homocysteine-induced neurotransmitter deficiency and depression of mood hypothesis to quality of life in older patients. *Int. J. Geriatr. Psychiatry* **2013**, *28*, 878–879. [CrossRef] [PubMed]
17. Almeida, O.P.; McCaul, K.; Hankey, G.J.; Norman, P.; Jamrozik, K.; Flicker, L. Homocysteine and depression in later life. *Arch. Gen. Psychiatry* **2008**, *65*, 1286–1294. [CrossRef] [PubMed]
18. Homocysteine Lowering Trialist's Collaboration. Dose-dependent effects of folic acid on blood concentrations of homocysteine: A meta-analysis of the randomized trials. *Am. J. Clin. Nutr.* **2005**, *82*, 806–812.
19. Almeida, O.P.; Marsh, K.; Alfonso, H.; Flicker, L.; Davis, T.M.; Hankey, G.J. B-vitamins reduce the long-term risk of depression after stroke: The VITATOPS-DEP trial. *Ann. Neurol.* **2010**, *68*, 503–510. [CrossRef] [PubMed]
20. Andreeva, V.A.; Latarche, C.; Hercberg, S.; Briancon, S.; Galan, P.; Kesse-Guyot, E. B vitamin and/or *n*-3 fatty acid supplementation and health-related quality of life: Ancillary findings from the SU.FOL.OM3 randomized trial. *PLoS ONE* **2014**, *9*, e84844. [CrossRef] [PubMed]
21. Bryan, J.; Calvaresi, E.; Hughes, D. Short-term folate, vitamin B-12 or vitamin B-6 supplementation slightly affects memory performance but not mood in women of various ages. *J. Nutr.* **2002**, *132*, 1345–1356. [PubMed]
22. Ford, A.H.; Flicker, L.; Alfonso, H.; Thomas, J.; Clarnette, R.; Martins, R.; Almeida, O.P. Vitamins B(12), B(6), and folic acid for cognition in older men. *Neurology* **2010**, *75*, 1540–1547. [CrossRef] [PubMed]
23. Hvas, A.M.; Juul, S.; Nexo, E.; Ellegaard, J. Vitamin B-12 treatment has limited effect on health-related quality of life among individuals with elevated plasma methylmalonic acid: A randomized placebo-controlled study. *J. Intern. Med.* **2003**, *253*, 146–152. [CrossRef] [PubMed]
24. Van Uffelen, J.G.; Chin A Paw, M.J.; Hopman-Rock, M.; van Mechelen, W. The effect of walking and vitamin B supplementation on quality of life in community-dwelling adults with mild cognitive impairment: A randomized, controlled trial. *Qual. Life Res.* **2007**, *16*, 1137–1146. [CrossRef] [PubMed]

25. Papakostas, G.I.; Cassiello, C.F.; Iovieno, N. Folates and *S*-adenosylmethionine for major depressive disorder. *Can. J. Psychiatry* **2012**, *57*, 406–413. [PubMed]
26. Reynolds, E.H.; Carney, M.W.; Toone, B.K. Methylation and mood. *Lancet* **1984**, *2*, 196–198. [CrossRef]
27. Bottiglieri, T.; Laundy, M.; Crellin, R.; Toone, B.K.; Carney, M.W.; Reynolds, E.H. Homocysteine, folate, methylation, and monoamine metabolism in depression. *J. Neurol. Neurosurg. Psychiatry* **2000**, *69*, 228–232. [CrossRef] [PubMed]
28. Van Wijngaarden, J.P.; Dhonukshe-Rutten, R.A.; van Schoor, N.M.; van der Velde, H.; Swart, K.M.A.; Enneman, A.W.; van Dijk, S.C.; Brouwer-Brolsma, E.M.; Zillikens, M.C.; van Meurs, J.B.J.; et al. Rationale and design of the B-PROOF study, a randomized controlled trial on the effect of supplemental intake of vitamin B_{12} and folic acid on fracture incidence. *BMC Geriatr.* **2011**, *11*, 80. [CrossRef] [PubMed]
29. Van Wijngaarden, J.P.; Swart, K.M.; Enneman, A.W.; Dhonukshe-Rutten, R.A.M.; van Dijk, S.C.; Ham, A.C.; Brouwer-Brolsma, E.M.; van der Zwaluw, N.L.; Sohl, E.; van Meurs, J.B.J.; et al. Effect of daily vitamin B-12 and folic acid supplementation on fracture incidence in elderly individuals with an elevated plasma homocysteine concentration: B-PROOF, a randomized controlled trial. *Am. J. Clin. Nutr.* **2014**, *100*, 1578–1586. [CrossRef] [PubMed]
30. Yesavage, J.A.; Brink, T.L.; Rose, T.L.; Lum, O.; Huang, V.; Adey, M.; Leirer, V.O. Development and validation of a geriatric depression screening scale: A preliminary report. *J. Psychiatr. Res.* **1982**, *17*, 37–49. [CrossRef]
31. Bijl, D.; van Marwijk, H.W.J.; Ader, H.J.; Beekman, A.T.F.; de Haan, M. Test-Characteristics of the GDS-15 in Screening for Major Depression in Elderly Patients in General Practice. *Clin. Gerontol.* **2005**, *29*, 1–9. [CrossRef]
32. Almeida, O.P.; Almeida, S.A. Short versions of the geriatric depression scale: A study of their validity for the diagnosis of a major depressive episode according to ICD-10 and DSM-IV. *Int. J. Geriatr. Psychiatry* **1999**, *14*, 858–865. [CrossRef]
33. Kind, P.; Dolan, P.; Gudex, C.; Williams, A. Variations in population health status: Results from a United Kingdom national questionnaire survey. *BMJ* **1998**, *316*, 736–741. [CrossRef] [PubMed]
34. De Smedt, D.; Clays, E.; Annemans, L.; De Bacquer, D. EQ-5D versus SF-12 in coronary patients: Are they interchangeable? *Value Health* **2014**, *17*, 84–89. [CrossRef] [PubMed]
35. Ware, J.; Snow, K.; Gandek, K.M. *SF-36 Health Survey: Manual and Interpretation Guide*; The Health Institute, New England Medical Center: Boston, MA, USA, 1993.
36. Lamers, L.M.; Stalmeier, P.F.; McDonnell, J.; Krabbe, P.F.; van Busschbach, J.J. Measuring the quality of life in economic evaluations: The Dutch EQ-5D tariff. *Ned. Tijdschr. Geneeskd.* **2005**, *149*, 1574–1578. (In Dutch) [PubMed]
37. Garretsen, H. *Probleemdrinken, Prevalentiebepaling, Beinvloedende Factoren en Preventiemogelijkheden: Theoretische Overwegingen en Onderzoek in Rotterdam*; Swets & Zeitlinger: Lisse, The Netherlands, 1983. (In Dutch)
38. Stel, V.S.; Smit, J.H.; Pluijm, S.M.; Visser, M.; Deeg, D.J.; Lips, P. Comparison of the LASA Physical Activity Questionnaire with a 7-day diary and pedometer. *J. Clin. Epidemiol.* **2004**, *57*, 252–258. [CrossRef] [PubMed]
39. Folstein, M.F.; Folstein, S.E.; McHugh, P.R. "Mini-mental state". A practical method for grading the cognitive state of patients for the clinician. *J. Psychiatr. Res.* **1975**, *12*, 189–198. [CrossRef]
40. Barros, A.J.; Hirakata, V.N. Alternatives for logistic regression in cross-sectional studies: An empirical comparison of models that directly estimate the prevalence ratio. *BMC Med. Res. Methodol.* **2003**, *3*, 21. [CrossRef] [PubMed]
41. Jacques, P.F.; Bostom, A.G.; Wilson, P.W.; Rich, S.; Rosenberg, I.H.; Selhub, J. Determinants of plasma total homocysteine concentration in the Framingham Offspring Cohort. *Am. J. Clin. Nutr.* **2001**, *73*, 613–621. [PubMed]
42. Raggi, A.; Corso, B.; Minicuci, N.; Quintas, R.; Sattin, D.; De Torres, L.; Chatterji, S.; Frisoni, G.B.; Haro, J.M.; Koskinen, S.; et al. Determinants of quality of life in ageing populations: Results from a cross-sectional study in Finland, Poland and Spain. *PLoS ONE* **2016**, *11*, e0159293. [CrossRef] [PubMed]
43. Allen, L.H. How common is vitamin B-12 deficiency? *Am. J. Clin. Nutr.* **2009**, *89*, 693S–696S. [CrossRef] [PubMed]
44. Seppala, J.; Koponen, H.; Kautiainen, H.; Eriksson, J.G.; Kampman, O.; Leiviskä, J.; Männistö, S.; Mäntyselkä, P.; Oksa, H.; Ovaskainen, Y.; et al. Association between vitamin B_{12} levels and melancholic depressive symptoms: A Finnish population-based study. *BMC Psychiatry* **2013**, *13*, 145. [CrossRef] [PubMed]
45. Ng, T.P.; Feng, L.; Niti, M.; Kua, E.H.; Yap, K.B. Folate, vitamin B_{12}, homocysteine, and depressive symptoms in a population sample of older Chinese adults. *J. Am. Geriatr. Soc.* **2009**, *57*, 871–876. [CrossRef] [PubMed]

46. Gilbody, S.; Lightfoot, T.; Sheldon, T. Is low folate a risk factor for depression? A meta-analysis and exploration of heterogeneity. *J. Epidemiol. Community Health* **2007**, *61*, 631–637. [CrossRef] [PubMed]
47. Penninx, B.W.; Guralnik, J.M.; Ferrucci, L.; Fried, L.P.; Allen, R.H.; Stabler, S.P. Vitamin B(12) deficiency and depression in physically disabled older women: Epidemiologic evidence from the Women's Health and Aging Study. *Am. J. Psychiatry* **2000**, *157*, 715–721. [CrossRef] [PubMed]
48. Kim, J.M.; Stewart, R.; Kim, S.W.; Yang, S.J.; Shin, I.S.; Yoon, J.S. Predictive value of folate, vitamin B_{12} and homocysteine levels in late-life depression. *Br. J. Psychiatry* **2008**, *192*, 268–274. [CrossRef] [PubMed]
49. Hintikka, J.; Tolmunen, T.; Tanskanen, A.; Viinamäki, H. High vitamins B_{12} level and good treatment outcome may be associated in major depressive disorder. *BMC Psychiatry* **2003**, *3*, 17. [CrossRef] [PubMed]
50. Ford, A.H.; Flicker, L.; Thomas, J.; Norman, P.; Jamrozik, K.; Almeida, O.P. Vitamins B_{12}, B6, and folic acid for onset of depressive symptoms in older men: Results from a 2-year placebo-controlled randomized trial. *J. Clin. Psychiatry* **2008**, *69*, 1203–1209. [CrossRef] [PubMed]
51. Hvas, A.M.; Juul, S.; Lauritzen, L.; Nexo, E.; Ellegaard, J. No effect of vitamin B-12 treatment on cognitive function and depression: A randomized placebo controlled study. *J. Affect. Disord.* **2004**, *81*, 269–273. [CrossRef]
52. Gerhards, S.A.; Huibers, M.J.; Theunissen, K.A.; de Graaf, L.E.; Widdershoven, G.A.; Evers, S.M. The responsiveness of quality of life utilities to change in depression: A comparison of instruments (SF-6D, EQ-5D, and DFD). *Value Health* **2011**, *14*, 732–739. [CrossRef] [PubMed]
53. Johnson, J.A.; Coons, S.J. Comparison of the EQ-5D and SF-12 in an adult US sample. *Qual. Life Res.* **1998**, *7*, 155–166. [CrossRef] [PubMed]
54. Shaffer, J.A.; Edmondson, D.; Wasson, L.T.; Falzon, L.; Homma, K.; Ezeokoli, N.; Li, P.; Davidson, K.W. Vitamin D supplementation for depressive symptoms: A systematic review and meta-analysis of randomized controlled trials. *Psychosom. Med.* **2014**, *76*, 190–196. [CrossRef] [PubMed]
55. Rafiq, R.; Swart, K.M.; van Schoor, N.M.; Deeg, D.J.; Lips, P.; de Jongh, R.T. Associations of serum 25-hydroxyvitamin D concentrations with quality of life and self-rated health in an older population. *J. Clin. Endocrinol. Metab.* **2014**, *99*, 3136–3143. [CrossRef] [PubMed]
56. Vidal-Alaball, J.; Butler, C.C.; Cannings-John, R.; Goringe, A.; Hood, K.; McCaddon, A.; McDowell, I.; Papaioannou, A. Oral vitamin B_{12} versus intramuscular vitamin B_{12} for vitamin B_{12} deficiency. *Cochrane Database Syst. Rev.* **2005**, *3*, CD004655.
57. Lachner, C.; Steinle, N.I.; Regenold, W.T. The neuropsychiatry of vitamin B_{12} deficiency in elderly patients. *J. Neuropsychiatry Clin. Neurosci.* **2012**, *24*, 5–15. [CrossRef] [PubMed]

4

Vitamin B12 among Vegetarians: Status, Assessment and Supplementation

Gianluca Rizzo [1], Antonio Simone Laganà [2,*], Agnese Maria Chiara Rapisarda [3], Gioacchina Maria Grazia La Ferrera [4], Massimo Buscema [5], Paola Rossetti [5], Angela Nigro [5], Vincenzo Muscia [5], Gaetano Valenti [3], Fabrizio Sapia [3], Giuseppe Sarpietro [3], Micol Zigarelli [3] and Salvatore Giovanni Vitale [2]

1. Vico Sant'andrea 5, Ritiro, Messina 98152, Italy; gianlucarizzo@email.it
2. Unit of Gynecology and Obstetrics, Department of Human Pathology in Adulthood and Childhood, "G. Barresi", University of Messina, Via Consolare Valeria 1, Messina 98125, Italy; vitalesalvatore@hotmail.com
3. Department of General Surgery and Medical Surgical Specialties, University of Catania, Via S. Sofia 78, Catania 95124, Italy; agni.rap@live.it (A.M.C.R.); valentigaetano@gmail.com (G.V.); fabrizio.sapia@libero.it (F.S.); peppe_sarpietro@hotmail.com (G.S.); micolziga@gmail.com (M.Z.)
4. Department of Gastroenterology and Digestive Endoscopy Maddalena Raimondi San Cataldo, Via Forlanini 5, San Cataldo, Caltanissetta 93017, Italy; giolaferrera@libero.it
5. Unit of Diabetology and Endocrino-Metabolic Diseases, Hospital for Emergency Cannizzaro, Via Messina 829, Catania 95126, Italy; buscemamassimo@gmail.com (M.B.); paolarossetti@alice.it (P.R.); ang.nigro@gmail.com (A.N.); vince80@alice.it (V.M.)

* Correspondence: antlagana@unime.it

Abstract: Cobalamin is an essential molecule for humans. It acts as a cofactor in one-carbon transfers through methylation and molecular rearrangement. These functions take place in fatty acid, amino acid and nucleic acid metabolic pathways. The deficiency of vitamin B12 is clinically manifested in the blood and nervous system where the cobalamin plays a key role in cell replication and in fatty acid metabolism. Hypovitaminosis arises from inadequate absorption, from genetic defects that alter transport through the body, or from inadequate intake as a result of diet. With the growing adoption of vegetarian eating styles in Western countries, there is growing focus on whether diets that exclude animal foods are adequate. Since food availability in these countries is not a problem, and therefore plant foods are sufficiently adequate, the most delicate issue remains the contribution of cobalamin, which is poorly represented in plants. In this review, we will discuss the status of vitamin B12 among vegetarians, the diagnostic markers for the detection of cobalamin deficiency and appropriate sources for sufficient intake, through the description of the features and functions of vitamin B12 and its absorption mechanism.

Keywords: cobalamin; vitamin B12; vegetarian; vegan; food sources; deficiency; cardiovascular disease; neurological symptoms; supplements; diagnostic markers

---

1. Introduction

Recently, the vegetarian eating style has increased in popularity, with 10% of the population opting to exclude animal foods from their diet [1]. The decision to undertake such a choice depends primarily on ethical and ecological aspects, but also on health reasons. However, when the reasons are ethical, this may result in a reduced interest in the knowledge of the nutritional aspects of such a choice [2]. The scientific literature shows that the reduction or exclusion of animal foods may reduce the risk of Coronary Heart Disease (CHD) and Type 2 Diabetes (T2D) through modifiable factors such as body mass, serum glucose, blood pressure and serum lipid profile. These disorders contribute to a high mortality rate in Western countries [3–7]. Nevertheless, the risk of possible nutritional deficiencies in a non-balanced vegetarian diet, due to the absence of nutrients that can nullify these health benefits [8], should not be underestimated. In the European Prospective Investigation into Cancer and Nutrition-Oxford (EPIC-Oxford) cohort study, all-cause mortality among vegetarians in comparison with non-vegetarians was not significantly different [9]. In five prospective study analyses of 24,000 vegetarians among a total of 76,000 men and women, mortality from ischemic heart disease was lower in lacto-ovo-vegetarians than in vegans [10].

In the 2010 American Dietary Guidelines, the United States Department of Agriculture (USDA) proposed vegetarian adaptation patterns, including proposals for a balanced vegan diet [11]. Since 1988, and recently with the position paper of 2009, the American Dietetic Association has established that vegetarian diets are sustainable and safe for all age groups and in all physiological conditions, from childhood to old age, in athletes, and during pregnancy and lactation [12,13]. Sustainability relates to vegetarian diets that do not exclude dairy and eggs, as well as a vegan diet. However, it should be focused on proper planning and supplementation.

Vitamin B12, also called cobalamin (Cbl), is a water-soluble vitamin found in substantial quantities only in animal foods. If the consumption of animal foods is very low or absent, its scarce presence in plant foods makes its introduction essential, either through supplements or fortified foods. This deficiency is common among vegetarians and is the result of a very low intake [14]. Lower Cbl blood concentration can promote hematological shortages, resulting in increased mean corpuscular red cell volume (MCV) and anemia through the alteration of erythropoiesis [15]. Cbl also plays a key role in neuronal health, and a severe deficiency would inhibit the physiological formation of the myelin sheath, altering correct nerve transmission [15]. The slowing down of the degradation pathway of odd-chain fatty acids leads to an unusual incorporation of large quantities of C15 and C17 fatty acids in the nerve sheaths. This is due to an alteration of glial cell synthesis resulting in myelin modification [16].

There is no shared diagnostic consensus for Cbl deficiency, and blood Cbl cutoffs vary from one group to another. In addition, the concentration of Cbl in the blood may not be sensitive enough to detect early signs of a deficiency and should be accompanied by other markers in order to reach a correct diagnosis.

2. Background

Among vegetarians, there are differing styles that are categorized according to the level of animal food exclusion. Vegetarianism can be classified into different plant-based subgroups: lacto-ovo-vegetarian (LOV) which excludes animal flesh but includes eggs and dairy products; ovo-vegetarian (OV), similar to LOV but excluding dairy products; lacto-vegetarian (LV), similar to LOV but excluding eggs; or vegan (VN), which excludes all animal foods, dairy products and eggs. In common language, the term vegetarian is interpreted differently depending on the country (i.e., LOV in Italy or LV in India).

Unbalanced vegetarian diets could be lacking in nutrients that are poorly represented in vegetal foodstuffs or with a low bioavailability (e.g., iron, zinc, vitamin D, ω3 polyunsaturated fatty acids) [17]. However, only Cbl seems to be virtually absent in vegetables and its shortage can have serious implications.

A common mistake is to think that the presence of dairy products and eggs in the diet, as in LOV, can still ensure a proper intake of Cbl, despite excluding animal flesh. In reality, consumption of such foods, despite containing significant amounts of Cbl, would be sufficient neither on a daily basis nor in order to meet vitamin requirements [18]. A Dietary Reference Intake (DRI) of 2.4 μg/day for Cbl in adults is a common chosen value [19,20]. Such an amount is apparently exceeded by American adults, with a mean intake ranging from 4.6 to 6.3 μg/day [21]. However, it is not uncommon to see a moderate deficiency among omnivores in Western countries [22,23]. A recent report by the European Food Safety Authority (EFSA) Panel on Dietetic Products, Nutrition and Allergies established an

Adequate Intake (AI) of 4 µg/day for adults, with a mean intake in European countries ranging between 4.2 and 8.6 µg/day [24].

The main source of consumption in the general population comes from animal foods with a significant contribution from milk and dairy products [25]. Losses of up to 50% can occur through food processing which involves cooking, pasteurization and exposure to fluorescent light. This limits its availability, together with a drop in absorption capacity and an increase in Cbl concentration in food [26]. Some researchers claim that the currently recommended intake levels may not be sufficient for an adequate daily intake, with particular regard to aging and the physiological reduction in absorptive capacity [27]. With senescence, the epithelial cells of the stomach reduce their ability to biosynthesize the transporter proteins of Cbl. The gastric secretion ability is necessary both for the dissociation of Cbl from foods and for the binding to the carriers [28]. For these reasons, the American Institute of Medicine recommends a supplementation of Cbl for people of 50 years of age and older [19]. The development of blood and cognitive disorders are rather common aspects found among the elderly population [29].

In the vegetarian diet, there are few sources of Cbl, whilst supplement use is frequently resisted.

Although some plant foods seem to represent a significant source of Cbl [30,31], data in the literature are still insufficient to determine whether Cbl is found in the active form, and whether regular consumption of these foods can be sustainable when the variability in the production processes is taken into account.

3. Chemical Properties of Cobalamin and Vitamin Activity

The synthesis of Cbl is a prerogative of some bacteria and archaea [32]. Its presence in animal foodstuffs depends on the process of biomagnification through food chains [30]. Small quantities found in plants and derived from biofilms bound by Cbl cannot be synthesized by either animals or plants [33]. Cbl is the vitamin with the largest steric hindrance (1355.4 Da) [34]. It consists of a tetrapyrrolic corrin ring core with a central cobalt atom, grouped with four nitrogen, one nucleotide base group and one upper ligand. The cobalt atom accepts different ligands on the upper surface: hydroxyl (Hydroxycobalamin-*H*-Cbl), deoxy-5′-adenosine (Deoxy-5′-adenosylcobalamin-Ado-Cbl), metyl (methylcobalamin-Me-Cbl), cyanide (Cyanocobalamin Cn-Cbl). Me-Cbl and Ado-Cbl are the active forms of vitamins used as coenzymes in the cell [35,36]. On the lower surface of the ring, the cobalt atom binds a 5,6-dimethylimidazole nucleotide base (DMB). Naturally occurring corrinoids without vitamin activity bind lower ligands different from DMB such as 2-methyladenylcobamide, methylmercaptoadenylcobamide-2,5-methoxybenzimidazolylcobamide, benzimidazolylcobamide, 5-hydroxybenzimidazolylcobamide, *p*-cresolylcobamide [30].

Me-Cbl is the cofactor of the enzyme methionine synthase participating in the metabolic homocysteine pathway (HCY), which is processed into methionine with the involvement of vitamin B6 and folate [37]. The reaction takes place in the cytosolic environment and the deficiency of vitamin cofactors leads to an increase in HCY blood concentration [38]. This pathway is critical in the regeneration of the methyl donor *S*-adenosylmethionine (SAM) and its dysfunction creates a shortage, affecting DNA synthesis and the physiological processes that require intense cell replication, such as hematopoietic process of the erythrocytes. Ado-Cbl is the vitamin cofactor of the methylmalonyl-CoA mutase enzyme. It works within the mitochondria, in the metabolism of branched-chain amino acids and fatty acid with an odd number of carbon atoms. These atoms are not subject to degradation by a beta-oxidation pathway accepting only two carbon units [39,40]. The shortage of Ado-Cbl leads to an accumulation of methylmalonic acid (MMA), an intermediate molecule of this pathway. A deficiency of this vitamin form is due primarily to neurological effects. The myelin sheaths of neurons are highly dependent on fatty acid metabolism and the low bioavailability of Ado-Cbl in neurons leads to the depletion of the myelin layer with dysfunctional nerve transmission. The role of Cbl in neuropathological lesions seems to be due to interactions with neurotrophic molecules such as Myelinolytic Tumor Necrosis Factor α (TNF-α), Epidermal Grow Factor (EGF) and Interleukin-6 (IL6) [41]. HCY itself appears to show a neurotoxic effect on synaptic receptors [42].

Cn-Cbl and H-Cbl are provitamin forms that require activation in cofactors Me-Cbl or Ado-Cbl to be utilized by the cells. Cn-Cbl is the form of Cbl first isolated and, although an artifact, it was initially identified as an anti-pernicious anemia factor [43]. Cobalamin performs a secondary function, that of removing potentially harmful molecules from the body. As a result, a small amount of Cbl in the blood stream is present in the Cn-Cbl form that binds cyanide residues. Cyanide is normally present in trace amounts in foods such as cassava, bitter almonds and apricot kernels (responsible for the bitter taste) [44]. H-Cbl is a form of cobalamin highly represented as a physiological intermediate [35]. Other corrinoids are non-vitamin analogs which are capable of engaging the carriers. These become less available to bind the vitamin forms, with an overall antinutrient outcome [45].

In the cell, the Cbl isoforms are metabolized inside the peroxisome by the reactions of dealkylation, decyanation and reduction, and then released in the specific cell compartment as coenzyme Me-Cbl and Ado-Cbl, according to their cytosolic or mitochondrial fate, respectively [46]. This step is crucial in the activation of the provitamin forms. Other corrinoid compounds do not fulfill the vitamin functions, in all probability due to the binding power of the lower ligand with the cobalt, which does not allow peroxisome activation [45]. It seems that all isoforms, provitamins and coenzymes should follow a mandatory route before being assigned to the appropriate cell district. However, the H-Cbl form may be more reactive, and its use can be facilitated by a number of enzymatic processes through non-specific cellular reactions [47]. If this mechanism were confirmed, the use of already active Cbl cofactors would not represent any provitamin advantage [45]. In 1982, Gimsing et al. analyzed Cbl in tissues from patients with pernicious anemia. After administration of H-Cbl or Cn-Cbl, they found that detected plasma Cbl was dependent on the form administered, dominant in the blood pattern. Results from erythrocytes and liver biopsies showed no differences, irrespective of the Cbl form used, indicating that administered Cbl preparations are converted in vivo to the necessary coenzymes [48]. Although current studies have many limitations and altogether there are no significant differences, the retention percentage after oral ingestion may change between different forms [49]. Following the ingestion of 1 μg of Cbl, the retention of Ado-Cbl and H-Cbl is 34% and 56%, respectively. Following the ingestion of 5 μg of Cbl, the retention of Ado-Cbl and Cn-Cbl is 13% and 20%, respectively. Following the ingestion of 25 μg of Cbl, the retention of Cn-Cbl and Ado-Cbl is 6% and 8%, respectively [50]. Updated data are not currently available.

4. Absorption and Transport

The absorption and transport of Cbl occurs via a complex network of proteins, which perform the task of optimizing the management of Cbl through the body districts. The study of rare genetic defects in carriers provided an opportunity to improve our understanding of the transport system and cellular trafficking of cobalamins [47,51]. Cbl is primarily associated with foodstuff proteins, such as Me-Cbl and Ado-Cbl. Free form, called crystalline or protein-unbound, is less represented and derived predominantly from supplements and fortified foods [25]. Transporters accept provitamin and coenzyme forms indifferently [52,53]. Following ingestion, the Cbl binds to the first salivary carrier R-binder or transcobalamin I, belonging to the corrin family of proteins. Its binding is non-specific and it binds various types of corrinoids, including antinutrient forms [52]. The increase of salivation promotes the secretion of R-binder and so the binding to the carrier that will occur after the dissociation from food proteins [54]. The gastric epithelial cells secrete hydrochloric acid and pepsin, responsible for the dissociation of Cbl from food proteins that enables binding to R-binder. The parietal cells also produce intrinsic factor (IF), another much more specific transporter for vitamin forms that binds Cbl released into the duodenum after cleavage from the R-binder through the use of trypsin and other pancreatic enzymes [55]. Thanks to the differing binding specificity, inactive analogs remain linked to R-binder and are excreted, while the vitamin forms continue on the route of absorption [56]. Binding to IF is critical for absorption into the terminal ileum, which is brought about by the membrane protein cubilin as part of the cubam receptor complex along with an amnion-less protein. The IF-Cbl complex is internalized by receptor-mediated endocytosis on the luminal side of the polarized enterocyte [57]. Inside the enterocyte, the IF-Cbl complex is degraded into the peroxisome with the recycling of cubam protein on the apical side, degrading IF and releasing Cbl from the baseline side due to the MRP1 transport protein. Here Cbl is readily associated with blood carriers [58]. In the blood stream, the cobalamins are transported by the trans-cobalamin II carrier (TCII) in a complex defined as holotranscobalamin II (HTCII) and considered the active Cbl form circulating in blood, as this transporter is highly specific to the molecules with vitamin activity [59]. Presumably, the TCII is secreted by endothelial cells of the cardiovascular system [60]. HTCII represents only a small percentage of the circulating Cbl (5%–20%). The remaining Cbl is linked to another more aspecific carrier named haptocorrin or transcobalamin III (HC), an isoform of the R-binder molecule [61]. While all cells have a specific receptor for HTCII called TCb1R, HC receptors have been discovered only in hepatocytes. It is thought that the function of this transporter is inactive analog removal through reverse transport to the liver and intestinal release from bile salts [62]. The HTCII complex that is not removed from the blood stream by the cell membrane protein TCb1R is filtered by the kidney, and reabsorbed in the proximal tubule through megalin protein-mediated reuptake [63]. The binding specificity of the different carriers for vitamin, high for IF and TCII and low for R-binder and HC, is necessary to reduce the absorption of a non-vitamin or degraded Cbl molecules that may saturate the transport system and affect vitamin absorption. Thus, the function of some carriers acquires the role of scavenger of the non-active corrinoid analogs. The TCb1R-HTCII complex is internalized in peripheral cells and degraded in the peroxisome with receptor recycling and proteolysis of TCII, including the release of Cbl in the cytosol due to transporters LMBD1 and ABCD4 [51,64,65]. Here, chaperon CblC removes upper ligands (methyl, hyroxyl, cyanide, or adenosyl), preparing Cbl for methylation and adenosylation [37,66,67].

Active absorption is severely limited. It is estimated that the absorptive capacity of Cbl is 1.5–2 µg per meal and depends on the maximum saturation of the cubam pool [68]. Conditions that reduce the secretion or binding efficiency can inhibit this amount significantly, as occurs with aging, with the chronic use of proton pump inhibitors (PPI) in Gastro-Esophageal Reflux Disease (GERD) or with gastric dysfunctions such as atrophic gastritis [69]. There is, however, a passive diffusion across the mucosal epithelium. This system is concentration-dependent and it is estimated that about 1% of Cbl follows this route. The aspecific transport is gradient-dependent and may be significant in the use of high oral doses (0.5–1 mg), with a good efficacy also in persons with limited capacity for active absorption, such as in cases of pernicious anemia or gastric atrophy [70,71]. Enterohepatic circulation is essential for the efficient absorption of Cbl. In fact, an excess of Cbl not internalized by cells is also secreted with bile and reabsorbed by the IF transport pathway [72]. Infants born to mothers with an adequate intake of Cbl show reserves of about 25 µg at birth [73]. Due to the intense activity of cell replication in tissue expansion, breast milk should continue to provide Cbl linked to a corrin, from which it becomes separated through the proteolytic action of the child's gastrointestinal enzymes [74].

5. Assessment and Diagnostic Markers

There is no reference method or gold standard regarding Cbl deficiency and the clinical signs could be hematological, neurological and/or biochemical [75]. The deficiency of Cbl is defined by the serum concentrations <110 pmol/L [76,77], <127 pmol/L [78], <148 pmol/L [79,80], <150 pmol/L [81–83], <156 pmol/L [84,85], <220 pmol/L [86], <250 pmol/L [8]. The Institute of Medicine defined 120–180 pmol/L as a depletion range [25]. With such heterogeneous deficiency criteria, there is a risk of ignoring conditions of medical relevance. Moreover, even at concentrations above the cutoffs of 156 pmol/L (a commonly used cutoff), deficiency conditions may already be present [18,87]. The predictive strength of blood concentration of total Cbl is very low and insufficient for a diagnosis of deficiency, which may result in loss of memory, personality disturbance, emotional liability and psychosis even with a low-normal Cbl blood concentration [88]. In fact, total Cbl does not take into account the ratio between HTCII and Cbl bound to haptocorrin. The detection of HTCII can provide useful information on the immediate availability of dietary Cbl [63]. The blood concentration of HTCII, like those of total Cbl, respond quickly to increased intake and thus can be misleading regardless of cellular restoration while using supplements [75]. HTCII is a more effective diagnostic marker compared to total Cbl but may be affected by the use of contraceptives as well as kidney or liver disease [89,90]. The sufficiency cutoff for HTCII is more homogeneously defined in literature as a plasma concentration above 35 pmol/L [18,82,84,91]. A Cbl deficiency at the cellular level is manifested through an accumulation of the intermediate products of the metabolic pathways, in which it participates as a coenzyme. The increased plasma concentration of HCY and urinary or serum MMA can provide more detailed information on the deficiency condition. As for serum Cbl, the criteria for an excess of HCY are heterogeneous: >15 µmol/L [78,80,81,83,85,92], >12 µmol/L [18,76,77,84,86,91,93,94], >10 µmol/L [8]. In addition, there are different criteria of deficiency for serum MMA cutoffs ranging from >271 nmol/L to >376 nmol/L, with the former being most prevalent [18,81,82,84,85,93–95]. Both blood markers, MMA and HCY, may be altered by renal failure and it is therefore useful to test glomerular function with creatinine [96]. The use of urinary MMA standardized for creatinine, although used less, may reduce the risk of an incorrect diagnosis [97]. Normally, the cutoff used for the assessment of Cbl deficiency by urinary MMA is >4 µg per mg of creatinine [98,99]. The increase of MMA can also be caused by intestinal bacterial overgrowth through the conversion of propionic acid produced by the human intestinal microbiota [100]. Given the high intake of vegetables in a vegetarian diet, it is unlikely that a rise of HCY is dependent on folate deficiency. It is likely that in fortification areas, where flour is enriched with folic acid, the main reason for the rise in plasma HCY is Cbl depletion [79]. The EFSA defined Cbl deficiency with serum Cbl below 140 pmol/L, serum MMA above 750 nmol/L, plasma HCY above 15 µmol/L and serum HTCII below 21–45 pmol/L [24]. In the Third National Health and Nutrition Examination Survey (NHANES III), the cutoffs for the diagnosis of hyperhomocysteinemia were defined as HCY above 11.4 µmol/L and 10.4 µmol for men and women, respectively [101]. The different values of diagnostic markers discussed are summarized in Tables 1–3.

Table 1. Vitamin B12 deficiency criteria.

Value	Country	References
<110 pmol/L	Austria	[76,77]
<127 pmol/L	Italy	[78]
<148 pmol/L	USA	[79]
<148 pmol/L	India	[80]
<150 pmol/L	India	[81]
<150 pmol/L	USA	[82]
<150 pmol/L	Turkey	[83]
<156 pmol/L	Germany/The Netherlands	[84]
<156 pmol/L	Germany	[85]
<220 pmol/L	Slovakia	[86]
<250 pmol/L	Germany	[8]

Table 2. Hyperhomocysteinemia criteria.

Value	Country	References
>15 μmol/L	Italy	[78]
>15 μmol/L	India	[80,81]
>15 μmol/L	Turkey	[83]
>15 μmol/L	Germany	[85]
>15 μmol/L	Taiwan	[92]
>12 μmol/L	Germany/The Netherlands	[18,84,94]
>12 μmol/L	Austria	[76,77]
>12 μmol/L	Slovakia	[86]
>12 μmol/L	Germany	[91,93]
>10 μmol/L	Germany	[8]

Table 3. Methylmalonic acid values for vitamin B12 deficiency.

Value	Country	References
>260 nmol/L	India	[81]
>271 nmol/L	Germany/The Netherlands	[18,84,94]
>271 nmol/L	Germany	[85,93]
>271 nmol/L	Germany/Oman	[95]
>376 nmol/L	USA	[82]

Some hematological markers can help to identify a shortage of vitamins, discriminating against red cell disorders as iron deficiency anemia, heterozygous thalassemia or other chronic diseases. The MCV and red cell distribution width (RDW) may increase in case of reduced availability of Cbl because of underlying hematopoietic alterations [102,103].

Herbert defined various stages of deficiency with the use of multiple markers as summarized in Table 4 [72]:

Table 4. Herbert's stratification for vitamin B12 deficiency [72].

Stage	Markers	Interpretation
I	HTCII	Blood and cellular reserves reduced with low HTCII
II	HC	Low concentrations of HC
III	HCY/MMA	Functional unbalanced with high concentrations of HCY and MMA
IV	MCV/Hb [1]	Clinical signs like high MCV, low Hb and macroovalocytosis

[1] Hb: Hemoglobin.

Unfortunately, some of the markers listed are not part of routine laboratory investigations and it is often difficult to locate diagnostic facilities that can perform all these tests.

Deficiency states could be boosted by impaired absorption. The Schilling test is a method, now rarely used, that was developed in 1953 (thanks to the availability of labeled Cbl) and applied in the diagnosis of food Cbl malabsorption [104]. This method quantifies the fraction of orally ingested labeled Cbl excreted in urine. Even if the Schilling test was considered the gold standard in the diagnosis of a Cbl deficiency, the use of radioactive material and misleading results in patients with antibodies against IF make it less suitable for clinical practice [105].

6. Status among Vegetarians

In Western countries, the intake of Cbl in the general population appears to be above the estimated requirements [19,21,24]. Its need during pregnancy and lactation increase due to the expansion of tissues and delivery to the fetus or the newborn. Thus the recommended dietary allowance has been determined at 2.6 μg/day and 2.8 μg/day for pregnancy and lactation, respectively [19,20].

The EFSA, however, settled on a safer amount of AI at 4.5 μg/day and 5 μg/day for pregnant and breastfeeding women, respectively [24]. A Cbl deficiency may occur by absorption alteration or nutritional insufficiency. Deficiencies are common in the elderly as a result of secondary hypochlorhydria due to drug treatment or a physiological alteration of the gastrointestinal mucosa itself [106]. The malabsorption can take place in cases of gastric or ileal resections, inflammatory bowel disease or for genetic defects in transport and cellular trafficking proteins [47,51,107]. The shortage of Cbl for low or no intake from food has been documented in low-income populations with poor nutritional status or in the case of vegetarians, with the first reports among vegetarian Indian people and Seventh-Day Adventist Church members [108,109]. Recent studies reported low serum cobalamin among vegetarians [103]. A deficiency in 11%–90% of elderly, 62% of pregnant women, 25%–86% of children, and 21%–41% of adolescents has been documented [110]. In a systematic review of literature based on the blood concentration of Cbl among vegetarians, a deficiency was present ranging from 0% to 86.5% among adults and elderly, up to 45% in infants, from 0% to 33.3% in children and adolescents, and from 17% to 39% among pregnant women [111]. The use of supplements or fortified foods seems to prevent deficiencies, indicating that a well-planned plant-based diet has proven to be adequate and sustainable [112,113]. However, despite the use of fortified foods, deficiency over a period of five years could occur, demonstrating a continuing insufficient intake or a possible decline in the absorptive capacity due to aging [114]. In all likelihood, even when supplementation occurs, it is possible that concentrations sufficient to avoid the reduction of body stock in the liver, blood and kidney cannot be reached. The liver is the main reservoir with a capacity of around 1–1.5 mg of Cbl [114].

Supplementation is often avoided due to preconceptions and aversion to products which are thought to be artificial, or due to the myth that the shortage will manifest itself only in rare cases after many years of ceased intake, an idea also supported by some researchers [115]. Although the shortage is documented in the macrobiotic community, many feel reluctant to use supplements, fortified foods, and more generally, processed foodstuffs [116].

The concomitant use of more specific markers enables a more detailed diagnosis. In adult German vegetarians, Cbl deficiency was present in 58%–66% or 61%–72% of participants if both criteria HTCII/MMA or HTCII alone were adopted, respectively [84,91,93,95]. Cbl deficiency leads to the accumulation of HCY, a molecule linked independently to the risk of cardiovascular disease (CVD), endothelial dysfunction and diabetes [117,118]. For each increment of 5 μmol/L of plasma HCY, there was a 20% increase in the risk of coronary heart disease (CHD) [119]. Concentrations of HCY among vegetarians seem to be higher and this correlates negatively with cardiovascular risk [54,76,103]. In a qualitative and quantitative review of the literature, it emerged that hyperhomocysteinemia with or without Cbl hipovitaminosis is a compelling risk factor for dementia [120]. In a meta-analysis on the status of vegetarians compared with omnivores by plasma HCY, six cohort case studies and 11 cross-sectional studies with a total of 3230 participants were analyzed, and an inverse relationship between HCY and Cbl for all diets was detected. Gradual worsening of both markers was evident from omnivores to VN with intermediate values in LV/LOV [54]. The HCY mechanisms of action are still unclear, but several theories have been proposed, including the initiation of the atherogenic process of reactive oxygen species (ROS) formation, inhibition of nitric oxide (NO) synthesis and influences on aortic calcification [121–123]. A recent meta-analysis of genome-wide association studies examined 18 single-nucleotide polymorphisms associated with total HCY concentrations [124]. A Mendelian randomization strategy was used to find no association between total HCY and the risk of coronary artery disease in genetic variants. These data may mitigate a causal correlation between HCY and CVD, but total blood HCY could be a useful marker for Cbl deficiency. When HCY, HTCII or MMA were used alone as diagnostic markers, the prevalence of deficiencies was greater in VN than in LOV/LV [18,76,77,85,91]. Although in the past it was thought that only the VN were at risk of vitamin deficiencies, recent studies indicate that even the LOV are at risk [125–127]. Herrmann et al. found that deficiency rates among LOV/LV and VN were 32% and 43%, respectively [85]. Supplementation in LOV/LV was effective in reducing deficiency rates from 68% to 31%, but the amounts were still insufficient [18]. Also the increase of MCV and RDW, associated with the lack of Cbl, leads to the increased cardiovascular risk [128,129]. Neurological manifestations of vitamin deficiency can also occur in the absence of anemia [130]. If the repletion comes late, the myelin degeneration caused by deficiency can also be irreversible [131]. In a review of 89 case studies of Cbl deficiency, 13 of which were vegetarianism related, neurological manifestations included progressive spastic paraparesis, acute onset of irrelevant speech and inability to comprehend, involuntary movements of the upper extremities, unsteady gait, acute onset of dizziness, ataxia, vomiting, mildly impaired cognitive functions, disorientation in time and short-term memory loss [132]. Psychiatric abnormalities and dermatological and oral manifestations were also found [132]. In the absence of Cbl sources, the decline of Cbl in blood is already evident during the first five years after the adoption of a vegetarian diet even without taking into account more specific markers, dispelling the myth that the shortage appears only after a very long time [101]. The first signs of a deficiency can occur as early as two years after Cbl intake has ceased [95,97]. The risks related to shortage are also frequent in children born to vegetarian mothers with inadequate reserves [133]. A depleted status among vegetarian women may be responsible for Cbl deficiency in infants, as well as a failure to thrive, low acceptability of solid foods and delays in neurodevelopment [74]. Moreover, there are indications that an inadequate Cbl status during pregnancy will affect fetal programming mechanisms, resulting in an increase of adiposity and insulin resistance in the offspring at six years, as well as for the mother herself [134,135]. The role of one-carbon metabolism of non-communicable diseases in fetal growth has been discussed [136]. The influence of Cbl deficiency during pregnancy and breastfeeding is so considerable that even a dietary restriction in the short term can result in an inadequate state in the infant [137]. In a pooled analysis of 48 cases of infant deficiency, there was a remarkable similarity in clinical symptoms between maternal veganism and maternal pernicious anemia [74].

7. Supplementation and Fortification

Supplements have been demonstrated as efficient in the restoration of Cbl blood concentration [97,138]. Currently, the official position of associations and government agencies is categorical and unequivocal: in the case of a vegetarian diet, including LOV, LV and OV, supplementation of Cbl is required [11,13]. Cbl concentration per 100 g of cow's milk, dairy products and chicken eggs ranged from 0.5 to 0.4 μg, from 4.2 to 3.6 μg, and from 2.5 to 1.1 μg, respectively [139,140]. Taking into account the losses during cooking and the specific absorption rate, these quantities are not sufficient to ensure the daily intake in a balanced diet [141]. The microorganisms generally used for large-scale productions of cobalamin are *Propionibacterium freudenreichii*, *P. shermanii* and *Pseudomonas dentrificans* [142]. The World Health Organization (WHO) and the Food and Agriculture Organization (FAO) Expert Consultation have jointly released a guide for nutrient calculation procedures for the necessary quantities when fortifying foods [143]. In some countries, certain foods are fortified, such as breakfast cereals, with Cbl. However, the quantities used are quite variable and the consumption of such foods cannot guarantee sufficiency in the absence of other sources [25,139]. Some researchers show that the daily intake levels used are insufficient to ensure proper Cbl intake in population subgroups at risk, and they recommended a mandatory program of fortification of flour with folic acid, as is currently the norm in Canada and the USA [144,145]. Although folic acid in the blood seems high among vegetarians, it can bring about a subcellular deficiency as a result of the "folate trap" mechanism, in which the absence of Cbl blocks folate in the form of 5-methyltetrahydrofolate. This occurrence results in the blockage of the methyl group transfer to the substrate. The folate trap can mask a possible silent functional deficiency of folic acid, even with high folate serum concentration [146]. The vegetarian diet, rich in folacin, may mask hematological symptoms, so Cbl deficiency may only be evident due to neurological signs in the late stages, such as neuropsychiatric abnormalities, neuropathy, dementia and, albeit rarely, atrophy of optic nerves [85,130]. Usually hematologic manifestations and anemia precede neurologic signs, which are more severe and mostly irreversible [147,148]. The response to treatment is inversely proportional to the severity of the deficiency state and to the latency of intervention [130]. Cbl used in fortified foodstuffs and in supplements is in crystalline form. There are different products containing Me-Cbl, Ado-Cbl and H-Cbl, either as a supplement or as pharmaceutical compositions.

Cn-Cbl is the most used form due to its high stability, cost effectiveness and safety of use [45]. At present, a tolerable upper intake level (TUIL) for Cbl from food or supplements was not defined, as the published data are insufficient in determining toxicity events. An accumulation and an excess of absorption are highly unlikely, in fact Cbl is a water-soluble molecule that requires a specific transport system which is easily saturated [19,149]. Its safety has been demonstrated through the use of an ultra-high parenteral dose of 25 mg daily for 10 days followed by 25 mg monthly for five months [150]. Cn-Cbl is the most common form used in the literature and in supplement formulation. Furthermore, it is the only compatible form in fortification thanks to its decent stability when heated [30]. In rare cases of genetic defects in peroxisome activation enzymes, the use of provitamin forms may not be recommendable [45]. At high doses such as 1–2 mg, about 10 μg is absorbed through non-specific internalization, functioning also in malabsorption diseases [151]. The therapeutic administration of oral Cbl has proven to be as effective as intramuscular administration [152]. This is very useful, as intramuscular administration is far more expensive and rather painful for the patient, as well as not being free from complications [153]. Recently, it was debated whether the coenzymes Me-Cbl and Ado-Cbl can be more efficient; that is, as a ready-to-use form that does not require a prior conversion [154,155]. The use of these more expensive formulations is not necessarily justified. In the literature, evidence of efficacy and safety is scarce. Moreover, a more responsive and less stable H-Cbl isoform may not reach the target [45]. If all forms of Cbl follow the same path of reduction-oxidation in the cell, the potential superiority of the coenzyme forms will not exist [45]. Since the crystalline form of Cbl is not bound to food proteins, the bioavailability in supplements is equal, if not superior. The Institute of Medicine (IOM) considers that naturally occurring Cbl in food is absorbed by 50% in healthy adults [25].

The vegetarian diet is very high in fiber, which may reduce the ability to absorb some nutrients efficiently [156]. An excess of fiber in the diet could disrupt the re-absorption of the Cbl mechanism through enterohepatic circulation, although there is no evidence to confirm that this happens in humans [157]. While there is not a higher incidence of anemia among vegetarians than in omnivores, in some cases iron intake may be inadequate [158]. Due to the low bioavailability of inorganic iron, the Institute of Medicine decided that the iron requirement is 1.8 times higher in a vegetarian diet [19]. Lower concentrations of iron can act on the gastric mucosa which favors atrophic gastritis, reducing the absorption capacity of Cbl via the intrinsic factor [110,159]. Although bone fractures among vegetarians are not statistically more frequent than in omnivores, a plant-based diet can result in lower calcium intake, especially among the VN [160]. The internalization of the IF-Cbl complex takes place thanks to a mechanism that requires calcium to function properly. A lower intake of calcium in the diet can inhibit the Cbl endocytosis mechanism in the distal ileum [161]. It was proposed that the metformin pharmacological treatment can alter the Ca-dependent uptake absorption of Cbl [162]. There are some indications that there is a correlation between polyunsaturated fatty acids of the series 3 (n3PUFA), especially long-chain (LC), and blood concentrations of HCY [163,164]. From preliminary data, the increased intake of LC n3PUFAs reduced plasma HCY with statistical significance [165–167]. Frequently, the vegetarian diet provides a high intake of n6PUFA and reduced contributions from n3PUFA, especially LC n3PUFA [168]. In addition to the possible link with HCY, excess n6PUFA can directly increase cardiovascular risk through the generation of proinflammatory eicosanoids and platelet aggregation [169]. For the above reasons, vegetarians should not underestimate Cbl intake through the appropriate use of supplements, while maintaining a balanced diet according to individual needs.

Absorption of Cbl from supplements depends on the dose and frequency of the intake [170]. The absorption capacity depends on the saturable active transport and on the efficiency of the aspecific route. The consumption of oral doses of 1 μg, 10 μg, 50 μg, 500 μg, 1000 μg, are absorbed with an efficiency of 56%, 16%, 3%, 2%, 1.3%, respectively [151]. The presence of Cbl inside the human gut is not a sufficient amount in terms of a daily intake, since it cannot be absorbed through the specific transport that requires binding to the transporters. In addition, 98% of corrinoid compounds synthesized by the microbiota found in human feces appear to be inactive [171].

Using multivitamins can be inefficient and counterproductive for the supplementation of Cbl. The Cbl can be degraded in the presence of vitamin C and copper with the formation of inactive by-products. These compounds can inhibit the transport system interacting with transporter proteins [172,173]. Nutritional yeast fortified with Cbl is available in the USA, though its use may be less effective than supplements, in the case of deficiency [97].

8. Vegetable Sources of Vitamin B12 and Future Research

The quantification of the Cbl content in foodstuff can be performed by various analytical systems, some of which are not able to distinguish between active and pseudo-Cbl analog forms. The recent use of more accurate systems, such as gas chromatographic methods or IF-based chemiluminescence, clarified that often the content of Cbl in food may have been overestimated [26].

Vegetables like broccoli, asparagus and bean sprouts contain only traces of Cbl [174]. The presence of 0.1–1.2 μg/100 g in tea leaves is not enough to consider tea as an adequate source for daily intake [175]. The most commonly eaten mushrooms in Europe, such as porcini and *pleurotus*, do not contain relevant amounts of Cbl [31]. However, an Italian study has shown that selected types of oyster mushrooms grown in the southern areas of Italy show a wide range of concentrations of Cbl from 0.44 to 1.93 μg/100 g, as detected by ELISA immunoassay. The highest concentration was found in the species *Pleurotus nebrodalis*, typical of the mountain areas in central Sicily [176]. Less common mushrooms such as *Craterellus cornucopioides* or *Cantharellus cibarius* may contain 1.09–2.65 μg/100 g [177]. Shiitake mushrooms, popular among vegetarians, can contain up to 5.61 $\pm$ 3.9 μg of Cbl per 100 g of dry weight (mostly in active form), although with great variability [178]. Even in this case, although a portion of 50 g of dried shiitake could be adequate to achieve the daily requirement, it is unlikely that this will happen daily. Among the most widely used edible seaweeds, *Enteromorpha* sp. and *Porphyra* sp. (also known as nori) contain relevant amounts of Cbl ranging from 32.3 to 63.6 μg/100 g [179]. In vitro tests are promising, but there are not enough human clinical trials to consider the use of seaweed as favorable in vitamin provision [180,181]. In a clinical trial of six vegan children, the daily use of nori seaweed seemed to prevent Cbl deficiency, measured via serum Cbl [182]. In disagreement with these data, Dagnelie et al. found no positive effects in using nori seaweed and spirulina on Cbl-deficient children [183]. The Cbl content of other edible macroalgae is negligible and approximately zero [184]. In a pilot study, supplementation with Klamath microalgae (*Aphanizomenon flos-Aque*) improved Cbl status among 15 vegan subjects, assessed by serum Cbl and plasma HCY in a three-month open-label intervention [185]. Klamath contains about 32 μg/100 g of Cbl but Watanabe et al. extracted only a pseudovitamin analog from Klamath [186]. *Chlorella pyrenoidosa* is a microalgae frequently used as a supplement [187]. Corrinoid content in micro and macroalgae depends on an exogenous uptake due to the association with microorganisms responsible for the biosynthesis of Cbl [33]. In a pilot study of 17 LOV/VN, 9 g of *Chlorella* for 30–60 days were effective in mitigating Cbl deficiency, although these quantities are not compatible with a daily intake over the time period and the study was not independent [188]. Cbl in commercial preparations can be highly variable and still lack sufficient clinical trials on humans to verify the viability of use [189]. Several edible cyanobacteria, such as *Spirulina platensis* and *Nostoc* sp., contain significant amounts of corrinoids, many of which appear to be pseudovitamin [190]. Characterization with sensitive methods able to discriminate from different corrinoid compounds showed that the concentration of Cbl in spirulina was 127–244 μg per 100 g of dry weight, about 80% of which were non-vitamin compounds [191]. At present, cyanobacteria cannot be considered a reliable source of Cbl [190,192,193]. Some fermented vegetable foods, such as sauerkraut, natto and tempeh, can have significant amounts of Cbl. It is unlikely that their daily use in Western countries represents a stable source of Cbl. The presence of Cbl in these foods depends on environmental bacteria randomly present in the fermentative microorganism pool [194]. It is very difficult to standardize the content from one product to another as they are subject to wide variation. Tempeh, for example, during the fermentation of soy beans can develop Cbl in a range between 0.7 to 8 μg per 100 g [195]. Other fermented soy foodstuff has only trace amounts of Cbl [196,197]. In sauerkraut production, the addition of *Proprionibacteria* sp. to cabbage may boost Cbl concentration up to 7.2 μg/100 g [198]. The use of organic fertilizer can increase the content of Cbl in spinach leaves up to 0.14 μg/100 g. However, the quantity of spinach that needs to be ingested in order to satisfy the daily requirement would be prohibitive [199]. Treatment with cyanocobalamin during the sprouting of daikon or through hydroponic techniques in lettuce may increase retention of Cbl and delivery through plant foods [200,201]. Promising data has indicated production of soy yogurt with an enhanced production of Cbl up to 18 μg/L, as detected with the HPLC method [202]. Cbl content in vegetable foods are summarized in Table 5.

Table 5. Cobalamin content in vegetable foods.

Foods	μg/100 g	Assay	References
Tea leaves	0.1–1.2	Microbiological	[175]
Tea leaves	0.046–0.859	IF-Chemiluminescence	[175]
Mushrooms (*Porcini, Pleurotus*)	0.01–0.09	LC/ESI-MS/MS	[177]
Mushrooms (*C. cornucopioides, C. cibarius*)	1.09–2.65	LC/ESI-MS/MS	[177]
Mushrooms (*Pleurotus* spp. from Sicily)	0.44–1.93	ELISA	[176]
Mushrooms (Shiitake)	3.95–5.61	LC/ESI-MS/MS	[178]
Seaweed (Nori)	32.26–63.58	Microbiological	[179]
Seaweed (Nori)	25.07–69.20	IF-Chemiluminescence	[179]
Microalgae (Klamath)	31.06–34.27	IF-Chemiluminescence	[186]
Microalgae (*Chlorella*)	200.9–211.6	IF-Chemiluminescence	[189]
Cyanobacteria (Spirulina)	127.2–244.3	Microbiological	[191]
Cyanobacteria (Spirulina)	6.2–17.4	IF-Chemiluminescence	[191]
Cyanobacteria (*Nostoc*)	11	HPLC	[190]
Tempeh	0.7–8	Not specified	[195]
Tempeh	0.02–0.7	Microbiological	[196]
Sauerkraut	Up to 7.2	Microbiological	[198]

9. Conclusions

The choice of limiting or removing foods of animal origin from the diet is increasing in popularity due to ethical, environmental and health reasons, posing doubts over whether a number of these restrictions could be detrimental or useful [203]. The vegetarian diet can be sustainable at all stages of life and in all physiological conditions, including infancy, pregnancy, lactation, senescence and sports [13]. Compared to non-vegetarians, vegetarians have reduced body mass index (BMI), serum cholesterol, serum glucose and blood pressure with a lower mortality rate due to ischemic heart disease (IHD) [17,204]. However, underestimating the correct supplementation of cobalamin (Cbl) can nullify these benefits [103]. It is also necessary that the diet be balanced and nutritionally adequate to reduce the risks of other deficiencies which could indirectly affect the absorption of Cbl. Studies on the use of plant foods to increase the Cbl intake are promising, but still require more data. Some seaweed, mushrooms and fermented foods can be a useful source of Cbl, but the data are still insufficient and production is too heterogeneous. The standardization of Cbl-rich plant foods may be useful in preventing vitamin deficiency, overcoming the frequent ideological barriers on supplementation. The use of fortified toothpaste could be a promising alternative to the fortification of flour, resolving the possible reduction of vitamins during cooking [205]. Studies of efficacy in maintaining vitamin sufficiency with different Cbl forms are absent. More trials with vegetarian people using supplements or fortified foods are needed to better explain the efficacy of different strategies of cobalamin uptake, focusing on the best dosages, media or foods, if reliable. Future research on the half-life of Cbl in various human body districts after the intake of different vitamin B12 supplements (H-Cbl, Ado-Cbl, Me-Cbl, Cn-Cbl) would be very useful in helping us understand Cbl utilization and needs, especially in vegetarians. At present, there is no international consensus for supplementation in vegetarians. According to Carmel, a single oral dose of 50 μg, 500 μg or 1000 μg will be absorbed at an amount of 1.5 μg, 9.7 μg or 13 μg, respectively [151]. To meet the daily requirement of Cbl, one oral dose of 50–100 μg daily or 2000 μg weekly divided into two oral cyanocobalamin doses could be sufficient to meet the needs of 2.4 μg/day for healthy vegetarian adults, taking into account the efficiency of absorption and the passive route. In 1988, Herbert stated that vegetarians' Cbl requirements could be satisfied by 1 μg tablet of vitamin B12 per day, based on human reabsorption through enterohepatic circulation [32]. This quantity is fairly low in respect to the proposed values for Cbl Dietary Reference Intake (DRI) in the general population [19,20]. Cyanocobalamin is the most economical—and historically the most used form—rendering it suitable for safe daily use [45]. There were no apparent substantial differences between the absorption of sublingual and oral forms [152,206]. However, oral dissolution could be critical in the secretion of the salivary R-binder and its subsequent bond. Since the Cbl would not be dissolved, about 88% could be not absorbed [54]. Since the development of a Cbl deficiency can also be observed among the LOV, the use of a supplement is necessary, regardless of the type of vegetarian diet [110]. In cases of malabsorption, such as hypochlorhydria or functional deficit, such amounts might be insufficient [151,207]. With senescence, the lowering of gastric secretion reduces the direct absorption capacities due to reduced release of IF and the impairment of active transport, but not of the passive transport. At the same time, the natural gastric barrier decreases with consequent risk of gastrointestinal bacterial overgrowth and competing for the use of ingested Cbl [69]. If rare genetic defects of cellular trafficking and processing proteins exist, the choice of alternative forms of Cbl, such as Me-Cbl or H-Cbl could improve the effectiveness of supplementation [154,208–210]. It was speculated that the use of Cn-Cbl is unsuitable for supplementation among smokers, because it represents a form preferentially excreted for the purpose of hydrocyanic acid removal [211,212]. In these cases, the use of H-Cbl may be desirable, although it is yet to be confirmed [213,214]. The data currently available do not permit an estimate of a maximum intake level for cobalamin. High levels of administration in particular lead to rare adverse events, mostly dermatological, such as pruritus, rash and skin eruptions [215]. The sufficiency of bodily stocks should not be a reason to delay supplementation, in light of the fact that the manifestation of the deficiency can occur through often irreversible neurological signs. The current data do not support the theory that vitamin deficiency needs 20–30 years to be manifested [125]. Nevertheless, future studies should take into account the possibility of supplementation even in a subclinical condition, as was already done for other deficiencies [216,217], which may become overt during the time-period [218,219]. The use of multiple diagnostic markers can facilitate the correct assessment of the status and allow a more sound decision in relation to the administration plan. The habit of using only one or a few of the multiple markers available implies that the deficiency status of Cbl among vegetarians, as among omnivores, may have sometimes been underestimated. Moreover, cobalamin displays other functions, not strictly metabolic, that could be lacking when deficient. A vitamin B12 deficiency could be related to oxidative stress markers like plasma glutathione, malondialdehyde and serum total antioxidant capacity, which could contribute to a neurophysiological disturbance [220]. Furthermore, Cbl, particularly H-Cbl, can act as a detoxifying agent, removing potentially dangerous cyanide molecules from the body [212].

Author Contributions: Vincenzo Muscia, Giuseppe Sarpietro and Micol Zigarelli collected data from the available literature; Gioacchina Maria Grazia La Ferrera, Gaetano Valenti and Fabrizio Sapia analyzed and interpreted the data retrieved from literature search; Gianluca Rizzo, Angela Nigro and Paola Rossetti wrote the draft of the manuscript; Salvatore Giovanni Vitale and Agnese Maria Chiara Rapisarda revised the draft of the manuscript; Antonio Simone Laganà and Massimo Buscema supervised the review development.

References

1. EURISPES 2016. Available online: http://eurispes.eu/content/rapporto-italia-2016-la-sindrome-del-palio (accessed on 28 July 2016).
2. Larsson, C.L.; Johansson, G.K. Dietary intake and nutritional status of young vegans and omnivores in Sweden. *Am. J. Clin. Nutr.* **2002**, *76*, 100–106. [PubMed]

3. World Health Organization. *Global Status Report on Non Communicable Diseases 2014*; WHO: Geneva, Switzerland, 2014.
4. Ferdowsian, H.R.; Barnard, N.D. Effects of plant-based diets on plasma lipids. *Am. J. Cardiol.* **2009**, *104*, 947–956. [CrossRef] [PubMed]
5. Pettersen, B.J.; Anousheh, R.; Fan, J.; Jaceldo-Siegl, K.; Fraser, G.E. Vegetarian diets and blood pressure among white subjects: Results from the Adventist Health Study-2 (AHS-2). *Public Health Nutr.* **2012**, *15*, 1909–1916. [CrossRef] [PubMed]
6. Barnard, N.D.; Katcher, H.I.; Jenkins, D.J.; Cohen, J.; Turner-McGrievy, G. Vegetarian and vegan diets in type 2 diabetes management. *Nutr. Rev.* **2009**, *67*, 255–263. [CrossRef] [PubMed]
7. Tonstad, S.; Butler, T.; Yan, R.; Fraser, G.E. Type of vegetarian diet, body weight, and prevalence of type 2 diabetes. *Diabetes Care* **2009**, *32*, 791–796. [CrossRef] [PubMed]
8. Waldmann, A.; Koschizke, J.W.; Leitzmann, C.; Hahn, A. German vegan study: Diet, life-style factors, and cardiovascular risk profile. *Ann. Nutr. Metab.* **2005**, *49*, 366–372. [CrossRef] [PubMed]
9. Key, T.J.; Appleby, P.N.; Davey, G.K.; Allen, N.E.; Spencer, E.A.; Travis, R.C. Mortality in British vegetarians: Review and preliminary results from EPIC-Oxford. *Am. J. Clin. Nutr.* **2003**, *78*, S533–S538.
10. Key, T.J.; Fraser, G.E.; Thorogood, M.; Appleby, P.N.; Bera, V.; Reeves, G.; Burr, M.L.; Chang-Claude, J.; Frentzel-Beyme, R.; Kuzma, J.W.; et al. Mortality in vegetarians and nonvegetarians: Detailed findings from a collaborative analysis of 5 prospective studies. *Am. J. Clin. Nutr.* **1999**, *70*, S516–S524.
11. U.S. Department of Agriculture; U.S. Department of Health and Human Services. *Dietary Guidelines for Americans 2010*, 7th ed.; U.S. Government Printing Office: Washington, DC, USA, 2010.
12. American Dietetic Association. Position of the American Dietetic Association: Vegetarian diets. *J. Am. Diet. Assoc.* **1988**, *88*, 351.
13. Craig, W.J.; Mangels, A.R.; American Dietetic Association. Position of the American Dietetic Association: Vegetarian diets. *J. Am. Diet. Assoc.* **2009**, *109*, 1266–1282. [PubMed]
14. Allen, L.H. Causes of vitamin B12 and folate deficiency. *Food Nutr. Bull.* **2008**, *29*, S20–S37. [CrossRef] [PubMed]
15. O'Leary, F.; Samman, S. Vitamin B12 in health and disease. *Nutrients* **2010**, *2*, 299–316. [CrossRef] [PubMed]
16. Stollhoff, K.; Schulte, F.J. Vitamin B12 and brain development. *Eur. J. Pediatr.* **1987**, *146*, 201–205. [CrossRef] [PubMed]
17. Li, D. Chemistry behind Vegetarianism. *J. Agric. Food Chem.* **2011**, *59*, 777–784. [CrossRef] [PubMed]
18. Herrmann, W.; Schorr, H.; Obeid, R.; Geisel, J. Vitamin B-12 status, particularly holotranscobalamin II and methylmalonic acid concentrations, and hyperhomocysteinemia in vegetarians. *Am. J. Clin. Nutr.* **2003**, *78*, 131–136. [PubMed]
19. Otten, J.J.; Hellwig, J.P.; Meyers, L.D. *Dietary Reference Intakes: The Essential Guide to Nutrient Requirements*; Institute of Medicine of the National Academies: Washington, DC, USA, 2006.
20. Società Italiana di Nutrizione Umana. *LARN: Livelli di Assunzione di Riferimento di Nutrienti ed Energia per la Popolazione Italiana*; Società Italiana di Nutrizione Umana: Milano, Italy, 2014.
21. U.S. Department of Agriculture; Agricultural Research Service; Beltsville Human Nutrition Research Center; Food Surveys Research Group; U.S. Department of Health and Human Services; Centers for Disease Control and Prevention; National Center for Health Statistics. What We Eat in America, NHANES 2009–2010. Nutrient Intakes from Food: Mean Amounts Consumed per Individual, by Gender and Age, in United States, 2009–2010. Available online: https://www.ars.usda.gov/SP2UserFiles/Place/80400530/pdf/0910/tables_1-40_2009-2010.pdf (accessed on 28 July 2016).
22. Obeid, R.; Schorr, H.; Eckert, R.; Herrmann, W. Vitamin B12 status in the elderly as judged by available biochemical markers. *Clin. Chem.* **2004**, *50*, 238–241. [CrossRef] [PubMed]
23. Yetley, E.A.; Pfeiffer, C.M.; Phinney, K.W.; Bailey, R.L.; Blackmore, S.; Bock, J.L.; Brody, L.C.; Carmel, R.; Curtin, L.R.; Durazo-Arvizu, R.A.; et al. Biomarkers of vitamin B-12 status in NHANES: A roundtable summary. *Am. J. Clin. Nutr.* **2011**, *94*, S313–S321. [CrossRef] [PubMed]
24. Panel on Dietetic Products, Nutrition, and Allergies. Scientific opinion on dietary reference values for cobalamin (Vitamin B12). *EFSA J.* **2015**, *13*, 4150.
25. Institute of Medicine. *A Report of the Standing Committee on the Scientific Evaluation of Dietary Reference Intakes and Its Panel on Folate, Other B Vitamins, and Choline and Subcommittee on Upper Reference Levels of Nutrients, Food and Nutrition Board*; National Academy: Washington, DC, USA, 1998.

26. Watanabe, F. Vitamin B12 sources and bioavailability. *Exp. Biol. Med.* **2007**, *232*, 1266–1274. [CrossRef] [PubMed]
27. Bor, M.V.; Lydeking-Olsen, E.; Møller, J.; Nexø, E. A daily intake of approximately 6 microg vitamin B-12 appears to saturate all the vitamin B-12-related variables in Danish postmenopausal women. *Am. J. Clin. Nutr.* **2006**, *83*, 52–58. [PubMed]
28. Andrès, E.; Kurtz, J.E.; Perrin, A.E.; Maloisel, F.; Demangeat, C.; Goichot, B.; Schlienger, J.L. Oral cobalamin therapy for the treatment of patients with food-cobalamin malabsorption. *Am. J. Med.* **2001**, *111*, 126–129. [CrossRef]
29. Peters, R.; Burch, L.; Warner, J.; Beckett, N.; Poulter, R.; Bulpitt, C. Haemoglobin, anaemia, dementia and cognitive decline in the elderly, a systematic review. *BMC Geriatr.* **2008**, *8*, 18. [CrossRef] [PubMed]
30. Watanabe, F.; Yabuta, Y.; Tanioka, Y.; Bito, T. Biologically active vitamin B12 compounds in foods for preventing deficiency among vegetarians and elderly subjects. *J. Agric. Food Chem.* **2013**, *61*, 6769–6775. [CrossRef] [PubMed]
31. Watanabe, F.; Yabuta, Y.; Bito, T.; Teng, F. Vitamin B_{12}-containing plant food sources for vegetarians. *Nutrients* **2014**, *6*, 1861–1873. [CrossRef] [PubMed]
32. Herbert, V. Vitamin B-12: Plant sources, requirements, and assay. *Am. J. Clin. Nutr.* **1988**, *48*, 852–858. [PubMed]
33. Watanabe, F.; Abe, K.; Takenaka, S.; Tamura, Y.; Maruyama, I.; Nakano, Y. Occurrence of cobalamin coenzymes in the photosynthetic green alga, *Chlorella vulgaris*. *Biosci. Biotechnol. Biochem.* **1997**, *61*, 896–897. [CrossRef]
34. Smith, E.L. Purification of anti-pernicious anaemia factors from liver. *Nature* **1948**, *161*, 638. [CrossRef] [PubMed]
35. Randaccio, L.; Geremia, S.; Demitri, N.; Wuerges, J. Vitamin B12: Unique metalorganic compounds and the most complex vitamins. *Molecules* **2010**, *15*, 3228–3259. [CrossRef] [PubMed]
36. Quadros, E.V. Advances in the understanding of cobalamin assimilation and metabolism. *Br. J. Haematol.* **2010**, *148*, 195–204. [CrossRef] [PubMed]
37. Gherasim, C.; Lofgren, M.; Banerjee, R. Navigating the B(12) road: Assimilation, delivery, and disorders of cobalamin. *J. Biol. Chem.* **2013**, *288*, 13186–13193. [CrossRef] [PubMed]
38. Cooper, B.A.; Rosenblatt, D.S. Inherited defects of vitamin B12 metabolism. *Annu. Rev. Nutr.* **1987**, *7*, 291–320. [CrossRef] [PubMed]
39. Fenton, W.A.; Hack, A.M.; Willard, H.F.; Gertler, A.; Rosenberg, L.E. Purification and properties of methylmalonyl coenzyme A mutase from human liver. *Arch. Biochem. Biophys.* **1982**, *214*, 815–823. [CrossRef]
40. Marsh, E.N.; Meléndez, G.D. Adenosylcobalamin enzymes: Theory and experiment begin to converge. *Biochim. Biophys. Acta* **2012**, *1824*, 1154–1164. [CrossRef] [PubMed]
41. Scalabrino, G.; Carpo, M.; Bamonti, F.; Pizzinelli, S.; D'Avino, C.; Bresolin, N.; Meucci, G.; Martinelli, V.; Comi, G.C.; Peracchi, M. High tumor necrosis factor-α in levels in cerebrospinal fluid of cobalamin-deficient patients. *Ann. Neurol.* **2004**, *56*, 886–890. [CrossRef] [PubMed]
42. Lipton, S.A.; Kim, W.K.; Choi, Y.B.; Kumar, S.; D'Emilia, D.M.; Rayudu, P.V.; Arnelle, D.R.; Stamler, J.S. Neurotoxicity associated with dual actions of homocysteine at the *N*-methyl-D-aspartate receptor. *Proc. Natl. Acad. Sci. USA* **1997**, *94*, 5923–5928. [CrossRef] [PubMed]
43. Hodgkin, D.C.; Kamper, J.; Mackay, M.; Pickworth, J.; Trueblood, K.N.; White, J.G. Structure of vitamin B12. *Nature* **1956**, *178*, 64–66. [CrossRef] [PubMed]
44. Chaouali, N.; Gana, I.; Dorra, A.; Khelifi, F.; Nouioui, A.; Masri, W.; Belwaer, I.; Ghorbel, H.; Hedhili, A. Potential Toxic Levels of Cyanide in Almonds (*Prunus amygdalus*), Apricot Kernels (*Prunus armeniaca*), and Almond Syrup. *ISRN Toxicol.* **2013**, *2013*, 610648. [CrossRef] [PubMed]
45. Obeid, R.; Fedosov, S.N.; Nexo, E. Cobalamin coenzyme forms are not likely to be superior to cyano- and hydroxyl-cobalamin in prevention or treatment of cobalamin deficiency. *Mol. Nutr. Food Res.* **2015**, *59*, 1364–1372. [CrossRef] [PubMed]
46. Banerjee, R. B12 trafficking in mammals: A for coenzyme escort service. *ACS Chem. Biol.* **2006**, *1*, 149–159. [CrossRef] [PubMed]
47. Hannibal, L.; Kim, J.; Brasch, N.E.; Wang, S.; Rosenblatt, D.S.; Banerjee, R.; Jacobsen, D.W. Processing of alkylcobalamins in mammalian cells: A role for the MMACHC (cblC) gene product. *Mol. Genet. Metab.* **2009**, *97*, 260–266. [CrossRef] [PubMed]

48. Gimsing, P.; Hippe, E.; Helleberg-Rasmussen, I.; Moesgaard, M.; Nielsen, J.L.; Bastrup-Madsen, P.; Berlin, R.; Hansen, T. Cobalamin forms in plasma and tissue during treatment of vitamin B12 deficiency. *Scand. J. Haematol.* **1982**, *29*, 311–318. [CrossRef] [PubMed]
49. Herbert, V.; Sullivan, L.W. Activity of Coenzyme B12 in Man. *Ann. N. Y. Acad. Sci.* **1964**, *112*, 855–870. [CrossRef] [PubMed]
50. Adams, J.F.; Ross, S.K.; Mervyn, L.; Boddy, K.; King, P. Absorption of cyanocobalamin, coenzyme B 12, methylcobalamin, and hydroxocobalamin at different dose levels. *Scand. J. Gastroenterol.* **1971**, *6*, 249–252. [CrossRef] [PubMed]
51. Gailus, S.; Höhne, W.; Gasnier, B.; Nürnberg, P.; Fowler, B.; Rutsch, F. Insights into lysosomal cobalamin trafficking: Lessons learned from cblF disease. *J. Mol. Med.* **2010**, *88*, 459–466. [CrossRef] [PubMed]
52. Wuerges, J.; Geremia, S.; Randaccio, L. Structural study on ligand specificity of human vitamin B12 transporters. *Biochem. J.* **2007**, *403*, 431–440. [CrossRef] [PubMed]
53. Gruber, K.; Puffer, B.; Kräutler, B. Vitamin B12-derivatives-enzyme cofactors and ligands of proteins and nucleic acids. *Chem. Soc. Rev.* **2011**, *40*, 4346–4363. [CrossRef] [PubMed]
54. Obersby, D.; Chappell, D.C.; Dunnett, A.; Tsiami, A.A. Plasma total homocysteine status of vegetarians compared with omnivores: A systematic review and meta-analysis. *Br. J. Nutr.* **2013**, *109*, 785–794. [CrossRef] [PubMed]
55. Mathews, F.S.; Gordon, M.M.; Chen, Z.; Rajashankar, K.R.; Ealick, S.E.; Alpers, D.H.; Sukumar, N. Crystal structure of human intrinsic factor: Cobalamin complex at 2.6-A resolution. *Proc. Natl. Acad. Sci. USA* **2007**, *104*, 17311–17316. [CrossRef] [PubMed]
56. Muir, M.; Chanarin, I. Separation of cobalamin analogues in human sera binding to intrinsic factor and to R-type vitamin B12 binders. *Br. J. Haematol.* **1983**, *54*, 613–621. [CrossRef] [PubMed]
57. Fyfe, J.C.; Madsen, M.; Højrup, P.; Christensen, E.I.; Tanner, S.M.; de la Chapelle, A.; He, Q.; Moestrup, S.K. The functional cobalamin (vitamin B12)-intrinsic factor receptor is a novel complex of cubilin and amnionless. *Blood* **2004**, *103*, 1573–1579. [CrossRef] [PubMed]
58. Beedholm-Ebsen, R.; van de Wetering, K.; Hardlei, T.; Nexø, E.; Borst, P.; Moestrup, S.K. Identification of multidrug resistance protein 1 (MRP1/ABCC1) as a molecular gate for cellular export of cobalamin. *Blood* **2010**, *115*, 1632–1639. [CrossRef] [PubMed]
59. Hippe, E.; Olesen, H. Nature of vitamin B 12 binding. 3. Thermodynamics of binding to human intrinsic factor and transcobalamins. *Biochim. Biophys. Acta* **1971**, *243*, 83–88. [CrossRef]
60. Quadros, E.V.; Rothenberg, S.P.; Jaffe, E.A. Endothelial cells from human umbilical vein secrete functional transcobalamin II. *Am. J. Physiol.* **1989**, *256*, C296–C303. [PubMed]
61. Herzlich, B.; Herbert, V. Depletion of serum holotranscobalamin II. An early sign of negative vitamin B12 balance. *Lab. Investig.* **1988**, *58*, 332–337. [PubMed]
62. Ashwell, G.; Morell, A. The dual role of sialic acid in the hepatic recognition and catabolism of serum glycoproteins. *Biochem. Soc. Symp.* **1974**, *40*, 117–124.
63. Moestrup, S.K.; Birn, H.; Fischer, P.B.; Petersen, C.M.; Verroust, P.J.; Sim, R.B.; Christensen, E.I.; Nexø, E. Megalin-mediated endocytosis of transcobalamin-vitamin-B12 complexes suggests a role of the receptor in vitamin-B12 homeostasis. *Proc. Natl. Acad. Sci. USA* **1996**, *93*, 8612–8617. [CrossRef] [PubMed]
64. Nielsen, M.J.; Rasmussen, M.R.; Andersen, C.B.; Nexø, E.; Moestrup, S.K. Vitamin B12 transport from food to the body's cells—A sophisticated, multistep pathway. *Nat. Rev. Gastroenterol. Hepatol.* **2012**, *9*, 345–354. [CrossRef] [PubMed]
65. Rutsch, F.; Gailus, S.; Miousse, I.R.; Suormala, T.; Sagné, C.; Toliat, M.R.; Nürnberg, G.; Wittkampf, T.; Buers, I.; Sharifi, A.; et al. Identification of a putative lysosomal cobalamin exporter altered in the cblF defect of vitamin B12 metabolism. *Nat. Genet.* **2009**, *41*, 234–239. [CrossRef] [PubMed]
66. Li, Z.; Gherasim, C.; Lesniak, N.A.; Banerjee, R. Glutathione-dependent one-electron transfer reactions catalyzed by a B12 trafficking protein. *J. Biol. Chem.* **2014**, *289*, 16487–16497. [CrossRef] [PubMed]
67. Koutmos, M.; Gherasim, C.; Smith, J.L.; Banerjee, R. Structural basis of multifunctionality in a vitamin B12-processing enzyme. *J. Biol. Chem.* **2011**, *286*, 29780–29787. [CrossRef] [PubMed]
68. Scott, J.M. Bioavailability of vitamin B12. *Eur. J. Clin. Nutr.* **1997**, *51*, S49–S53. [PubMed]
69. Baik, H.W.; Russell, R.M. Vitamin B12 deficiency in the elderly. *Annu. Rev. Nutr.* **1999**, *19*, 357–377. [CrossRef] [PubMed]

70. Berlin, H.; Berlin, R.; Brante, G. Oral treatment of pernicious anemia with high doses of vitamin B12 without intrinsic factor. *Acta Med. Scand.* **1968**, *184*, 247–258. [CrossRef] [PubMed]
71. Elia, M. Oral or parenteral therapy for B12 deficiency. *Lancet* **1998**, *352*, 1721–1722. [CrossRef]
72. Herbert, V. Staging vitamin B-12 (cobalamin) status in vegetarians. *Am. J. Clin. Nutr.* **1994**, *59*, S1213–S1222.
73. McPhee, A.J.; Davidson, G.P.; Leahy, M.; Beare, T. Vitamin B12 deficiency in a breast fed infant. *Arch. Dis. Child* **1988**, *63*, 921–923. [CrossRef] [PubMed]
74. Dror, D.K.; Allen, L.H. Effect of vitamin B12 deficiency on neurodevelopment in infants: Current knowledge and possible mechanisms. *Nutr. Rev.* **2008**, *66*, 250–255. [CrossRef] [PubMed]
75. Schneede, J.; Ueland, P.M. Novel and established markers of cobalamin deficiency: Complementary or exclusive diagnostic strategies. *Semin. Vasc. Med.* **2005**, *5*, 140–155. [CrossRef] [PubMed]
76. Elmadfa, I.; Singer, I. Vitamin B-12 and homocysteine status among vegetarians: A global perspective. *Am. J. Clin. Nutr.* **2009**, *89*, S1693–S1698. [CrossRef] [PubMed]
77. Majchrzak, D.; Singer, I.; Männer, M.; Rust, P.; Genser, D.; Wagner, K.H.; Elmadfa, I. B-vitamin status and concentrations of homocysteine in Austrian omnivores, vegetarians and vegans. *Ann. Nutr. Metab.* **2006**, *50*, 485–491. [CrossRef] [PubMed]
78. Bissoli, L.; Di Francesco, V.; Ballarin, A.; Mandragona, R.; Trespidi, R.; Brocco, G.; Caruso, B.; Bosello, O.; Zamboni, M. Effect of vegetarian diet on homocysteine levels. *Ann. Nutr. Metab.* **2002**, *46*, 73–79. [CrossRef] [PubMed]
79. Green, R.; Miller, J.W. Vitamin B12 deficiency is the dominant nutritional cause of hyperhomocysteinemia in a folic acid-fortified population. *Clin. Chem. Lab. Med.* **2005**, *43*, 1048–1051. [CrossRef] [PubMed]
80. Naik, S.; Bhide, V.; Babhulkar, A.; Mahalle, N.; Parab, S.; Thakre, R.; Kulkarni, M. Daily milk intake improves vitamin B-12 status in young vegetarian Indians: An intervention trial. *Nutr. J.* **2013**, *12*, 136. [CrossRef] [PubMed]
81. Refsum, H.; Yajnik, C.S.; Gadkari, M.; Schneede, J.; Vollset, S.E.; Orning, L.; Guttormsen, A.B.; Joglekar, A.; Sayyad, M.G.; Ulvik, A.; et al. Hyperhomocysteinemia and elevated methylmalonic acid indicate a high prevalence of cobalamin deficiency in Asian Indians. *Am. J. Clin. Nutr.* **2001**, *74*, 233–241. [PubMed]
82. Haddad, E.H.; Berk, L.S.; Kettering, J.D.; Hubbard, R.W.; Peters, W.R. Dietary intake and biochemical, hematologic, and immune status of vegans compared with nonvegetarians. *Am. J. Clin. Nutr.* **1999**, *70*, S586–S593.
83. Karabudak, E.; Kiziltan, G.; Cigerim, N. A comparison of some of the cardiovascular risk factors in vegetarian and omnivorous Turkish females. *J. Hum. Nutr. Diet.* **2008**, *21*, 13–22. [CrossRef] [PubMed]
84. Herrmann, W.; Obeid, R.; Schorr, H.; Geisel, J. Functional vitamin B12 deficiency and determination of holotranscobalamin in populations at risk. *Clin. Chem. Lab. Med.* **2003**, *41*, 1478–1488. [CrossRef] [PubMed]
85. Herrmann, W.; Schorr, H.; Purschwitz, K.; Rassoul, F.; Richter, V. Total homocysteine, vitamin B(12), and total antioxidant status in vegetarians. *Clin. Chem.* **2001**, *47*, 1094–1101. [PubMed]
86. Krivosíková, Z.; Krajcovicová-Kudlácková, M.; Spustová, V.; Stefíková, K.; Valachovicová, M.; Blazícek, P.; Němcová, T. The association between high plasma homocysteine levels and lower bone mineral density in Slovak women: The impact of vegetarian diet. *Eur. J. Nutr.* **2010**, *49*, 147–153. [CrossRef] [PubMed]
87. Herrmann, W.; Geisel, J. Vegetarian lifestyle and monitoring of vitamin B-12 status. *Clin. Chim. Acta* **2002**, *326*, 47–59. [CrossRef]
88. Lindenbaum, J.; Healton, E.B.; Savage, D.G.; Brust, J.C.; Garrett, T.J.; Podell, E.R.; Marcell, P.D.; Stabler, S.P.; Allen, R.H. Neuropsychiatric disorders caused by cobalamin deficiency in the absence of anemia or macrocytosis. *N. Engl. J. Med.* **1988**, *318*, 1720–1728. [CrossRef] [PubMed]
89. Riedel, B.; Bjørke Monsen, A.L.; Ueland, P.M.; Schneede, J. Effects of oral contraceptives and hormone replacement therapy on markers of cobalamin status. *Clin. Chem.* **2005**, *51*, 778–781. [CrossRef] [PubMed]
90. Carmel, R. Measuring and interpreting holo-transcobalamin (holo-transcobalamin II). *Clin. Chem.* **2002**, *48*, 407–409. [PubMed]
91. Herrmann, W.; Obeid, R.; Schorr, H.; Geisel, J. The usefulness of holotranscobalamin in predicting vitamin B12 status in different clinical settings. *Curr. Drug Metab.* **2005**, *6*, 47–53. [CrossRef] [PubMed]
92. Huang, Y.C.; Chang, S.J.; Chiu, Y.T.; Chang, H.H.; Cheng, C.H. The status of plasma homocysteine and related B-vitamins in healthy young vegetarians and nonvegetarians. *Eur. J. Nutr.* **2003**, *42*, 84–90. [CrossRef] [PubMed]
93. Geisel, J.; Schorr, H.; Bodis, M.; Isber, S.; Hübner, U.; Knapp, J.P.; Obeid, R.; Herrmann, W. The vegetarian

lifestyle and DNA methylation. *Clin. Chem. Lab. Med.* **2005**, *43*, 1164–1169. [CrossRef] [PubMed]

94. Obeid, R.; Geisel, J.; Schorr, H.; Hübner, U.; Herrmann, W. The impact of vegetarianism on some haematological parameters. *Eur. J. Haematol.* **2002**, *69*, 275–279. [CrossRef] [PubMed]
95. Herrmann, W.; Obeid, R.; Schorr, H.; Hübner, U.; Geisel, J.; Sand-Hill, M.; Ali, N.; Herrmann, M. Enhanced bone metabolism in vegetarians—The role of vitamin B12 deficiency. *Clin. Chem. Lab. Med.* **2009**, *47*, 1381–1387. [CrossRef] [PubMed]
96. Stabler, S.P.; Lindenbaum, J.; Allen, R.H. The use of homocysteine and other metabolites in the specific diagnosis of vitamin B-12 deficiency. *J. Nutr.* **1996**, *126*, S1266–S1272.
97. Donaldson, M.S. Metabolic vitamin B12 status on a mostly raw vegan diet with follow-up using tablets, nutritional yeast, or probiotic supplements. *Ann. Nutr. Metab.* **2000**, *44*, 229–234. [CrossRef] [PubMed]
98. Kwok, T.; Cheng, G.; Lai, W.K.; Poon, P.; Woo, J.; Pang, C.P. Use of fasting urinary methylmalonic acid to screen for metabolic vitamin B12 deficiency in older persons. *Nutrition* **2004**, *20*, 764–768. [CrossRef] [PubMed]
99. Miller, D.R.; Specker, B.L.; Ho, M.L.; Norman, E.J. Vitamin B-12 status in a macrobiotic community. *Am. J. Clin. Nutr.* **1991**, *53*, 524–529. [PubMed]
100. Lindenbaum, J.; Savage, D.G.; Stabler, S.P.; Allen, R.H. Diagnosis of cobalamin deficiency: II. Relative sensitivities of serum cobalamin, methylmalonic acid, and total homocysteine concentrations. *Am. J. Hematol.* **1990**, *34*, 99–107. [CrossRef] [PubMed]
101. Selhub, J.; Jacques, P.F.; Rosenberg, I.H.; Rogers, G.; Bowman, B.A.; Gunter, E.W.; Wright, J.D.; Johnson, C.L. Serum total homocysteine concentrations in the third National Health and Nutrition Examination Survey (1991–1994): Population reference ranges and contribution of vitamin status to high serum concentrations. *Ann. Intern. Med.* **1999**, *131*, 331–339. [CrossRef] [PubMed]
102. Bessman, J.D.; Gilmer, P.R., Jr.; Gardner, F.H. Improved classification of anemias by MCV and RDW. *Am. J. Clin. Pathol.* **1983**, *80*, 322–326. [CrossRef] [PubMed]
103. Pawlak, R. Is vitamin B12 deficiency a risk factor for cardiovascular disease in vegetarians? *Am. J. Prev. Med.* **2015**, *48*, e11–e26. [CrossRef] [PubMed]
104. Schilling, R.F. Intrinsic factor studies II. The effect of gastric juice on the urinary excretion of radioactivity after the oral administration of radioactive vitamin B12. *J. Lab. Clin. Med.* **1953**, *42*, 860–866. [CrossRef] [PubMed]
105. Chanarin, I. Historical review: A history of pernicious anaemia. *Br. J. Haematol.* **2000**, *111*, 407–415. [CrossRef] [PubMed]
106. Herrmann, W.; Obeid, R. Causes and early diagnosis of vitamin B12 deficiency. *Dtsch. Arztebl. Int.* **2008**, *105*, 680–685. [PubMed]
107. Headstrom, P.D.; Rulyak, S.J.; Lee, S.D. Prevalence of and risk factors for vitamin B(12) deficiency in patients with Crohn's disease. *Inflamm. Bowel Dis.* **2008**, *14*, 217–223. [CrossRef] [PubMed]
108. Banerjee, D.K.; Chatterjea, J.B. Serum vitamin B12 in vegetarians. *Br. Med. J.* **1960**, *2*, 992–994. [CrossRef] [PubMed]
109. Armstrong, B.K.; Davis, R.E.; Nicol, D.J.; van Merwyk, A.J.; Larwood, C.J. Hematological, vitamin B 12, and folate studies on Seventh-day Adventist vegetarians. *Am. J. Clin. Nutr.* **1974**, *27*, 712–718. [PubMed]
110. Pawlak, R.; Parrott, S.J.; Raj, S.; Cullum-Dugan, D.; Lucus, D. How prevalent is vitamin B(12) deficiency among vegetarians? *Nutr. Rev.* **2013**, *71*, 110–117. [CrossRef] [PubMed]
111. Pawlak, R.; Lester, S.E.; Babatunde, T. The prevalence of cobalamin deficiency among vegetarians assessed by serum vitamin B12: A review of literature. *Eur. J. Clin. Nutr.* **2014**, *68*, 541–548. [CrossRef] [PubMed]
112. Schüpbach, R.; Wegmüller, R.; Berguerand, C.; Bui, M.; Herter-Aeberli, I. Micronutrient status and intake in omnivores, vegetarians and vegans in Switzerland. *Eur. J. Nutr.* **2015**. [CrossRef] [PubMed]
113. Mądry, E.; Lisowska, A.; Grebowiec, P.; Walkowiak, J. The impact of vegan diet on B-12 status in healthy omnivores: Five-year prospective study. *Acta Sci. Pol. Technol. Aliment.* **2012**, *11*, 209–212. [PubMed]
114. Rappazzo, M.E.; Salmi, H.A.; Hall, C.A. The content of vitamin B12 in adult and foetal tissue: A comparative study. *Br. J. Haematol.* **1970**, *18*, 425–433. [CrossRef] [PubMed]
115. Rizzo, N.S.; Jaceldo-Siegl, K.; Sabate, J.; Fraser, G.E. Nutrient profiles of vegetarian and nonvegetarian dietary patterns. *J. Acad. Nutr. Diet.* **2013**, *113*, 1610–1619. [CrossRef] [PubMed]

116. Van Dusseldorp, M.; Schneede, J.; Refsum, H.; Ueland, P.M.; Thomas, C.M.; de Boer, E.; van Staveren, W.A. Risk of persistent cobalamin deficiency in adolescents fed a macrobiotic diet in early life. *Am. J. Clin. Nutr.* **1999**, *69*, 664–671. [PubMed]
117. Van Guldener, C.; Stehouwer, C.D. Diabetes mellitus and hyperhomocysteinemia. *Semin. Vasc. Med.* **2002**, *2*, 87–95. [CrossRef] [PubMed]
118. Homocysteine Studies Collaboration. Homocysteine and risk of ischemic heart disease and stroke: A meta-analysis. *JAMA* **2002**, *288*, 2015–2022.
119. Humphrey, L.L.; Fu, R.; Rogers, K.; Freeman, M.; Helfand, M. Homocysteine level and coronary heart disease incidence: A systematic review and meta-analysis. *Mayo Clin. Proc.* **2008**, *83*, 1203–1212. [CrossRef] [PubMed]
120. Werder, S.F. Cobalamin deficiency, hyperhomocysteinemia, and dementia. *Neuropsychiatr. Dis. Treat.* **2010**, *6*, 159–195. [CrossRef] [PubMed]
121. Welch, G.N.; Loscalzo, J. Homocysteine and atherothrombosis. *N. Engl. J. Med.* **1998**, *338*, 1042–1050. [PubMed]
122. Shargorodsky, M.; Boaz, M.; Pasternak, S.; Hanah, R.; Matas, Z.; Fux, A.; Beigel, Y.; Mashavi, M. Serum homocysteine, folate, vitamin B12 levels and arterial stiffness in diabetic patients: Which of them is really important in atherogenesis? *Diabetes Metab. Res. Rev.* **2009**, *25*, 70–75. [CrossRef] [PubMed]
123. Mahalle, N.; Kulkarni, M.V.; Garg, M.K.; Naik, S.S. Vitamin B12 deficiency and hyperhomocysteinemia as correlates of cardiovascular risk factors in Indian subjects with coronary artery disease. *J. Cardiol.* **2013**, *61*, 289–294. [CrossRef] [PubMed]
124. Van Meurs, J.B.; Pare, G.; Schwartz, S.M.; Hazra, A.; Tanaka, T.; Vermeulen, S.H.; Cotlarciuc, I.; Yuan, X.; Mälarstig, A.; Bandinelli, S.; et al. Common genetic loci influencing plasma homocysteine concentrations and their effect on risk of coronary artery disease. *Am. J. Clin. Nutr.* **2013**, *98*, 668–676. [CrossRef] [PubMed]
125. Allen, L.H. How common is vitamin B-12 deficiency? *Am. J. Clin. Nutr.* **2009**, *89*, S693–S696. [CrossRef] [PubMed]
126. Stabler, S.P.; Allen, R.H. Vitamin B12 deficiency as a worldwide problem. *Annu. Rev. Nutr.* **2004**, *24*, 299–326. [CrossRef] [PubMed]
127. Antony, A.C. Vegetarianism and vitamin B-12 (cobalamin) deficiency. *Am. J. Clin. Nutr.* **2003**, *78*, 3–6. [PubMed]
128. Tonelli, M.; Sacks, F.; Arnold, M.; Moye, L.; Davis, B.; Pfeffer, M.; for the Cholesterol and Recurrent Events (CARE) Trial Investigators. Relation between Red Blood Cell Distribution Width and Cardiovascular Event Rate in People with Coronary Disease. *Circulation* **2008**, *117*, 163–168. [CrossRef] [PubMed]
129. Dabbah, S.; Hammerman, H.; Markiewicz, W.; Aronson, D. Relation between red cell distribution width and clinical outcomes after acute myocardial infarction. *Am. J. Cardiol.* **2010**, *105*, 312–317. [CrossRef] [PubMed]
130. Ralapanawa, D.M.; Jayawickreme, K.P.; Ekanayake, E.M.; Jayalath, W.A. B12 deficiency with neurological manifestations in the absence of anaemia. *BMC Res. Notes* **2015**, *8*, 458. [CrossRef] [PubMed]
131. Brocadello, F.; Levedianos, G.; Piccione, F.; Manara, R.; Pesenti, F.F. Irreversible subacute sclerotic combined degeneration of the spinal cord in a vegan subject. *Nutrition* **2007**, *23*, 622–624. [CrossRef] [PubMed]
132. Rusher, D.R.; Pawlak, R. A Review of 89 Published Case Studies of Vitamin B12 Deficiency. *J. Hum. Nutr. Food Sci.* **2013**, *1*, 1008.
133. Koebnick, C.; Hoffmann, I.; Dagnelie, P.C.; Heins, U.A.; Wickramasinghe, S.N.; Ratnayaka, I.D.; Gruendel, S.; Lindemans, J.; Leitzmann, C. Long-term ovo-lacto vegetarian diet impairs vitamin B-12 status in pregnant women. *J. Nutr.* **2004**, *134*, 3319–3326. [PubMed]
134. Yajnik, C.S.; Deshmukh, U.S. Maternal nutrition, intrauterine programming and consequential risks in the offspring. *Rev. Endocr. Metab. Disord.* **2008**, *9*, 203–211. [CrossRef] [PubMed]
135. Knight, B.A.; Shields, B.M.; Brook, A.; Hill, A.; Bhat, D.S.; Hattersley, A.T.; Yajnik, C.S. Lower Circulating B12 Is Associated with Higher Obesity and Insulin Resistance during Pregnancy in a Non-Diabetic White British Population. *PLoS ONE* **2015**, *10*, e0135268. [CrossRef] [PubMed]
136. Yajnik, C.S.; Deshmukh, U.S. Fetal programming: Maternal nutrition and role of one-carbon metabolism. *Rev. Endocr. Metab. Disord.* **2012**, *13*, 121–127. [CrossRef] [PubMed]
137. Rosenblatt, D.S.; Whitehead, V.M. Cobalamin and folate deficiency: Acquired and hereditary disorders in children. *Semin. Hematol.* **1999**, *36*, 19–34. [PubMed]
138. Evatt, M.L.; Terry, P.D.; Ziegler, T.R.; Oakley, G.P. Association between vitamin B12-containing supplement

consumption and prevalence of biochemically defined B12 deficiency in adults in NHANES III (third national health and nutrition examination survey). *Public Health Nutr.* **2010**, *13*, 25–31. [CrossRef] [PubMed]
139. USDA National Nutrient Database for Standard Reference. USDA Food Composition Database. Available online: https://ndb.nal.usda.gov (accessed on 28 July 2016).
140. Banca Dati Di Composizione Degli Alimenti per Gli Studi Epidemiologici in Italia (BDA). Available online: http://www.bda-ieo.it (accessed on 28 July 2016).
141. Doscherholmen, A.; McMahon, J.; Ripley, D. Vitamin B12 absorption from eggs. *Proc. Soc. Exp. Biol. Med.* **1975**, *149*, 987–990. [CrossRef] [PubMed]
142. Dubey, R.C.; Maheshwari, D.K. *A Textbook of Microbiology*; S Chand & Company Ltd.: New Delhi, India, 2013.
143. Allen, L.; de Benoist, B.; Dary, O.; Hurrell, R. *Guidelines on Food Fortification with Micronutrients*; World Health Organization; Food and Agriculture Organization: Geneva, Switzerland, 2006.
144. Green, R. Is it time for vitamin B-12 fortification? What are the questions? *Am. J. Clin. Nutr.* **2009**, *89*, S712–S716. [CrossRef] [PubMed]
145. Allen, L.H.; Rosenberg, I.H.; Oakley, G.P.; Omenn, G.S. Considering the case for vitamin B12 fortification of flour. *Food Nutr. Bull.* **2010**, *31*, S36–S46. [CrossRef] [PubMed]
146. Stover, P.J. Physiology of folate and vitamin B12 in health and disease. *Nutr. Rev.* **2004**, *62*, S3–S13. [CrossRef] [PubMed]
147. Bhuiyan, A.; Dash, S.; Shahriar, S.; Nahid, F.; Arefin, S. A case of sub-acute combined degeneration of the spinal cord with associated pernicious anaemia. *Pulse* **2011**, *5*, 57–60. [CrossRef]
148. Tan, L.T.H.; Ho, K.K.F.; Fong, G.C.Y.; Ong, K.L. Subacute combined degeneration of the spinal cord. *Hong Kong J. Emerg. Med.* **2010**, *17*, 79–81.
149. EFSA Panel on Dietetic Products, Nutrition, and Allergies (NDA). *Tolerable Upper Intake Levels for Vitamins and Minerals*; EFSA: Parma, Italy, 2016.
150. Shibuya, K.; Misawa, S.; Nasu, S.; Sekiguchi, Y.; Beppu, M.; Iwai, Y.; Mitsuma, S.; Isose, S.; Arimura, K.; Kaji, R.; et al. Safety and efficacy of intravenous ultra-high dose methylcobalamin treatment for peripheral neuropathy: A phase I/II open label clinical trial. *Intern. Med.* **2014**, *53*, 1927–1931. [CrossRef] [PubMed]
151. Carmel, R. How I treat cobalamin (vitamin B12) deficiency. *Blood* **2008**, *112*, 2214–2221. [CrossRef] [PubMed]
152. Sharabi, A.; Cohen, E.; Sulkes, J.; Garty, M. Replacement therapy for vitamin B12 deficiency: Comparison between the sublingual and oral route. *Br. J. Clin. Pharmacol.* **2003**, *56*, 635–638. [CrossRef] [PubMed]
153. Van Walraven, C.; Austin, P.; Naylor, C.D. Vitamin B12 injections versus oral supplements. How much money could be saved by switching from injections to pills? *Can. Fam. Physician* **2001**, *47*, 79–86. [PubMed]
154. Thakkar, K.; Billa, G. Treatment of vitamin B12 deficiency-methylcobalamine? Cyancobalamine? Hydroxocobalamin?-clearing the confusion. *Eur. J. Clin. Nutr.* **2015**, *69*, 1–2. [CrossRef] [PubMed]
155. Zhang, Y.F.; Ning, G. Mecobalamin. *Expert Opin. Investig. Drugs* **2008**, *17*, 953–964. [CrossRef] [PubMed]
156. Institute of Medicine. *Dietary Reference Intakes for Energy, Carbohydrate, Fiber, Fat, Fatty Acids, Cholesterol, Protein, and Amino Acids (Macronutrients)*; National Academies: Washington, DC, USA, 2005.
157. Doi, K.; Matsuura, M.; Kawara, A.; Tanaka, T.; Baba, S. Influence of dietary fiber (konjac mannan) on absorption of vitamin B12 and vitamin E. *Tohoku J. Exp. Med.* **1983**, *141*, 677–681. [CrossRef] [PubMed]
158. Alexander, D.; Ball, M.J.; Mann, J. Nutrient intake and haematological status of vegetarians and age-sex matched omnivores. *Eur. J. Clin. Nutr.* **1994**, *48*, 538–546. [PubMed]
159. Herbert, V. Everyone should be tested for iron disorders. *J. Am. Diet. Assoc.* **1992**, *92*, 1502–1509. [PubMed]
160. Appleby, P.; Roddam, A.; Allen, N.; Key, T. Comparative fracture risk in vegetarians and nonvegetarians in EPIC-Oxford. *Eur. J. Clin. Nutr.* **2007**, *61*, 1400–1406. [CrossRef] [PubMed]
161. Herzlich, B.; Herbert, V. The role of the pancreas in cobalamin (vitamin B12) absorption. *Am. J. Gastroenterol.* **1984**, *79*, 489–493. [PubMed]
162. Bauman, W.A.; Shaw, S.; Jayatilleke, E.; Spungen, A.M.; Herbert, V. Increased intake of calcium reverses vitamin B12 malabsorption induced by metformin. *Diabetes Care* **2000**, *23*, 1227–1231. [CrossRef] [PubMed]
163. Li, D.; Yu, X.M.; Xie, H.B.; Zhang, Y.H.; Wang, Q.; Zhou, X.Q.; Yu, P.; Wang, L.J. Platelet phospholipid n-3 PUFA negatively associated with plasma homocysteine in middle-aged and geriatric hyperlipaemia patients. *Prostaglandins Leukot. Essent. Fat. Acids* **2007**, *76*, 293–297. [CrossRef] [PubMed]
164. Kulkarni, A.; Mehendale, S.; Pisal, H.; Kilari, A.; Dangat, K.; Salunkhe, S.; Taralekar, V.; Joshi, S. Association of omega-3 fatty acids and homocysteine concentrations in pre-eclampsia. *Clin. Nutr.* **2011**, *30*, 60–64. [CrossRef] [PubMed]

165. Grundt, H.; Nilsen, D.W.; Mansoor, M.A.; Hetland, Ø.; Nordøy, A. Reduction in homocysteine by n-3 polyunsaturated fatty acids after 1 year in a randomised double-blind study following an acute myocardial infarction: No effect on endothelial adhesion properties. *Pathophysiol. Haemost. Thromb.* **2003**, *33*, 88–95. [CrossRef] [PubMed]
166. Pooya, S.H.; Jalali, M.D.; Jazayery, A.D.; Saedisomeolia, A.; Eshraghian, M.R.; Toorang, F. The efficacy of omega-3 fatty acid supplementation on plasma homocysteine and malondialdehyde levels of type 2 diabetic patients. *Nutr. Metab. Cardiovasc. Dis.* **2010**, *20*, 326–331. [CrossRef] [PubMed]
167. Zeman, M.; Zák, A.; Vecka, M.; Tvrzická, E.; Písaríková, A.; Stanková, B. *N*-3 fatty acid supplementation decreases plasma homocysteine in diabetic dyslipidemia treated with statin-fibrate combination. *J. Nutr. Biochem.* **2006**, *17*, 379–384. [CrossRef] [PubMed]
168. Rosell, M.S.; Lloyd-Wright, Z.; Appleby, P.N.; Sanders, T.A.; Allen, N.E.; Key, T.J. Long-chain *n*-3 polyunsaturated fatty acids in plasma in British meat-eating, vegetarian, and vegan men. *Am. J. Clin. Nutr.* **2005**, *82*, 327–334. [PubMed]
169. Li, D.; Turner, A.; Sinclair, A.J. Relationship between platelet phospholipid FA and mean platelet volume in healthy men. *Lipids* **2002**, *37*, 901–906. [CrossRef] [PubMed]
170. Adams, J.F. The urinary excretion and tissue retention of Cyanocobalamin by subjects given repeated parenteral doses. *J. Clin. Pathol.* **1964**, *17*, 31–38. [CrossRef] [PubMed]
171. Allen, R.H.; Stabler, S.P. Identification and quantitation of cobalamin and cobalamin analogues in human feces. *Am. J. Clin. Nutr.* **2008**, *87*, 1324–1335. [PubMed]
172. Kondo, H.; Binder, M.J.; Kolhouse, J.F.; Smythe, W.R.; Podell, E.R.; Allen, R.H. Presence and formation of cobalamin analogues in multivitamin-mineral pills. *J. Clin. Investig.* **1982**, *70*, 889–898. [CrossRef] [PubMed]
173. Takenaka, S.; Sugiyama, S.; Watanabe, F.; Abe, K.; Tamura, Y.; Nakano, Y. Effects of Carnosine and Anserine on the Destruction of Vitamin B12 with Vitamin C in the Presence of Copper. *Biosci. Biotechnol. Biochem.* **1997**, *61*, 2137–2139. [CrossRef] [PubMed]
174. Miyamoto, E.; Kittaka-Katsura, H.; Adachi, S.; Watanabe, F. Assay of vitamin B12 in edible bamboo shoots. *Vitamins* **2005**, *79*, 329–332.
175. Kittaka-Katsura, H.; Watanabe, F.; Nakano, Y. Occurrence of vitamin B12 in green, blue, red, and black tea leaves. *J. Nutr. Sci. Vitaminol.* **2004**, *50*, 438–440. [CrossRef] [PubMed]
176. La Guardia, M.; Venturella, G.; Venturella, F. On the chemical composition and nutritional value of pleurotus taxa growing on umbelliferous plants (*Apiaceae*). *J. Agric. Food Chem.* **2005**, *53*, 5997–6002. [CrossRef] [PubMed]
177. Watanabe, F.; Schwarz, J.; Takenaka, S.; Miyamoto, E.; Ohishi, N.; Nelle, E.; Hochstrasser, R.; Yabuta, Y. Characterization of vitamin B_{12}compounds in the wild edible mushrooms black trumpet (*Craterellus cornucopioides*) and golden chanterelle (*Cantharellus cibarius*). *J. Nutr. Sci. Vitaminol.* **2012**, *58*, 438–441. [CrossRef] [PubMed]
178. Bito, T.; Teng, F.; Ohishi, N.; Takenaka, S.; Miyamoto, E.; Sakuno, E.; Terashima, K.; Yabuta, Y.; Watanabe, F. Characterization of vitamin B12 compounds in the fruiting bodies of shiitake mushroom (*Lentinula edodes*) and bed logs after fruiting of the mushroom. *Mycoscience* **2014**, *55*, 462–468. [CrossRef]
179. Watanabe, F.; Takenaka, S.; Katsura, H.; Masumder, S.A.; Abe, K.; Tamura, Y.; Nakano, Y. Dried green and purple lavers (Nori) contain substantial amounts of biologically active vitamin B(12) but less of dietary iodine relative to other edible seaweeds. *J. Agric. Food Chem.* **1999**, *47*, 2341–2343. [CrossRef] [PubMed]
180. Miyamoto, E.; Yabuta, Y.; Kwak, C.S.; Enomoto, T.; Watanabe, F. Characterization of vitamin B12 compounds from Korean purple laver (*Porphyra* sp.) products. *J. Agric. Food Chem.* **2009**, *57*, 2793–2796. [CrossRef] [PubMed]
181. Yamada, S.; Shibata, Y.; Takayama, M.; Narita, Y.; Sugawara, K.; Fukuda, M. Content and characteristics of vitamin B12 in some seaweeds. *J. Nutr. Sci. Vitaminol.* **1996**, *42*, 497–505. [CrossRef] [PubMed]
182. Suzuki, H. Serum vitamin B12 levels in young vegans who eat brown rice. *J. Nutr. Sci. Vitaminol.* **1995**, *41*, 587–594. [CrossRef] [PubMed]
183. Dagnelie, P.C.; van Staveren, W.A.; van den Berg, H. Vitamin B-12 from algae appears not to be bioavailable. *Am. J. Clin. Nutr.* **1991**, *53*, 695–697. [PubMed]
184. Watanabe, F.; Takenaka, S.; Kittaka-Katsura, H.; Ebara, S.; Miyamoto, E. Characterization and bioavailability of vitamin B12-compounds from edible algae. *J. Nutr. Sci. Vitaminol.* **2002**, *48*, 325–331. [CrossRef] [PubMed]
185. Baroni, L.; Scoglio, S.; Benedetti, S.; Bonetto, C.; Pagliarani, S.; Benedetti, Y.; Rocchi, M.; Canestrari, F. Effect of

a Klamath algae product ("AFA-B12") on blood levels of vitamin B12 and homocysteine in vegan subjects: A pilot study. *Int. J. Vitam. Nutr. Res.* **2009**, *79*, 117–123. [CrossRef] [PubMed]

186. Miyamoto, E.; Tanioka, Y.; Nakao, T.; Barla, F.; Inui, H.; Fujita, T.; Watanabe, F.; Nakano, Y. Purification and characterization of a corrinoid-compound in an edible cyanobacterium *Aphanizomenon flos-aquae* as a nutritional supplementary food. *J. Agric. Food Chem.* **2006**, *54*, 9604–9607. [CrossRef] [PubMed]
187. Pulz, O.; Gross, W. Valuable products from biotechnology of microalgae. *Appl. Microbiol. Biotechnol.* **2004**, *65*, 635–648. [CrossRef] [PubMed]
188. Merchant, R.E.; Phillips, T.W.; Udani, J. Nutritional Supplementation with *Chlorella pyrenoidosa* Lowers Serum Methylmalonic Acid in Vegans and Vegetarians with a Suspected Vitamin B_{12} Deficiency. *J. Med. Food* **2015**, *18*, 1357–1362. [CrossRef] [PubMed]
189. Kittaka-Katsura, H.; Fujita, T.; Watanabe, F.; Nakano, Y. Purification and characterization of a corrinoid compound from *Chlorella* tablets as an algal health food. *J. Agric. Food Chem.* **2002**, *50*, 4994–4997. [CrossRef] [PubMed]
190. Watanabe, F.; Tanioka, Y.; Miyamoto, E.; Fujita, T.; Takenaka, H.; Nakano, Y. Purification and characterization of corrinoid-compounds from the dried powder of an edible cyanobacterium, *Nostoc commune* (Ishikurage). *J. Nutr. Sci. Vitaminol.* **2007**, *53*, 183–186. [CrossRef] [PubMed]
191. Watanabe, F.; Katsura, H.; Takenaka, S.; Fujita, T.; Abe, K.; Tamura, Y.; Nakatsuka, T.; Nakano, Y. Pseudovitamin B(12) is the predominant cobamide of an algal health food, spirulina tablets. *J. Agric. Food Chem.* **1999**, *47*, 4736–4741. [CrossRef] [PubMed]
192. Herbert, V.; Drivas, G. Spirulina and vitamin B 12. *JAMA* **1982**, *248*, 3096–3097. [CrossRef] [PubMed]
193. Tanioka, Y.; Yabuta, Y.; Miyamoto, E.; Inui, H.; Watanabe, F. Analysis of vitamin B12 in food by silica gel 60 TLC and bioautography with vitamin B12-dependent *Escherichia coli* 215. *J. Liq. Chromatogr. Relat. Technol.* **2008**, *31*, 1977–1985. [CrossRef]
194. Denter, J.; Bisping, B. Formation of B-vitamins by bacteria during the soaking process of soybeans for tempe fermentation. *Int. J. Food Microbiol.* **1994**, *22*, 23–31. [CrossRef]
195. Nout, M.J.R.; Rombouts, F.M. Recent developments in tempe research. *J. Appl. Bacteriol.* **1990**, *69*, 609–633. [CrossRef]
196. Okada, N.; Hadioetomo, P.S.; Nikkuni, S.; Katoh, K.; Ohta, T. Vitamin B12 content of fermented foods in the tropics. *Rep. Natl. Food Res. Inst.* **1983**, *43*, 126–129.
197. Kwak, C.S.; Hwang, J.Y.; Watanabe, F.; Park, S.C. Vitamin B12 contents in some Korean fermented foods and edible seaweeds. *Korean Nutr.* **2008**, *41*, 439–447.
198. Babuchowski, A.; Laniewska-Moroz, L.; Warminska-Radyko, I. Propionibacteria in fermented vegetables. *Lait* **1999**, *79*, 113–124. [CrossRef]
199. Mozafar, A. Enrichment of some B-vitamins in plants with application of organic fertilizers. *Plant Soil* **1994**, *167*, 305–311. [CrossRef]
200. Sato, K.; Kudo, Y.; Muramatsu, K. Incorporation of a high level of vitamin B12 into a vegetable, kaiware daikon (Japanese radish sprout), by the absorption from its seeds. *Biochim. Biophys. Acta* **2004**, *1672*, 135–137. [CrossRef] [PubMed]
201. Bito, T.; Ohishi, N.; Hatanaka, Y.; Takenaka, S.; Nishihara, E.; Yabuta, Y.; Watanabe, F. Production and characterization of cyanocobalamin-enriched lettuce (*Lactuca sativa* L.) grown using hydroponics. *J. Agric. Food Chem.* **2013**, *61*, 3852–3858. [CrossRef] [PubMed]
202. Gu, Q.; Zhang, C.; Song, D.; Li, P.; Zhu, X. Enhancing vitamin B12 content in soy-yogurt by *Lactobacillus reuteri*. *Int. J. Food Microbiol.* **2015**, *206*, 56–59. [CrossRef] [PubMed]
203. Rizzo, G.; Baroni, L. Health and ecological implications of fish consumption: A deeper insight. *Med. J. Nutr. Metab.* **2016**, *9*, 7–22. [CrossRef]
204. Craig, W.J. Nutrition concerns and health effects of vegetarian diets. *Nutr. Clin. Pract.* **2010**, *25*, 613–620. [CrossRef] [PubMed]
205. Clinical Trials NCT02679833. Available online: https://clinicaltrials.gov/ct2/show/NCT02679833 (accessed on 28 July 2016).
206. Yazaki, Y.; Chow, G.; Mattie, M. A single-center, double-blinded, randomized controlled study to evaluate the relative efficacy of sublingual and oral vitamin B-complex administration in reducing total serum homocysteine levels. *J. Altern. Complement. Med.* **2006**, *12*, 881–885. [CrossRef] [PubMed]
207. Vidal-Alaball, J.; Butler, C.C.; Cannings-John, R.; Goringe, A.; Hood, K.; McCaddon, A.; McDowell, I.;

Papaioannou, A. Oral vitamin B12 versus intramuscular vitamin B12 for vitamin B12 deficiency. *Cochrane Database Syst. Rev.* **2005**, *3*, CD004655.

208. Oladipo, O.; Rosenblatt, D.S.; Watkins, D.; Miousse, I.R.; Sprietsma, L.; Dietzen, D.J.; Shinawi, M. Cobalamin F disease detected by newborn screening and follow-up on a 14-year-old patient. *Pediatrics* **2011**, *128*, e1636–e1640. [CrossRef] [PubMed]
209. Waggoner, D.J.; Ueda, K.; Mantia, C.; Dowton, S.B. Methylmalonic aciduria (*cblF*): Case report and response to therapy. *Am. J. Med. Genet.* **1998**, *79*, 373–375. [CrossRef]
210. Andersson, H.C.; Shapira, E. Biochemical and clinical response to hydroxocobalamin versus cyanocobalamin treatment in patients with methylmalonic acidemia and homocystinuria (*cblC*). *J. Pediatr.* **1998**, *132*, 121–124. [CrossRef]
211. Linnell, J.C.; Smith, A.D.; Smith, C.L.; Wilson, J.; Matthews, D.M. Effects of smoking on metabolism and excretion of vitamin B12. *Br. Med. J.* **1968**, *2*, 215–216. [CrossRef] [PubMed]
212. Shepherd, G.; Velez, L.I. Role of hydroxocobalamin in acute cyanide poisoning. *Ann. Pharmacother.* **2008**, *42*, 661–669. [CrossRef] [PubMed]
213. Freeman, A.G. Cyanocobalamin—A case for withdrawal: Discussion paper. *J. R. Soc. Med.* **1992**, *85*, 686–687. [PubMed]
214. Freeman, A.G. Hydroxocobalamin versus cyanocobalamin. *J. R. Soc. Med.* **1996**, *89*, 659. [PubMed]
215. Balta, I.; Ozuguz, P. Vitamin B12-induced acneiform eruption. *Cutan. Ocul. Toxicol.* **2014**, *33*, 94–95. [CrossRef] [PubMed]
216. Cianci, A.; Colacurci, N.; Paoletti, A.M.; Perino, A.; Cicinelli, E.; Maffei, S.; Di Martino, M.; Daguati, R.; Stomati, M.; Pilloni, M.; et al. Soy isoflavones, inulin, calcium, and vitamin D3 in post-menopausal hot flushes: An observational study. *Clin. Exp. Obstet. Gynecol.* **2015**, *42*, 743–745. [PubMed]
217. Cignini, P.; Mangiafico, L.; Padula, F.; D'Emidio, L.; Dugo, N.; Aloisi, A.; Giorlandino, C.; Vitale, S.G. Supplementation with a dietary multicomponent (Lafergin®) based on Ferric Sodium EDTA (Ferrazone®): Results of an observational study. *J. Prenat. Med.* **2015**, *9*, 1–7. [CrossRef] [PubMed]
218. Colonese, F.; Laganà, A.S.; Colonese, E.; Sofo, V.; Salmeri, F.M.; Granese, R.; Triolo, O. The pleiotropic effects of vitamin D in gynaecological and obstetric diseases: An overview on a hot topic. *Biomed. Res. Int.* **2015**, *2015*, 986281. [CrossRef] [PubMed]
219. Laganà, A.S.; Vitale, S.G.; Nigro, A.; Sofo, V.; Salmeri, F.M.; Rossetti, P.; Rapisarda, A.M.; La Vignera, S.; Condorelli, R.A.; Rizzo, G.; et al. Pleiotropic Actions of Peroxisome Proliferator-Activated Receptors (PPARs) in Dysregulated Metabolic Homeostasis, Inflammation and Cancer: Current Evidence and Future Perspectives. *Int. J. Mol. Sci.* **2016**, *17*, E999. [CrossRef] [PubMed]
220. Misra, U.K.; Kalita, J.; Singh, S.K.; Rahi, S.K. Oxidative stress markers in vitamin B12 deficiency. *Mol. Neurobiol.* **2016**, 1–7. [CrossRef] [PubMed]

5

Organ-Specific Gene Expression Changes in the Fetal Liver and Placenta in Response to Maternal Folate Depletion

Jill A. McKay [1], Long Xie [2], Michiel Adriaens [3], Chris T. Evelo [4], Dianne Ford [5] and John C. Mathers [2,*]

1 Human Nutrition Research Centre, Institute for Health & Society, Newcastle University, Sir James Spence Institute, Royal Victoria Infirmary, Queen Victoria Road, Newcastle upon Tyne NE1 4LP, UK; jill.mckay@ncl.ac.uk
2 Human Nutrition Research Centre; Institute of Cellular Medicine, Newcastle University, Newcastle upon Tyne NE4 5PL, UK; long.xie@ncl.ac.uk
3 Maastricht Centre for Systems Biology, MaCSBio, Maastricht University, Maastricht 6200 MD, The Netherlands; michiel.adriaens@maastrichtuniversity.nl
4 Department of Bioinformatics, BiGCaT, Maastricht University, Maastricht 6200 MD, The Netherlands; chris.evelo@maastrichtuniversity.nl
5 Faculty of Health and Life Sciences, Northumbria University, Newcastle upon Tyne NE1 8ST, UK; dianne.ford@northumbria.ac.uk
* Correspondence: john.mathers@ncl.ac.uk

Abstract: Growing evidence supports the hypothesis that the in utero environment can have profound implications for fetal development and later life offspring health. Current theory suggests conditions experienced in utero prepare, or "programme", the fetus for its anticipated post-natal environment. The mechanisms responsible for these programming events are poorly understood but are likely to involve gene expression changes. Folate is essential for normal fetal development and inadequate maternal folate supply during pregnancy has long term adverse effects for offspring. We tested the hypothesis that folate depletion during pregnancy alters offspring programming through altered gene expression. Female C57BL/6J mice were fed diets containing 2 mg or 0.4 mg folic acid/kg for 4 weeks before mating and throughout pregnancy. At 17.5 day gestation, genome-wide gene expression was measured in male fetal livers and placentas. In the fetal liver, 989 genes were expressed differentially (555 up-regulated, 434 down-regulated) in response to maternal folate depletion, with 460 genes expressed differentially (250 up-regulated, 255 down-regulated) in the placenta. Only 25 differentially expressed genes were common between organs. Maternal folate intake during pregnancy influences fetal gene expression in a highly organ specific manner which may reflect organ-specific functions.

Keywords: transcriptome; programming; developmental origins of health and disease; pregnancy; diet

---

1. Introduction

The developmental origins of health and disease (DOHaD) hypothesis proposes that in utero and early life exposures can lead to altered programming of offspring. Such programming events can cause permanent changes in organ development, physiology and metabolism leading to altered disease risk in later life. Suboptimal nutrition, both under- and over-nutrition, during fetal and neonatal development increases susceptibility to a wide range of diseases [1]. These observations indicate a degree of plasticity during development, in which the fetal phenotype may be altered due to environment cues [2] to prepare it for the anticipated post-natal environment [3]. The biological mechanisms underlying this "programming" effect of nutrition during early life are poorly understood, but are likely to involve changes in gene expression.

The protective effect of adequate dietary folate intake and of folic acid supplementation during pregnancy on risk of neural tube defects (NTDs) is well established [4,5]. Further, epidemiological evidence suggests that adequate dietary folate intake or supplementation with folic acid during pregnancy may reduce the risk of other congenital defects [6] and adverse pregnancy outcomes [7], as well enhancing neurodevelopment [8] and reducing the risk of severe language delay [9], autism [10,11] and some cancers (leukaemia [12–14], brain tumours [15,16] and neuroblastoma [17]) [18] in children. In rodent models, folate deficiency during pregnancy can cause spontaneous abortion, teratogenic effects in offspring, reduced litter number, and altered offspring body weight [19,20]. Sufficient maternal folate intake during pregnancy is essential for successful pregnancy outcomes/normal fetal development and for the long-term health of the offspring.

Folate, a B vitamin, is central to one-carbon metabolism which, in addition to formation of the universal methyl donor, *S*-adenosyl-methionine (SAM), interacts with several other cellular pathways including amino acid metabolism and biosynthesis of purine and pyrimidines [21]. SAM is critical for the methylation of biological molecules including DNA, lipids and proteins. Epigenetic mechanisms (including methylation of DNA and of histones) which regulate gene expression are susceptible to modification via altered SAM availability in response to changes in folate intake (reviewed in [22]). Therefore, we hypothesised that inadequate folate supply during pregnancy alters programming of the offspring via changes in gene expression and that this is responsible for the observed adverse effects of this maternal nutritional insult on pregnancy outcomes and offspring health in later life. Mammals respond to inadequate nutrient supply by prioritising allocation of nutrients to specific purposes [23,24] which may result in cell, tissue and organ differences in gene expression. Little is known about such inter-organ differences in fetal gene expression in response to restricted folate supply. We hypothesised that the fetal liver and placenta, which represent organs with long and short-term consequences for the developing animal, would be subject to distinctly different responses to folate depletion. To test these hypotheses, we quantified genome-wide gene expression patterns in fetal liver and placenta in response to maternal folate depletion before, and throughout, pregnancy.

2. Experimental Section

2.1. Animal Husbandry and Experimental Diets

All animal procedures were approved by the Newcastle University Ethics Review Committee and the UK Home Office (Project Licence number 60/3979) and have been described previously [25]. Animals were housed in the Comparative Biology Centre, Newcastle University at 20–22 °C and with 12 h light and dark cycles. Fresh water was available ad libitum. Female C57BL/6J mice were allocated at random to either a low folate (0.4 mg folic acid/kg diet) or normal folate diet (2 mg folic acid/kg diet) (6 g of allocated diet was offered to each mouse per day), and maintained on this diet for 4 weeks prior to mating. Diet compositions were modified from AIN-93G [26] and have been described previously [25]. L-amino acids were used as a protein substitute. All ingredients, other than folic acid, were included in both diets at the same concentrations to avoid potential confounding through other dietary factors. The degree of folate depletion induced by feeding the diet containing 0.4 mg folic acid/kg was sufficient to impose a nutritional stress (evidenced by reduced circulating concentrations of folate) but not so severe as to limit reproduction. The normal folate diet contained 2 mg folic acid/kg diet which is considered sufficient to support breeding and maintenance in this species. Mice were time mated i.e., a male was added to a cage containing two females overnight and removed the following morning. Pregnant females, identified by the presence of a vaginal plug, were re-caged and offered 10 g/day of allocated diet throughout pregnancy. At 17.5 days gestation, dams were killed for collection of blood and organs.

2.2. Sample Collection

Animals were anesthetised using gaseous isoflurane, blood was removed by cardiac puncture and animals were killed by cervical dislocation. Blood was collected and stored in EDTA tubes.

Whole blood 5-methyltetrahydrofolate (THF) and 5–10-methylTHF concentrations were measured by liquid chromatography-tandem mass spectrometry (LC-MS/MS) and data reported previously [25]. The uterus, containing all fetuses and placentas, was removed and placed immediately in ice cold PBS. The liver and placenta of each fetus were removed, weighed and snap frozen in liquid nitrogen and stored at −80 °C until required for RNA extraction.

2.3. RNA Extraction

To avoid any potential influence of sex on resultant data, only male tissues were analysed. Fetal sex was determined by polymerase chain reaction (PCR) of the sex determining region-Y (*SRY*) gene using DNA extracted from embryonic tail tissue [25,27]. RNA was extracted from whole fetal livers and placentas of males only using Tri-reagent (Sigma-Aldrich, Gillingham, Dorset, SP8 4XT, UK) and following the manufacturer's instructions. Briefly, 50 mg tissue was homogenised in 500 μL Tri-reagent on ice. A further 500 μL Tri-reagent and 200 μL chloroform were added, then the sample was mixed by inversion and incubated on ice for 5 min. Samples were then centrifuged at 13,500 rpm for 15 min at 4 °C. The upper aqueous phase was removed, RNA was precipitated by incubation on ice with 500 μL isopropanol for 10 min, after which it was collected by centrifugation at 13,500 rpm for 10 min at 4 °C. The supernatant fluid was removed and the pellet was washed with 1 mL 75% ethanol for 10 min before centrifuging at 6000 rpm for 5 min at 4 °C. The supernatant fluid was removed, and the pellet was allowed to dry for 10 min before resuspending the RNA in 40 μL water. Contaminating DNA was removed using RQ1 DNase (Promega, Southampton, Hampshire, SO16 7NS, UK). RNA integrity was checked on an agarose gel and concentration and purity were measured using a Nanodrop spectrophotometer (Thermo Fisher, Waltham, MA, USA).

2.4. Gene Expression Arrays

RNA from each tissue was pooled for three male fetuses per litter (5 μg/fetus with a final concentration of 500 ng/μL) and hybridised to a single array for a total of 12 litters ($n = 6$ per dietary group) for each organ. Where a litter had more than three male fetuses, the three fetuses with weights closest to the mean litter weight were analysed.

Genome-wide transcript abundance was determined by ServiceXS (Plesmanlaan 1/D, 2333 BZ Leiden, The Netherlands) on the Affymetrix GeneChip platform with the NuGO mouse array (NuGO_Mm1a520177). This array comprises over 24,000 probe sets, covering the majority of established genes. Before the labelling process, the integrity of all RNA samples (RNA Integrity Number (RIN) > 8) was confirmed using the Agilent 2100 Bioanalyser (Agilent Technologies, Stockport, Cheshire, SK8 3GY, UK). Output data were supplied as Affymetrix CEL files and imported into R (version 2.15.3) using the Affy package [28]. Data from liver and placenta were pre-processed separately using gcRMA background correction and quantile normalisation [29] to correct for batch effects and other technical confounders. To maximize sensitivity and specificity, updated Entrez gene probe-set annotation was used from the BrainArray project [30] (version 14.1.0) resulting in 16,270 re-annotated probesets mapping to unique transcripts. Statistical analysis comparing the two diet groups was performed separately for each organ using the empirical Bayes approach of the Limma package [31] which performs a moderated t-test. On filtering genes for significant changes using False Discovery Rate (FDR) values calculated using the Benjamini and Hochberg method (FDR < 0.05), no genes remained statistically significant. Pathway analysis can in part replace FDR corrections by testing for the regulation of related genes, which suffers less from oversampling. Genes were, therefore, considered to show a differential expression relevant for further analysis in enrichment analysis in response to maternal folate depletion if there was a significant ($p < 0.05$) increase or reduction of at least 1.2 fold. DAVID [32] was used to carry out Gene Ontology enrichment analysis and to investigate KEGG pathways affected by maternal folate depletion. The threshold for significance for Gene Ontology enrichment analysis was set at $p < 0.05$ (corrected for multiple testing), and at $p < 0.05$ (uncorrected) for KEGG pathway enrichment analysis. Additional pathway analysis was carried out using PathVisio 3.2.0 and the curated pathway collection of WikiPathways (download date: 1 September 2015), applying the same parameters for significant fold-change as stated above, imposing a Z score of 1.9 for significance to filter for probable changed pathways. All raw and processed microarray data have been deposited in the ArrayExpress database (accession ID E-MTAB-3940).

2.5. Validation of Gene Expression Changes Using Real-Time PCR

To confirm the gene expression changes observed in the microarray analysis, real-time PCR was performed on each individual (i.e., not pooled) fetal RNA sample that was analysed by microarray hybridisation, focusing on 13 gene targets. Target genes were selected on the basis of being the most up or down regulated in the liver and placenta. Gene transcripts analysed in placental RNA were *Cyp21a1*, *Hbb-y*, *Slco1b2*, *Ptgs2*, *Vcan*, *Lrrn4*, and *Mettl7b* and in fetal liver RNA were *Asgr1*, *Hamp*, *Actc1*, *Ckm*, *Tnnc2* and *Smpx*.

RNA (1 μg) was reverse transcribed using Quantitect Reverse Transcription kit (Qiagen, Cat No. 205313) according to the manufacturer's instructions. Briefly, 1 μg of RNA was incubated with 2 μL genomic DNA Wipeout buffer in a reaction volume of 14 μL at 42 °C for 2 min to remove any genomic DNA. The mixture was then placed immediately on ice. RNA was incubated with 1 μL Quantiscript reverse transcriptase, 1 μL RT primer mix and 4 μL Quantiscript RT buffer for 15 min at 42 °C, after which time it was incubated at 95 °C for 3 min. The cDNA samples generated were then diluted 1:9 with water for use in real time PCR.

Prior to sample analysis, expression values, linearity and efficiency of each assay were determined through cDNA standard curves completed for each transcript measured. Transcript levels of the genes of interest were measured on a Roche Lightcycler 480 (Roche Applied Science, Burgess Hill, West Sussex, RH15 9RY, UK) in a total reaction volume of 25 μL using 2.5 μL Quantitect sybr green transcript specific primers (Qiagen, see Supplementary Materials Table S1 for details of manufacturer's individual catalogue numbers), 12.5 μL Quantitect SYBR green mix (Qiagen Cat. No. 204145), 1 μL diluted cDNA and 9 μL water and cycling parameters 95 °C for 5 min (1 cycle); 95 °C for 10 s followed by 60 °C for 30 s (40 cycles); followed by a final melt curve analysis and cooling to 40 °C. Using the delta CT method, transcript levels of the genes of interest were normalised to *GAPDH* transcript levels which were determined using the same procedure and parameters described.

2.6. In Silico Analysis of Gene Promoter Regions for Transcription Factor (TF) Binding Sites

Genomatix software (https://www.genomatix.de/v3.5 24 July 2015) was employed to obtain promoter sequences for genes of interest using the Gene2Promoter function. Promoter sequences were analysed for common transcription factor binding sites using the Common TFs function. Lists of TFs belonging to the transcription factor binding site families identified were downloaded from Genomatix and compared with fetal liver gene expression data.

2.7. Statistical Analysis

Statistical analysis of array data is described above. For all other datasets, data distributions were examined by the Kolmogorov-Smirnov test and all datasets were normally distributed. Analysis of variance (Statistical Package for the Social Sciences (SPSS) version 21, IBM, Armonk, New York 10504, NY, USA) was used to examine the effects of diet on placental weight, placental efficiency and gene expression analysis on data obtained from RT PCR analysis. $p < 0.05$ was considered statistically significant.

3. Results

3.1. Influence of Maternal Folate Intake during Pregnancy on Fetal Weight, Liver Weight, Placental Weight and Placental Efficiency

Data on the effects of maternal folate depletion on fetal weight and fetal liver weight have been presented previously [25]. In addition, exposure to the Low Folate diet reduced maternal whole blood

5′methyl THF concentration significantly ($p < 0.001$) with values of 666 (40.9) and 378 (50.0) nmol/L for Normal and Low Folate diets respectively [25]. Maternal folate depletion increased fetal weight but had no effect on weight of the fetal liver. There was no significant influence of maternal folate intake during pregnancy on placental weight (mean placental weights were 107.0 mg and 107.3 mg for normal ($n = 56$) and low ($n = 37$) folate groups respectively ($p = 0.945$)). Placental efficiency, calculated by dividing fetal weight by placental weight, was not influenced by maternal folate depletion (mean placental efficiencies were 7.9 and 9.1 for normal ($n = 56$) and low ($n = 37$) folate groups respectively ($p = 0.200$)).

3.2. *Influence of Maternal Folate Intake during Pregnancy on Gene Expression in the Fetal Liver*

In the fetal liver, 989 genes were differentially expressed in response to maternal folate depletion, comprising 555 up-regulated genes and 434 down-regulated genes (Supplementary Materials Table S2). All raw and processed microarray data have been deposited in the ArrayExpress database (accession ID E-MTAB-3940). Seventy three (7.4%) of these differentially expressed genes code for known transcription factor proteins (see Supplementary Materials Table S3 for list of genes). Although the majority (95.3%) of the gene expression changes were small (i.e., ranging from a fold change of 1.2–2), the expression of 47 genes was changed by greater than two-fold (Table 1).

Whilst gene ontology analysis found no statistically significant influence on biological processes, KEGG pathway analysis revealed that "Lysosome" and "Tight Junction" pathways were significantly affected in the fetal liver in response to maternal folate depletion (Table 2). Analysis of WikiPathways using PathVisio found 13 pathways in which a significant number of genes had altered expression in the fetal liver in response to maternal folate depletion (Table 3).

3.3. *Influence of Maternal Folate Intake during Pregnancy on Gene Expression in the Placenta*

In the placenta, 460 genes were differentially expressed (250 up-regulated and 255 down-regulated) in response to maternal folate depletion (Supplementary Materials Table S4). All raw and processed microarray data have been deposited in the ArrayExpress database (accession ID E-MTAB-3940). Twenty two (4.8%) of these differentially expressed genes code for known transcription factor proteins (see Supplementary Materials Table S5 for list of genes). Of all the genes expressed differentially, only three had a change in expression of greater than two-fold (Table 4), with the vast majority (99.4%) of changes being small (i.e., ranging from 1.2 to 2 fold change).

Whilst gene ontology analysis found no statistically significant effects on biological processes in placenta, KEGG pathway analysis revealed that "Amino sugar and nucleotide sugar metabolism", "Valine, leucine and isoleucine degradation" and "Complement and coagulation cascades" pathways were significantly affected in the placenta in response to maternal folate depletion (Table 5). Interrogation of WikiPathways using PathVisio found 13 pathways which were altered significantly in response to maternal folate depletion (Table 6).

3.4. *Comparison of Gene Expression Changes in the Placenta and Fetal Liver in Response to Maternal Folate Depletion*

More genes in the fetal liver than in the placenta had altered expression in response to maternal folate intake during pregnancy ($n = 989$ and 460 respectively). Only 25 genes were common to the data-sets for fetal liver and placenta (see Table 7 for gene list). The expected overlap between two random subsets with elements of 989 and 460 respectively picked from a set of 16270 elements (the total number of measured genes) is 28, hence the observed overlap of 25 genes is likely due to chance. Of the genes found to respond to maternal folate in both placenta and fetal liver, only four displayed the same direction of change in both organs, with 21 showing the opposite direction of change (Figure 1), which suggests that finding expression changes in the same genes in the two organs may be due to chance.

Table 1. Genes with greater than two-fold expression change in fetal liver in response to maternal folate depletion [1,2].

Gene Symbol	Gene Name	Ensembl ID	Direction of Change	Fold Change	*p* Value	FDR
Actc1	actin, alpha, cardiac muscle 1	ENSMUSG00000068614	Down	20.5	0.001	0.379
Ckm	creatine kinase, muscle	ENSMUSG00000030399	Down	14.8	0.001	0.379
Tnnc2	troponin C2, fast	ENSMUSG00000017300	Down	14.0	0.015	0.458
Smpx	small muscle protein, X-linked	ENSMUSG00000041476	Down	13.4	0.001	0.379
Tnni2	troponin I, skeletal, fast 2	ENSMUSG00000031097	Down	9.1	0.016	0.460
Actn2	actinin alpha 2	ENSMUSG00000052374	Down	8.6	0.001	0.379
Atp1b4	ATPase, $(Na^{+})/K^{+}$ transporting, beta 4 polypeptide	ENSMUSG00000016327	Down	7.9	0.009	0.443
Tnnt3	troponin T3, skeletal, fast	ENSMUSG00000061723	Down	7.6	0.016	0.461
Eno3	enolase 3, beta muscle	ENSMUSG00000060600	Down	7.5	0.003	0.379
Tnni1	troponin I, skeletal, slow 1	ENSMUSG00000026418	Down	7.2	0.008	0.435
Myh8	myosin, heavy polypeptide 8, skeletal muscle, perinatal	ENSMUSG00000055775	Down	6.9	0.024	0.487
Casq2	calsequestrin 2	ENSMUSG00000027861	Down	6.7	0.001	0.379
Mybpc1	myosin binding protein C, slow-type	ENSMUSG00000020061	Down	6.6	0.022	0.477
Myh3	myosin, heavy polypeptide 3, skeletal muscle, embryonic	ENSMUSG00000020908	Down	6.6	0.015	0.458
Ldb3	LIM domain binding 3	ENSMUSG00000021798	Down	6.3	0.002	0.379
Mylpf	myosin light chain, phosphorylatable, fast skeletal muscle	ENSMUSG00000030672	Down	6.1	0.021	0.477
Sln	Sarcolipin	ENSMUSG00000042045	Down	6.0	0.017	0.465
Myl4	myosin, light polypeptide 4	ENSMUSG00000061086	Down	5.4	0.005	0.407
Ckmt2	creatine kinase, mitochondrial 2	ENSMUSG00000021622	Down	4.9	0.007	0.435
Myot	Myotilin	ENSMUSG00000024471	Down	4.6	0.014	0.451
Csrp3	cysteine and glycine-rich protein 3	ENSMUSG00000030470	Down	4.3	0.017	0.465
Srl	Sarcalumenin	ENSMUSG00000022519	Down	4.1	0.005	0.407
Pgam2	phosphoglycerate mutase 2	ENSMUSG00000020475	Down	3.6	0.015	0.458
Atp2a1	ATPase, Ca++ transporting, cardiac muscle, fast twitch 1	ENSMUSG00000030730	Down	3.6	0.042	0.545
Tnnt1	troponin T1, skeletal, slow	ENSMUSG00000064179	Down	3.4	0.023	0.481
Sh3bgr	SH3-binding domain glutamic acid-rich protein	ENSMUSG00000040666	Down	3.1	0.002	0.379
Itgb1bp2	integrin beta 1 binding protein 2	ENSMUSG00000031312	Down	2.9	0.023	0.481
Cdh11	cadherin 11	ENSMUSG00000031673	Down	2.6	0.012	0.447
Crh	corticotropin releasing hormone	ENSMUSG00000049796	Down	2.5	0.036	0.529
Fhl1	four and a half LIM domains 1	ENSMUSG00000023092	Down	2.5	0.002	0.379
Apobec2	apolipoprotein B mRNA editing enzyme, catalytic polypeptide 2	ENSMUSG00000040694	Down	2.4	0.009	0.442
Egfl6	EGF-like-domain, multiple 6	ENSMUSG00000000402	Down	2.4	0.004	0.395
Myom1	myomesin 1	ENSMUSG00000024049	Down	2.4	0.029	0.498
Mlf1	myeloid leukemia factor 1	ENSMUSG00000048416	Down	2.3	0.020	0.476
Cav2	caveolin 2	ENSMUSG00000000058	Down	2.3	0.001	0.379
Shh	sonic hedgehog	ENSMUSG00000002633	Down	2.2	0.019	0.465
Slit2	slit homolog 2 (Drosophila)	ENSMUSG00000031558	Down	2.2	0.003	0.379

Table 1. *Cont.*

Gene Symbol	Gene Name	Ensembl ID	Direction of Change	Fold Change	*p* Value	FDR
Rps6ka6	ribosomal protein S6 kinase polypeptide 6	ENSMUSG00000025665	Down	2.1	0.034	0.526
Scn7a	sodium channel, voltage-gated, type VII, alpha	ENSMUSG00000034810	Down	2.1	0.020	0.476
Sparcl1	SPARC-like 1	ENSMUSG00000029309	Down	2.1	0.012	0.447
Nr1h4	nuclear receptor subfamily 1, group H, member 4	ENSMUSG00000047638	Up	2.0	0.001	0.379
Pemt	phosphatidylethanolamine *N*-methyltransferase	ENSMUSG00000000301	Up	2.1	0.021	0.477
Serpine1	serine (or cysteine) peptidase inhibitor, clade E, member 1	ENSMUSG00000037411	Up	2.1	0.001	0.379
LOC100503019	hypothetical protein LOC100503019	NA	Up	2.5	0.018	0.465
Cyp2e1	cytochrome P450, family 2, subfamily e, polypeptide 1	ENSMUSG00000025479	Up	2.7	0.012	0.443
Asgr1	asialoglycoprotein receptor 1	ENSMUSG00000020884	Up	2.8	0.010	0.443
Hamp	hepcidin antimicrobial peptide	ENSMUSG00000050440	Up	3.3	0.001	0.379

[1] The Low and Normal folate diets contained 0.4 and 2.0 mg folic acid/kg diet respectively; [2] For each comparison, data were obtained from three male fetuses from each of six litters from dams fed either the Low or Normal folate diets.

Table 2. KEGG pathways in the fetal liver altered by maternal folate depletion during pregnancy [1].

KEGG Pathway Term	Pathway Name	Total Genes on Pathway	Number of Altered Genes	Differentially Expressed Genes	*p* Value
mmu04142	Lysosome	119	12	*Ap3m1* (ENSMUSG00000021824), *Gm2a* (ENSMUSG00000000594)	0.031
				Atp6v0a1 (ENSMUSG00000019302), *Naga* (ENSMUSG00000022453)	
				Arsg (ENSMUSG00000020604), *Gba* (ENSMUSG00000028048)	
				Cd68 (ENSMUSG00000018774), *Ap3s2* (ENSMUSG00000063801)	
				Gla (ENSMUSG00000031266), *Dnase2b* (ENSMUSG00000028185)	
				Galns (ENSMUSG00000015027), *Gaa* (ENSMUSG00000025579)	
mmu04530	Tight junction	135	13	*Tjp1* (ENSMUSG00000030516), *B230120H23Rik* (ENSMUSG00000004085)	0.033
				Myh3 (ENSMUSG00000020908), *Hcls1* (ENSMUSG00000022831)	
				Gnai3 (ENSMUSG00000000001), *Myh8* (ENSMUSG00000055775)	
				Nras (ENSMUSG00000027852), *Actn2* (ENSMUSG00000052374)	
				Ppp2r1a (ENSMUSG00000007564), *Epb4.1l2* (ENSMUSG00000019978)	
				Mylpf (ENSMUSG00000030672), *Spnb2* (ENSMUSG00000020315),	
				Akt2 (ENSMUSG00000004056)	

[1] The Low and Normal folate diets contained 0.4 and 2.0 mg folic acid/kg diet respectively.

Table 3. WikiPathways in the fetal liver altered by maternal folate depletion during pregnancy [1,2] and identified using PathVisio.

Pathway	Number of Genes Altered on Pathway	Number of Genes Measured on Pathway	Total Number of Genes on Pathway	% Affected	Z Score	p-Value (Permuted)
Striated Muscle Contraction	16	32	46	50	9.35	<0.001
Adipogenesis genes	16	111	133	14	2.95	0.005
Fatty Acid Biosynthesis	5	21	26	24	2.93	0.011
Iron Homeostasis	3	10	16	30	2.77	0.013
TGF Beta Signaling Pathway	7	42	53	17	2.36	0.015
miR-1 in cardiac development	1	2	6	50	2.33	0.029
One carbon metabolism and related pathways	6	37	86	16	2.11	0.028
EPO Receptor Signaling	4	21	27	19	2.09	0.038
Spinal Cord Injury	11	85	110	13	2.04	0.035
Alanine and aspartate metabolism	2	8	43	25	1.94	0.038
Methylation	2	8	15	25	1.94	0.045
Osteoblast	2	8	14	25	1.94	0.040

[1] The Low and Normal folate diets contained 0.4 and 2.0 mg folic acid/kg diet respectively; [2] For each comparison, data were obtained from three male fetuses from each of six litters from dams fed either the Low or Normal folate diets.

Table 4. Genes with greater than two-fold expression change in the placenta in response to maternal low folate intake [1,2].

Gene Symbol	Gene Name	Ensembl ID	Direction of Change	Fold Change	p Value	FDR
Cyp21a1	cytochrome P450, family 21, subfamily a, polypeptide 1	ENSMUSG00000024365	Down	2.5	0.002	0.999
Hbb-y	hemoglobin Y, beta-like embryonic chain	ENSMUSG00000052187	Down	2.2	0.035	0.999
Slco1b2	solute carrier organic anion transporter family, member 1b2	ENSMUSG00000030236	Down	2.1	0.011	0.999

[1] The Low and Normal folate diets contained 0.4 and 2.0 mg folic acid/kg diet respectively; [2] For each comparison, data were obtained from three male fetuses from each of six litters from dams fed either the Low or Normal folate diets.

Table 5. KEGG pathways in the placenta altered by maternal folate depletion during pregnancy [1,2].

KEGG Pathway Term	Pathway Name	Total Genes on Pathway	Number of Altered Genes	Differentially Expressed Genes	*p* Value
mmu00520	Amino sugar and nucleotide sugar metabolism	44	5	*Gnpda2* (ENSMUSG00000029209), *Pgm2* (ENSMUSG00000025791), *Uap1* (ENSMUSG00000026670), *Gmppb* (ENSMUSG00000070284), *Pgm3* (ENSMUSG00000056131)	0.017
mmu00280	Valine, leucine and isoleucine degradation	46	5	*Mccc2* (ENSMUSG00000021646), *Oxct2a* (ENSMUSG00000076436), *Hsd17b10* (ENSMUSG00000025260), *Bckdhb* (ENSMUSG00000032263), *Abat* (ENSMUSG00000057880)	0.019
mmu04610	Complement and coagulation cascades	75	6	*Cd55* (ENSMUSG00000026399), *Serpina1b* (ENSMUSG00000071178), *F11* (ENSMUSG00000031645), *F2* (ENSMUSG00000027249), *C9* (ENSMUSG00000022149), *C3* (ENSMUSG00000024164)	0.026

[1] The Low and Normal folate diets contained 0.4 and 2.0 mg folic acid/kg diet respectively; [2] For each comparison, data were obtained from three male fetuses from each of six litters from dams fed either the Low or Normal folate diets.

Table 6. WikiPathways in the placenta altered by maternal folate depletion [1,2] during pregnancy and identified using PathVisio.

Pathway	Number of Genes Altered on Pathway	Number of Genes Measured on Pathway	Total Number of Genes on Pathway	% Affected	Z Score	*p*-Value (Permuted)
Complement Activation, Classical Pathway	3	13	19	23	3.77	0.002
Statin Pathway	3	16	29	19	3.26	>0.000
Alanine and aspartate metabolism	2	8	43	25	3.25	0.007
Glucocorticoid & Mineralocorticoid Metabolism	2	9	27	22	3	0.016
Selenium metabolism/Selenoproteins	3	18	49	17	2.98	0.015
Alzheimers Disease	6	54	91	11	2.98	0.006
Nuclear Receptors	4	31	38	13	2.79	0.015
Glucuronidation	2	10	33	20	2.78	0.012
Arachidonate Epoxygenase Epoxide Hydrolase	1	3	13	33	2.76	0.037
Polyol pathway	1	3	12	33	2.76	0.024
Complement and Coagulation Cascades	5	54	64	9	2.24	0.015
Acetylcholine Synthesis	1	5	18	20	1.97	0.050
Aflatoxin B1 metabolism	1	5	11	20	1.97	0.037

[1] The Low and Normal folate diets contained 0.4 and 2.0 mg folic acid/kg diet respectively; [2] For each comparison, data were obtained from three male fetuses from each of six litters from dams fed either the Low or Normal folate diets.

Table 7. Genes differentially expressed in both fetal liver and placental organs in response to maternal folate depletion [1,2,3].

Gene Symbol	Ensembl ID	Expression fold Change in Fetal Liver	*p* Value for Fetal Liver	Expression Fold Change in Placenta	*p* Value for Placenta
A830035A12RIK	NA	1.5	0.025	−1.5	0.019
Aadat	ENSMUSG00000057228	−1.3	0.033	−1.3	0.031
Akr7a5	ENSMUSG00000028743	1.2	0.023	−1.3	0.003
Apon	ENSMUSG00000051716	1.4	0.019	−1.4	0.021
Atp6v0a1	ENSMUSG00000019302	1.2	0.028	−1.3	0.007
Atrnl1	ENSMUSG00000054843	−1.3	0.013	1.3	0.008
Bcas3	ENSMUSG00000059439	1.2	0.034	−1.2	0.035
Col15a1	ENSMUSG00000028339	−1.3	0.013	−1.2	0.029
Cyld	ENSMUSG00000036712	−1.3	0.030	1.3	0.024
E130309D02RIK	ENSMUSG00000039244	1.2	0.015	−1.2	0.027
Fkbp8	ENSMUSG00000019428	1.2	0.045	−1.3	0.020
Inpp1	ENSMUSG00000026102	1.2	0.019	−1.2	0.026
Itgb4	ENSMUSG00000020758	1.3	0.027	−1.2	0.039
Med6	ENSMUSG00000002679	−1.4	0.009	1.3	0.029
Nubpl	ENSMUSG00000035142	1.6	0.014	1.5	0.040
Oxct2a	ENSMUSG00000076436	−1.3	0.024	1.5	0.004
Pgm3	ENSMUSG00000056131	1.2	0.045	−1.3	0.028
Prtg	ENSMUSG00000036030	1.3	0.026	1.2	0.048
Rbp2	ENSMUSG00000032454	1.5	0.036	−1.9	0.001
Sepx1	ENSMUSG00000075705	1.2	0.040	−1.3	0.026
Slc13a3	ENSMUSG00000018459	1.6	0.003	−1.4	0.018
Slc39a5	ENSMUSG00000039878	1.4	0.049	−1.4	0.037
Slc48a1	ENSMUSG00000081534	1.3	0.012	−1.2	0.041
Slc6a13	ENSMUSG00000030108	1.3	0.021	−1.2	0.048
Tomm40	ENSMUSG00000002984	1.4	0.021	−1.5	0.001

[1] The Low and Normal folate diets contained 0.4 and 2.0 mg folic acid/kg diet respectively; [2] For each comparison, data were obtained from three male fetuses from each of six litters from dams fed either the Low or Normal folate diets; [3] A negative fold change indicates lower expression in offspring from dams fed the Low folate diet.

No common KEGG pathways were significantly influenced by maternal folate intake in both the liver and placenta (Tables 2 and 5). Use of PathVisio to interrogate WikiPathways revealed that "Alanine and aspartate metabolism" may be altered in both the fetal liver and the placenta of offspring of folate depleted mothers (Tables 3 and 6). However, different genes in the pathway were differentially expressed in response to maternal folate depletion in the two tissues. In the fetal liver *Agxt* and *Pcx* were up-regulated in response to maternal folate depletion, whilst in the placenta *Abat* and *Asl* were down regulated.

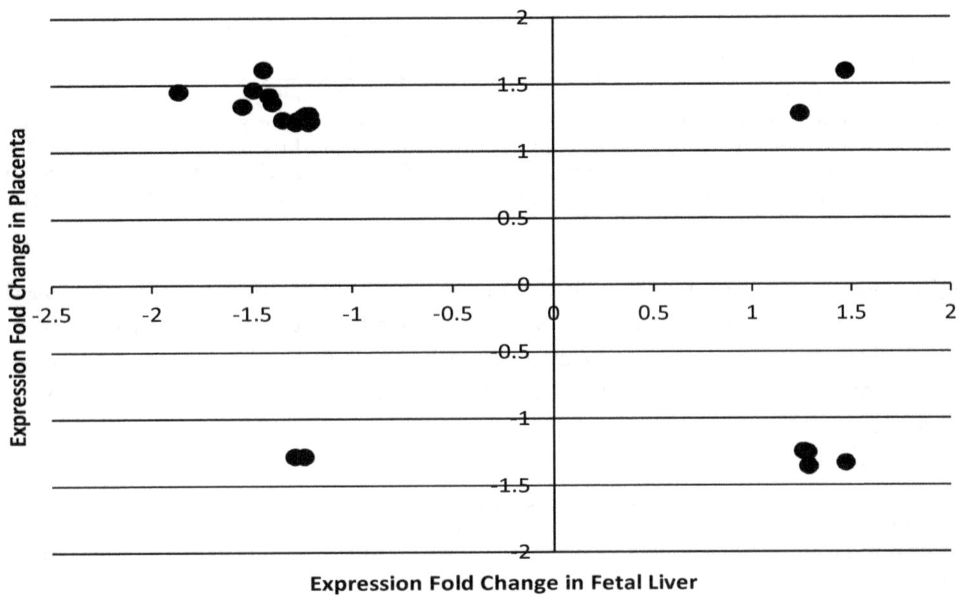

Figure 1. Scatterplot summarising the direction and level of fold change in expression of genes which were altered in both fetal liver and placenta by maternal folate depletion [1,2,3]. [1] The Low and Normal folate diets contained 0.4 and 2.0 mg folic acid/kg diet respectively; [2] For each comparison, data were obtained from three male fetuses from each of six litters from dams fed either the Low or Normal folate diets; [3] A negative fold change indicates lower expression in offspring from dams fed the Low folate diet.

3.5. Validation of Gene Expression Data from Array Analysis by RT-qPCR Analysis

For a subset of genes from both liver and placenta which showed altered expression in response to maternal folate depletion using microarray analysis, data were validated by RT-qPCR. For fetal liver, where the largest fold changes in response to maternal folate depletion were found in down regulated genes, we selected the four most down regulated genes i.e., *Actc1*, *Ckm*, *Tnn2* and *Smpx*. In addition, we analysed the two most up regulated genes i.e., *Hamp* and *Asgr1*. All genes showed the same direction of change using both methods (Table 8) but for 5/6 genes measured by RT-qPCR the change in expression was not statistically significant.

For placenta, fold changes in expression for up- and down-regulated genes in response to maternal folate depletion were similar and so the three genes with the largest fold changes in each direction were selected for validation analysis i.e., *Cyp21a1*, *Hbb-y* and *Slco1b2* for down-regulated genes and *Ptgs2*, *Vcan* and *Lrrn4* for up-regulated genes. In addition, a gene of particular interest, *Mettl7b*, was also selected for RT-PCR analysis. This gene encodes the protein methyltransferase-like 7B, and is likely to have methyltransferase activity (inferred through sequence similarity with other protein methyltransferases (http://www.uniprot.org/uniprot/Q6UX53)), and thus may have a role in epigenetic regulation of gene expression. All seven genes showed the same directional changes in expression in response to maternal folate depletion when assayed by RT-qPCR and by microarray but for 6/7 genes measured by RT-qPCR the change in expression was not statistically significant (Table 9).

Table 8. RT-qPCR expression analysis of selected genes which were differentially expressed in fetal liver in response to maternal folate depletion [1,2] when assayed by microarray.

Gene Name	Mean Expression Low Folate Group	SEM	Mean Expression Normal Folate Group	SEM	*p* Value	Direction of Change in Agreement with Array
Asgr1	0.35	0.07	0.12	0.07	0.050	Yes
Hamp	4.00	0.75	1.73	0.75	0.058	Yes
Actc1	3.63	3.04	8.29	3.04	0.305	Yes
Ckm	1.12	0.95	3.30	0.95	0.134	Yes
Tnnc2	0.51	0.66	2.39	0.66	0.073	Yes
Smpx	0.11	0.09	0.38	0.09	0.066	Yes

[1] The Low and Normal folate diets contained 0.4 and 2.0 mg folic acid/kg diet respectively; [2] For each comparison, data were obtained from three male fetuses from each of six litters from dams fed either the Low or Normal folate diets. Expression values are in arbitrary units calculated using the delta CT method; *GAPDH* was used as the reference gene. Expression levels were quantified in individual fetuses (n = 18 per group) with mean expression levels calculated for individuals litters (n = 6 per group) for use in statistical analyses to match procedures used for array data.

Table 9. RT-qPCR expression analysis of selected genes which were differentially expressed in placenta in response to maternal folate depletion [1,2] when assayed by microarray. Expression values are in arbitrary units calculated using the delta cycle threshold (CT) method. *GAPDH* was used as the reference gene. Expression levels were quantified in individual fetuses (n = 18 per group) with mean expression levels calculated for individuals litters (n = 6 per group) for use in statistical analyses to match procedures used for array data.

Gene Name	Mean Expression Low Folate Group	SEM	Mean Expression Normal Folate Group	SEM	*p* Value	Direction of Change in Agreement with Array
Cyp21a1	0.55	0.13	0.88	0.13	0.118	Yes
Hbb-y	0.39	0.16	0.83	0.16	0.076	Yes
Slco1b2	0.29	0.08	0.49	0.08	0.106	Yes
Ptgs2	0.31	0.03	0.22	0.03	0.030	Yes
Vcan	0.66	0.09	0.46	0.09	0.144	Yes
Lrrn4	0.05	0.01	0.03	0.01	0.118	Yes
Mettl7b	3.07	0.61	4.83	0.61	0.068	Yes

[1] The Low and Normal folate diets contained 0.4 and 2.0 mg folic acid/kg diet respectively; [2] For each comparison, data were obtained from three male fetuses from each of six litters from dams fed either the Low or Normal folate diet.

3.6. Comparison of Gene Expression Changes in Fetal Liver in Response to Maternal Folate Depletion with Similar Published Transcriptomic Studies

Previous studies have reported gene expression changes at the transcriptomic level in the liver of rodents in response to diets low in folate [33–35]. Although several aspects of design differ between studies (summarised in Table 10), to identify a key set of genes in the liver that respond to changes in folate intake (or more broadly, changes in one carbon metabolism), we compared reported changes in gene expression between our data and three other studies [33–35]. Of the 989 genes which were differentially expressed in the fetal liver in response to maternal folate depletion in our study, 4, 89, 90 and 239 genes were also found to be differentially expressed in CBA mice, BALB/c mice, CBA/Ca mice and Wistar rats respectively [33–35] (full list of these genes for individual studies are in Supplementary Materials Table S6). Comparison of the differentially expressed genes from all studies revealed a set of 21 key genes whose expression was affected by altered folate/methyl donor intake in at least four of the five data sets (see Table 11). Importantly, none of the 25 genes which we found were expressed differentially in both fetal liver and placenta in response to maternal folate depletion are in this list of 21 genes.

Table 10. Overview of experimental designs of studies investigating the influence of folate/methyl donor intake on genome wide gene expression in the liver.

Study	Model	Diets	Period of Exposure	Arrays
This study	Male C57Bl6J mice	2 mg folic acid/kg OR	4 weeks prior to mating to 17.5 days gestation	NuGO mouse array (NuGO_Mm1a520177)
		0.4 mg folic acid/kg		
Champier et al. [33]	Male CBA mice	8 mg folic acid + 10 g of succinylsulfathiazole/kg OR	8–12 weeks of age	CodeLinkUniset Mouse Whole Genome bioarrays
		0 mg folic acid + 10 g of succinylsulfathiazole/kg		
Glen et al. [35]	Male BALB/c & CBA/Ca mice	Low methionine (0.18%, w/w) & lacking choline & folic acid OR	4–12 weeks of age	NimbleGen 12 × 135 K Mouse Expression Array
		Low methionine (0.18%, w/w) & supplemented with choline & folic acid		
Chen et al. [34]	Wistar rats	Standard food OR	1 month before pregnancy to 21 days post-weaning	Agilent Arrays
		Diet without vitamin B_{12} & folate		

Table 11. Genes which were differentially expressed in response to low dietary folate/methyl donor intake in the liver across multiple studies [1].

Gene Symbol	Gene Differentially Expressed				
	McKay et al.	Champier et al. [33]	Glen et al. [35] (BALB/c Mice)	Glen et al. [35] (CBA/Ca Mice)	Chen et al. [34]
ACOT2	Y	N	Y	Y	Y
COL6A2	Y	N	Y	Y	Y
CSTB	Y	N	Y	Y	Y
DCTD	Y	N	Y	Y	Y
ENTPD2	Y	N	Y	Y	Y
FETUB	Y	N	Y	Y	Y
FGF21	N	Y	Y	Y	Y
IL7R	Y	N	Y	Y	Y
JUB	Y	N	Y	Y	Y
LTBP2	Y	N	Y	Y	Y
OXCT1	Y	N	Y	Y	Y
RHBDF1	Y	N	Y	Y	Y
RUNX3	Y	N	Y	Y	Y
SERPINE1	Y	N	Y	Y	Y
SLC15A3	Y	N	Y	Y	Y
SLC30A10	Y	N	Y	Y	Y
SLC39A5	Y	N	Y	Y	Y
SLC41A3	Y	N	Y	Y	Y
SLPI	Y	N	Y	Y	Y
SORCS2	Y	N	Y	Y	Y
TMIE	Y	N	Y	Y	Y

[1] For details of diet compositions, please see Table 10. Y = Yes; N = No.

3.7. *In Silico Analysis of Promoter Regions of Key Folate/Methyl Donor Responsive Genes for Transcription Factor Binding Sites*

For these 21 genes found to be affected robustly in liver by altered folate supply (Table 11), 76 unique promoter regions were found for 130 transcripts using the Gene2Promoter function in Genomatix (data not shown). Transcription factor binding sites for five families of transcription factors were present in 90% of the promoters investigated; ETS1 factors (ETSF), Kruppel like transcription factors (KLFS), Nuclear receptor subfamily 2 factors (NR2F), RXR heterodimer binding site (RXRF) and SOX/SRY sex/testis determining and related HMG box factors (SORY). Of these, the RXRF transcription factors had binding sites in all 76 analysed promoters. TFs belonging to the five identified families were compared with TFs found to be differentially expressed in the fetal liver and five TFs were found to overlap viz. *Elk3, Nr2c1, Nr2f1, Rxra, and Sox30.*

However the same analysis on randomly-selected sets of 21 genes that were affected by folate supply from each of the five studies plus two sets of 21 genes that did not respond to maternal folate supply revealed similar occurrence rates for these same transcription factor binding sites. Thus, this analysis identified no potential transcriptional regulatory mechanisms which may be responsible exclusively for coordinating the liver-specific changes in expression of these key genes in response to folate supply.

4. Discussion

Here we describe gene expression changes at the transcriptome level in the placenta and fetal liver in response to maternal folate depletion before mating and throughout pregnancy. Ames' triage theory posits that if availability of a specific nutrient is inadequate, Darwinian processes ensure that essential functions, i.e., those required for short-term survival and/or reproduction, dependent on that nutrient that are protected at the expense of those functions that are less essential i.e., where reduced function does not have short term negative consequences. However, such prioritisation of some most critical (short-term) functions may impact adversely on other functions which may have long-term insidious effects that increase risk of diseases associated with ageing [23,24]. In response to inadequate maternal folate intake during pregnancy, we hypothesised that, due to different organ-specific functions, individual fetal organs would implement differential prioritisation hierarchies and thus display differential gene expression changes in response to folate depletion. We chose to investigate gene expression in the liver and placenta as examples of organs with very different roles in mammalian function across the lifecourse. In addition, the liver represents a major site for folate storage and metabolism, whilst the placenta (containing both maternal and fetal cells) is the route for delivery of nutrients (including folate) from the dam to the fetus during development. Our observations support our hypothesis that specific fetal organs exhibit specific transcriptional responses to maternal folate depletion. It is plausible that these organ-specific changes in gene expression are due to differential pathway prioritisation in each organ which reflect their contrasting functions.

The primary function of the placenta is the transfer of nutrients to the fetus, so it is essential that this function is protected to support fetal growth and development. In response to maternal folate depletion, we saw no changes in pathways associated with nutrient transport, suggesting that placental transfer of nutrients to the fetus was protected despite the reduced maternal folate intake. We observed no teratogenic effects of this reduced nutrient supply on the offspring [25]. It is important to note that we analysed whole placental samples containing both maternal and fetal cell populations and so we are unable to determine the cellular origin of the observed expression changes.

The liver is a highly metabolic organ responsible for a wide range of functions that are important at all life stages and include defence of the body against xenobiotics, assisting with digestion and with metabolism of absorbed nutrients, regulating blood lipids, synthesis of a wide range of secreted proteins and hormonal regulation. As such, during periods of undernutrition, it may not be possible for the liver to maintain all important functions, so that those functions essential for short-term survival and/or reproduction may be prioritised. The sequela is that some functions not critical for short-term survival but which are important for long term health may be de-prioritised leading to impaired function which may have significant long-term adverse effects for the organism. We observed that maternal folate depletion altered several processes and pathways, each of which could impact adversely on long-term liver function and organismal health. These included "adipogenesis genes", "fatty acid biosynthesis" and "iron homeostasis" pathways. Whilst only one time point was investigated here (so that we are unable to comment on long-term gene expression changes or phenotypic outcomes), these observations are consistent with the fact that diets deficient in folate and choline can induce non-alcoholic fatty liver disease (NAFLD) in rodent models [36]. We observed up-regulation of genes involved in "fatty acid biosynthesis" (5/5 differentially expressed genes present on the pathway), and an abundance of up-regulated genes involved in the "adipogenesis genes" pathway (10/16 differentially expressed genes present on the pathway). Up-regulation of these genes may result in overall up-regulation of the pathways that potentially could result in altered hepatic fatty acid metabolism in offspring. Indeed, we observed that when the offspring of folate depleted dams were fed a high fat diet from weaning [37], they had significantly increased plasma triacylglycerol (TAG) concentrations whilst plasma TAG concentrations were unaffected in the offspring of folate replete dams [37]. Taken together, these data suggest that maternal folate depletion results in an altered response to high fat feeding which may be via programmed transcriptional changes in pathways associated with fat metabolism in the liver.

This analysis has focussed on the genes which were differentially expressed in the liver and in the placenta in response to maternal folate depletion. However, it is important to recognise that there are alternative explanations for genes which did not change in response to this nutritional insult. Whilst such unaltered genes may be components of pathways which are especially critical to that particular organ, it is also possible that these genes are simply unresponsive to folate supply. The present study design is unable to distinguish between these alternatives.

It is important to highlight that most of the gene expression changes observed in this study were relatively small and not statistically significant when applying the more stringent FDR value so that these data should be interpreted with caution. However, our observations are consistent with findings from other studies [33,34] and confirms the subtle, but pervasive, effects on gene expression of folate/methyl donor depletion. Furthermore, it is pertinent to point out that our gene expression studies were undertaken in male offspring only and it is possible, if theoretically unlikely, that effects could be different in females.

Whilst we show clearly that folate responsive gene expression changes are organ specific, the mechanisms behind the observed organ specific expression changes are less clear. A plausible mechanistic explanation could be based on inter-organ differences in expression of transcription factors (TFs) when exposed to inadequate folate intake. We tested this hypothesis by identifying all TFs which were differentially expressed in the liver and in the placenta in response to maternal folate depletion. In the fetal liver, we found that expression of 73 TFs differed in folate replete vs. folate depleted offspring, which accounted for 7.4% of the altered genes. In contrast, in the placenta only 22 TFs (4.8% of altered genes) displayed altered expression. Consistent with the idea that organ-specific changes in gene expression profiles are driven by organ-specific changes in TF expression, there was very little overlap between the TFs that were altered in liver and placenta—only one TF, *Med6*, was common between the organs.

It is plausible that changes in epigenetic processes are responsible for the organ-specific patterns in gene expression in response to folate depletion. Epigenetic marks, including DNA methylation, are modifiable by diet and other environmental factors and constitute an important and flexible system for regulating gene expression [38,39]. Folate is central to one-carbon metabolism and the formation of the universal methyl donor SAM, which is critical for the methylation of biological molecules including DNA. Indeed the influence of dietary folate intake on DNA methylation patterns has been reported widely [25,34,40–42] and may be responsible for the organ specific folate responsive gene expression changes observed here.

Although previous studies have reported gene specific expression changes in the rat placenta in response to increased levels of folate in the maternal diet [42,43], to the best of our knowledge this is the first report describing gene expression changes in response to low maternal folate (or methyl donor) intake in this organ, and the first study to investigate this at the transcriptomic level. However, previous studies have used transcriptomic approaches to investigate gene expression changes in the liver in response to low folate-containing diets [33–36,44,45] so we compared our data with outcomes from these studies. Whilst there were differences in gene expression profiles between studies, likely to be due to differences in rodent models, diet composition, duration and timing of the nutrient insult and the particular transcriptomic approaches employed (Table 10), we uncovered a key set of genes which were differentially expressed in the liver in response to low dietary folate/methyl donor intake across multiple studies (Table 11). Importantly, expression of none of these genes was altered in placenta by maternal folate depletion, indicating that these changes reflect a liver-specific response rather than being genes that are generally malleable in response to perturbation in folate supply. Moreover, this observation substantiates our suggestion that the transcriptome responses of fetal liver and placenta to folate restriction are distinct and physiologically-appropriate. Of the key set of 21 genes differentially expressed across multiple studies (Table 11), the use of DAVID [32] to carry out Gene Ontology enrichment analysis suggested that three genes are involved in wound healing i.e., *JUB*, *ENTPD2* and *SERPINE1* and, thus, altered transcription of genes associated with wound healing may help explain the observed association between low methyl donor intake and liver damage [36]. Furthermore, the discovery of these key folate responsive genes may provide candidate biomarkers for future studies of folate adequacy. Such studies should test the effects of different doses of folate without potential confounding from other dietary factors which may have been an issue in some of the studies included in Table 10.

To investigate potential mechanisms through which expression of these key genes in the liver are altered in response to methyl donor intake, the promoter regions were interrogated for the presence of common transcription factor binding sites. Whilst binding sites for five families of transcription factors were found to be highly represented in the promoters of these 21 genes, similar occurrence rates of these same transcription factor binding sites were also observed when seven randomly selected sets of genes were analysed. This suggests that this specific set of TFs is not responsible for co-ordinating transcriptional responses to maternal folate/methyl-donor supply in the liver. However, it is possible that there are regulatory regions outside the promoters of the genes investigated here which would merit investigation in future studies.

5. Conclusions

The data presented here suggest that maternal folate status during pregnancy influences gene expression in the fetus in a highly organ-specific manner. We hypothesise that this organ specificity is a rational response to limited nutrient supply which protects the most essential functions of each individual organ for short term survival (and reproduction), at the expense of less immediately essential processes which may lead to long-term adverse health sequelae. However, as we have noted above, there are viable alternative explanations for our observations. Our observations are consistent with the DOHaD hypothesis and suggest a plausible mechanism by which inadequate folate supply during early development leads to changes in gene expression to protect functions of the liver that are appropriate in this particular developmental and nutritional context, but that may contribute to the aetiology of cardiometabolic diseases if the postnatal environment is such that these changes become disadvantageous.

Supplementary Materials:
Table S1: Details of manufacturer's product codes for primers used to determine gene transcript levels by RT-qPCR, Table S2: List of genes differentially expressed in the fetal liver in reponse to low maternal folate. Genes were considered to be significantly differentially expressed in response to low maternal folate if (a) the p value for t-test between dietary groups was < 0.05 and (b) if there was a fold change of ±1.2, Table S3: List of genes encoding transcription factors differentially expressed in the fetal liver in reponse to low maternal folate. Genes were considered to be significantly differentially expressed in response to low maternal folate if (a) the p value for t-test between dietary groups was < 0.05 and (b) if there was a fold change of ±1.2. B1, Table S4: List of genes differentially expressed in the placenta in reponse to low maternal folate. Genes were considered to be significantly differentially expressed in response to low maternal folate if (a) the p value for t-test between dietary groups was < 0.05 and (b) if there was a fold change of ±1.2.D1, Table S5: List of genes encoding transcription factors differentially expressed in the placenta in reponse to low maternal folate. Genes were considered to be significantly differentially expressed in response to low maternal folate if (a) the p value for t-test between dietary groups was < 0.05 and (b) if there was a fold change of ±1.2, Table S6: Lists of genes found in in common with other published data sets. Genes found to be differentially expressed in response to maternal folate depletion in the fetal liver were compared to other published gene lists where diets low in folate were reported to alter gene expression in the liver.

Acknowledgments: We thank Sandra Hogg, CBC, Newcastle University for care of the animals. This project was funded by NuGO ('The European Nutrigenomics Organisation; linking genomics, nutrition and health research', NuGO; CT-2004-505944) and the BBSRC (BB/G007993/1), with additional salary support from the North of England Children's Cancer Research Fund (NECCR).

Author Contributions: J.A.M., D.F. & J.C.M. conceived and designed the experiments; J.A.M. and L.X. performed the experiments; J.A.M. and M.A. analysed the data; J.A.M., D.F., C.E. and J.C.M. contributed reagents/materials/analysis tools; J.A.M., D.F. and J.C.M. wrote the paper, with contributions from M.A., C.E. and L.X., J.A.M. and J.C.M. had primary responsibility for final content. All authors have read and approved the final manuscript.

References

1. Gluckman, P.D.; Hanson, M.A.; Cooper, C.; Thornburg, K.L. Effect of in utero and early-life conditions on adult health and disease. *N. Engl. J. Med.* **2008**, *359*, 61–73. [CrossRef] [PubMed]
2. Bateson, P.; Barker, D.; Clutton-Brock, T.; Deb, D.; D'Udine, B.; Foley, R.A.; Gluckman, P.; Godfrey, K.; Kirkwood, T.; Lahr, M.M.; et al. Developmental plasticity and human health. *Nature* **2004**, *430*, 419–421. [CrossRef] [PubMed]
3. Gluckman, P.D.; Hanson, M.A.; Morton, S.M.; Pinal, C.S. Life-long echoes-a critical analysis of the developmental origins of adult disease model. *Biol. Neonate* **2005**, *87*, 127–139. [CrossRef] [PubMed]

4. Blencowe, H.; Cousens, S.; Modell, B.; Lawn, J. Folic acid to reduce neonatal mortality from neural tube disorders. *Int. J. Epidemiol.* **2010**, *39* (Suppl. S1), i110–i121. [CrossRef] [PubMed]
5. De-Regil, L.M.; Fernandez-Gaxiola, A.C.; Dowswell, T.; Pena-Rosas, J.P. Effects and safety of periconceptional folate supplementation for preventing birth defects. *Cochrane Database Syst. Rev.* **2010**, Cd007950. [CrossRef]
6. Botto, L.D.; Olney, R.S.; Erickson, J.D. Vitamin supplements and the risk for congenital anomalies other than neural tube defects. *Am. J. Med. Genet. Part C Semin. Med. Genet.* **2004**, *125c*, 12–21. [CrossRef] [PubMed]
7. Bortolus, R.; Blom, F.; Filippini, F.; van Poppel, M.N.; Leoncini, E.; de Smit, D.J.; Benetollo, P.P.; Cornel, M.C.; de Walle, H.E.; Mastroiacovo, P. Prevention of congenital malformations and other adverse pregnancy outcomes with 4.0 mg of folic acid: Community-based randomized clinical trial in Italy and the Netherlands. *BMC Pregnancy Childbirth* **2014**, *14*, 166. [CrossRef] [PubMed]
8. Chatzi, L.; Papadopoulou, E.; Koutra, K.; Roumeliotaki, T.; Georgiou, V.; Stratakis, N.; Lebentakou, V.; Karachaliou, M.; Vassilaki, M.; Kogevinas, M. Effect of high doses of folic acid supplementation in early pregnancy on child neurodevelopment at 18 months of age: The mother-child cohort 'rhea' study in crete, greece. *Public Health Nutr.* **2012**, *15*, 1728–1736. [CrossRef] [PubMed]
9. Roth, C.; Magnus, P.; Schjolberg, S.; Stoltenberg, C.; Suren, P.; McKeague, I.W.; Davey, S.G.; Reichborn-Kjennerud, T.; Susser, E. Folic acid supplements in pregnancy and severe language delay in children. *JAMA* **2011**, *306*, 1566–1573. [CrossRef] [PubMed]
10. Schmidt, R.J.; Tancredi, D.J.; Ozonoff, S.; Hansen, R.L.; Hartiala, J.; Allayee, H.; Schmidt, L.C.; Tassone, F.; Hertz-Picciotto, I. Maternal periconceptional folic acid intake and risk of autism spectrum disorders and developmental delay in the charge (childhood autism risks from genetics and environment) case-control study. *Am. J. Clin. Nutr.* **2012**, *96*, 80–89. [CrossRef] [PubMed]
11. Suren, P.; Roth, C.; Bresnahan, M.; Haugen, M.; Hornig, M.; Hirtz, D.; Lie, K.K.; Lipkin, W.I.; Magnus, P.; Reichborn-Kjennerud, T.; et al. Association between maternal use of folic acid supplements and risk of autism spectrum disorders in children. *JAMA* **2013**, *309*, 570–577. [CrossRef] [PubMed]
12. Amigou, A.; Rudant, J.; Orsi, L.; Goujon-Bellec, S.; Leverger, G.; Baruchel, A.; Bertrand, Y.; Nelken, B.; Plat, G.; Michel, G.; et al. Folic acid supplementation, mthfr and mtrr polymorphisms, and the risk of childhood leukemia: The escale study (sfce). *Cancer Causes Control (CCC)* **2012**, *23*, 1265–1277. [CrossRef] [PubMed]
13. Bailey, H.D.; Miller, M.; Langridge, A.; de Klerk, N.H.; van Bockxmeer, F.M.; Attia, J.; Scott, R.J.; Armstrong, B.K.; Milne, E. Maternal dietary intake of folate and vitamins B6 and B12 during pregnancy and the risk of childhood acute lymphoblastic leukemia. *Nutr. Cancer* **2012**, *64*, 1122–1130. [CrossRef] [PubMed]
14. Metayer, C.; Milne, E.; Dockerty, J.D.; Clavel, J.; Pombo-de-Oliveira, M.S.; Wesseling, C.; Spector, L.G.; Schuz, J.; Petridou, E.; Ezzat, S.; et al. Maternal supplementation with folic acid and other vitamins and risk of leukemia in offspring: A childhood leukemia international consortium study. *Epidemiology* **2014**, *25*, 811–822. [CrossRef] [PubMed]
15. Greenop, K.R.; Miller, M.; de Klerk, N.H.; Scott, R.J.; Attia, J.; Ashton, L.J.; Dalla-Pozza, L.; Bower, C.; Armstrong, B.K.; Milne, E. Maternal dietary intake of folate and vitamins B6 and B12 during pregnancy and risk of childhood brain tumors. *Nutr. Cancer* **2014**, *66*, 800–809. [CrossRef] [PubMed]
16. Milne, E.; Greenop, K.R.; Bower, C.; Miller, M.; van Bockxmeer, F.M.; Scott, R.J.; de Klerk, N.H.; Ashton, L.J.; Gottardo, N.G.; Armstrong, B.K. Maternal use of folic acid and other supplements and risk of childhood brain tumors. *Cancer Epidemiol. Biomark. Prev.* **2012**, *21*, 1933–1941. [CrossRef] [PubMed]
17. French, A.E.; Grant, R.; Weitzman, S.; Ray, J.G.; Vermeulen, M.J.; Sung, L.; Greenberg, M.; Koren, G. Folic acid food fortification is associated with a decline in neuroblastoma. *Clin. Pharmacol. Ther.* **2003**, *74*, 288–294. [CrossRef]
18. Goh, Y.I.; Bollano, E.; Einarson, T.R.; Koren, G. Prenatal multivitamin supplementation and rates of pediatric cancers: A meta-analysis. *Clin. Pharmacol. Ther.* **2007**, *81*, 685–691. [CrossRef] [PubMed]
19. Burgoon, J.M.; Selhub, J.; Nadeau, M.; Sadler, T.W. Investigation of the effects of folate deficiency on embryonic development through the establishment of a folate deficient mouse model. *Teratology* **2002**, *65*, 219–227. [CrossRef] [PubMed]
20. Heid, M.K.; Bills, N.D.; Hinrichs, S.H.; Clifford, A.J. Folate deficiency alone does not produce neural tube defects in mice. *J. Nutr.* **1992**, *122*, 888–894. [PubMed]
21. Locasale, J.W. Serine, glycine and one-carbon units: Cancer metabolism in full circle. *Nat. Rev. Cancer* **2013**, *13*, 572–583. [CrossRef] [PubMed]

22. Anderson, O.S.; Sant, K.E.; Dolinoy, D.C. Nutrition and epigenetics: An interplay of dietary methyl donors, one-carbon metabolism and DNA methylation. *J. Nutr. Biochem.* **2012**, *23*, 853–859. [CrossRef] [PubMed]
23. Ames, B.N. Low micronutrient intake may accelerate the degenerative diseases of aging through allocation of scarce micronutrients by triage. *Proc. Natl. Acad. Sci. USA* **2006**, *103*, 17589–17594. [CrossRef] [PubMed]
24. McCann, J.C.; Ames, B.N. Adaptive dysfunction of selenoproteins from the perspective of the triage theory: Why modest selenium deficiency may increase risk of diseases of aging. *FASEB J. Off. Publ. Fed. Am. Soc. Exp. Biol.* **2011**, *25*, 1793–1814. [CrossRef] [PubMed]
25. McKay, J.A.; Wong, Y.K.; Relton, C.L.; Ford, D.; Mathers, J.C. Maternal folate supply and sex influence gene-specific DNA methylation in the fetal gut. *Mol. Nutr. Food Res.* **2011**, *55*, 1717–1723. [CrossRef] [PubMed]
26. Reeves, P.G.; Nielsen, F.H.; Fahey, G.C., Jr. Ain-93 purified diets for laboratory rodents: Final report of the American institute of nutrition ad hoc writing committee on the reformulation of the Ain-76a rodent diet. *J. Nutr.* **1993**, *123*, 1939–1951. [PubMed]
27. McClive, P.J.; Sinclair, A.H. Rapid DNA extraction and PCR-sexing of mouse embryos. *Mol. Reprod. Dev.* **2001**, *60*, 225–226. [CrossRef] [PubMed]
28. Gautier, L.; Cope, L.; Bolstad, B.M.; Irizarry, R.A. Affy—Analysis of affymetrix genechip data at the probe level. *Bioinformatics* **2004**, *20*, 307–315. [CrossRef] [PubMed]
29. Wu, Z.; Irizarry, R.A.; Gentleman, R.; Murillo, F.M.; Forrest, S. A model-based background adjustment for oligonucleotide expression arrays. *J. Am. Stat. Assoc.* **2004**, *99*, 909–917. [CrossRef]
30. Dai, M.; Wang, P.; Boyd, A.D.; Kostov, G.; Athey, B.; Jones, E.G.; Bunney, W.E.; Myers, R.M.; Speed, T.P.; Akil, H.; et al. Evolving gene/transcript definitions significantly alter the interpretation of genechip data. *Nucleic Acids Res.* **2005**, *33*, e175. [CrossRef] [PubMed]
31. Smyth, G.K. Linear models and empirical bayes methods for assessing differential expression in microarray experiments. *Stat. Appl. Genet. Mol. Biol.* **2004**, *3*. [CrossRef] [PubMed]
32. Sherman, B.T.; Huang, D.W.; Tan, Q.; Guo, Y.; Bour, S.; Liu, D.; Stephens, R.; Baseler, M.W.; Lane, H.C.; Lempicki, R.A. David knowledgebase: A gene-centered database integrating heterogeneous gene annotation resources to facilitate high-throughput gene functional analysis. *BMC Bioinform.* **2007**, *8*, 426. [CrossRef] [PubMed]
33. Champier, J.; Claustrat, F.; Nazaret, N.; Fevre, M.M.; Claustrat, B. Folate depletion changes gene expression of fatty acid metabolism, DNA synthesis, and circadian cycle in male mice. *Nutr. Res.* **2012**, *32*, 124–132. [CrossRef] [PubMed]
34. Chen, G.; Broseus, J.; Hergalant, S.; Donnart, A.; Chevalier, C.; Bolanos-Jimenez, F.; Gueant, J.L.; Houlgatte, R. Identification of master genes involved in liver key functions through transcriptomics and epigenomics of methyl donor deficiency in rat: Relevance to nonalcoholic liver disease. *Mol. Nutr. Food Res.* **2015**, *59*, 293–302. [CrossRef] [PubMed]
35. Glen, C.D.; McVeigh, L.E.; Voutounou, M.; Dubrova, Y.E. The effects of methyl-donor deficiency on the pattern of gene expression in mice. *Mol. Nutr. Food Res.* **2015**, *59*, 501–506. [CrossRef] [PubMed]
36. Tryndyak, V.; de Conti, A.; Kobets, T.; Kutanzi, K.; Koturbash, I.; Han, T.; Fuscoe, J.C.; Latendresse, J.R.; Melnyk, S.; Shymonyak, S.; et al. Interstrain differences in the severity of liver injury induced by a choline- and folate-deficient diet in mice are associated with dysregulation of genes involved in lipid metabolism. *FASEB J. Off. Publ. Fed. Am. Soc. Exp. Biol.* **2012**, *26*, 4592–4602. [CrossRef] [PubMed]
37. McKay, J.A.; Xie, L.; Manus, C.; Langie, S.A.; Maxwell, R.J.; Ford, D.; Mathers, J.C. Metabolic effects of a high-fat diet post-weaning after low maternal dietary folate during pregnancy and lactation. *Mol. Nutr. Food Res.* **2014**, *58*, 1087–1097. [CrossRef] [PubMed]
38. McKay, J.A.; Mathers, J.C. Diet induced epigenetic changes and their implications for health. *Acta Physiol.* **2011**, *202*, 103–118. [CrossRef] [PubMed]
39. Mathers, J.C.; Strathdee, G.; Relton, C.L. Induction of epigenetic alterations by dietary and other environmental factors. *Adv. Genet.* **2010**, *71*, 3–39. [PubMed]
40. McKay, J.A.; Waltham, K.J.; Williams, E.A.; Mathers, J.C. Folate depletion during pregnancy and lactation reduces genomic DNA methylation in murine adult offspring. *Genes Nutr.* **2011**, *6*, 189–196. [CrossRef] [PubMed]
41. McKay, J.A.; Xie, L.; Harris, S.; Wong, Y.K.; Ford, D.; Mathers, J.C. Blood as a surrogate marker for tissue-specific DNA methylation and changes due to folate depletion in post-partum female mice. *Mol. Nutr. Food Res.* **2011**, *55*, 1026–1035. [CrossRef] [PubMed]

42. Penailillo, R.; Guajardo, A.; Llanos, M.; Hirsch, S.; Ronco, A.M. Folic acid supplementation during pregnancy induces sex-specific changes in methylation and expression of placental 11beta-hydroxysteroid dehydrogenase 2 in rats. *PLoS ONE* **2015**, *10*, e0121098. [CrossRef] [PubMed]
43. Khot, V.; Kale, A.; Joshi, A.; Chavan-Gautam, P.; Joshi, S. Expression of genes encoding enzymes involved in the one carbon cycle in rat placenta is determined by maternal micronutrients (folic acid, vitamin b12) and omega-3 fatty acids. *BioMed Res. Int.* **2014**, *2014*, 613078. [CrossRef] [PubMed]
44. Christensen, K.E.; Wu, Q.; Wang, X.; Deng, L.; Caudill, M.A.; Rozen, R. Steatosis in mice is associated with gender, folate intake, and expression of genes of one-carbon metabolism. *J. Nutr.* **2010**, *140*, 1736–1741. [CrossRef] [PubMed]
45. Meher, A.; Joshi, A.; Joshi, S. Differential regulation of hepatic transcription factors in the wistar rat offspring born to dams fed folic acid, vitamin b12 deficient diets and supplemented with omega-3 fatty acids. *PLoS ONE* **2014**, *9*, e90209. [CrossRef] [PubMed]

6

Impact of Pre-Pregnancy BMI on B Vitamin and Inflammatory Status in Early Pregnancy

Anne-Lise Bjørke-Monsen [1,*], Arve Ulvik [2], Roy M. Nilsen [3], Øivind Midttun [2], Christine Roth [4,5], Per Magnus [4], Camilla Stoltenberg [4,6], Stein Emil Vollset [4,6], Ted Reichborn-Kjennerud [4,7] and Per Magne Ueland [1,8]

1 Laboratory of Clinical Biochemistry, Haukeland University Hospital, 5021 Bergen, Norway; per.ueland@ikb.uib.no
2 Bevital AS, 5021 Bergen, Norway; Arve.Ulvik@uib.no (A.U.); oivind.midttun@bevital.no (Ø.M.)
3 Centre for Clinical Research, Haukeland University Hospital, 5021 Bergen, Norway; Roy.Nilsen@uib.no
4 The Norwegian Institute of Public Health, 0403 Oslo, Norway; Christine.Roth@fhi.no (C.R.); Per.Magnus@fhi.no (P.M.); camilla.stoltenberg@fhi.no (C.S.); SteinEmil.Vollset@fhi.no (S.E.V.); Ted.Reichborn-Kjennerud@fhi.no (T.R.-K.)
5 Nic Waals Institute, Lovisenberg Hospital, Oslo 0456, Norway
6 Department of Public Health and Primary Health Care, University of Bergen, 5007 Bergen, Norway
7 Institute of Clinical Medicine, University of Oslo, 0313 Oslo, Norway
8 Department of Clinical Science, University of Bergen, 5007 Bergen, Norway
* Correspondance: almo@helse-bergen.no

Abstract: Maternal nutrition and inflammation have been suggested as mediators in the development of various adverse pregnancy outcomes associated with maternal obesity. We have investigated the relation between pre-pregnancy BMI, B vitamin status, and inflammatory markers in a group of healthy pregnant women. Cobalamin, folate, pyridoxal 5′-phosphate, and riboflavin; and the metabolic markers homocysteine, methylmalonic acid, and 3-hydroxykynurenine/xanthurenic acid ratio (HK/XA); and markers of cellular inflammation, neopterin and kynurenine/tryptophan ratio (KTR) were determined in pregnancy week 18 and related to pre-pregnancy body mass index (BMI), in 2797 women from the Norwegian Mother and Child Cohort Study (MoBa). Pre-pregnancy BMI was inversely related to folate, cobalamin, pyridoxal 5′-phosphate (PLP), and riboflavin ($p < 0.001$), and associated with increased neopterin and KTR levels ($p < 0.001$). Inflammation seemed to be an independent predictor of low vitamin B6 status, as verified by low PLP and high HK/XA ratio. A high pre-pregnancy BMI is a risk factor for low B vitamin status and increased cellular inflammation. As an optimal micronutrient status is vital for normal fetal development, the observed lower B vitamin levels may contribute to adverse pregnancy outcomes associated with maternal obesity and B vitamin status should be assessed in women with high BMI before they get pregnant.

Keywords: pregnancy; obesity; pre-pregnancy BMI; B vitamins; inflammation

1. Introduction

There is an increasing prevalence of obesity in most parts of the world, also affecting women of childbearing age [1]. Pre-pregnancy obesity is associated with an increased risk of adverse pregnancy outcomes for both mother and child, including subfertility, miscarriage, gestational diabetes, gestational hypertension, preeclampsia, macrosomia, preterm birth, congenital anomalies, and fetal death [2,3]. Epidemiological studies have revealed strong links between nutritional excess during pregnancy and later development of metabolic disease, such as type 2 diabetes and obesity, in adult life [4]. Maternal metabolic, nutritional, and inflammatory factors have been suggested as mediators in the development of the various negative pregnancy outcomes associated with maternal obesity.

A higher body mass index (BMI) has been associated with an adverse nutritional status in both non-pregnant adults [5–7] and children [8,9]. An inverse relation between pre-pregnancy BMI and several micronutrients like folate, vitamin D, carotenoids, zinc, and essential fatty acids have been reported in pregnant women, and negative pregnancy outcomes related to obesity might be related to impaired micronutrient status [10–13]. An adequate B vitamin status during pregnancy is important for maternal health and normal fetal development [14]. Deficiencies of folate, cobalamin, riboflavin, or vitamin B6 are associated with an increased risk of placental abruption, still-births, low birth weight, preterm deliveries, preeclampsia, as well as fetal malformations [14].

Obesity in itself results in an inflammatory state in metabolic tissues [15], and higher levels of the inflammatory markers C-reactive protein, neopterin, and kynurenine/tryptophan ratio (KTR) are seen in overweight and obese adults [16,17]. Inflammation has been associated with low circulating levels of several micronutrients [18], such as the active form of vitamin B_6, pyridoxal 5′-phosphate (PLP) [19], and vitamin D [20].

The objective of the study was to investigate whether BMI and inflammation are independent determinants of B vitamin status, we investigated the association of pre-pregnancy BMI with plasma B vitamin status and inflammatory markers in pregnancy week 18 in 2797 women from the Norwegian Mother and Child Cohort Study (MoBa).

2. Experimental Section

2.1. Study Population

This study is based on a subsample of 2825 women included in the Norwegian Mother and Child Cohort Study (MoBa), a long-term, prospective study conducted by the Norwegian Institute of Public Health and including more than 100,000 Norwegian pregnant women and their infants during 1999–2008 [21]. The women included in this sub-study of MoBa gave a singleton birth between July 2002 and December 2003, and returned a baseline questionnaire including data on height and pre-pregnancy weight and donated a blood sample in pregnancy week 18, and were registered in the Medical Birth Registry of Norway. A detailed description of this sub population and the sampling procedures has been published [22].

2.2. Ethics

Written informed consent was obtained from each participant, and the study was approved by the Regional Committee for Medical Research Ethics Sør-Øst A, 19/10-2011 (permission number 2009/2593a) and the Norwegian Data Inspectorate. All questions used in the MoBa can be found online at www.fhi.no/morogbarn.

2.3. Blood Sampling and Laboratory Analyses

Maternal non-fasting blood samples were collected in ethylenediamine tetraacetic acid (EDTA) tubes in median pregnancy week 18. The samples were centrifuged within 30 min after collection and stored at 4 °C until shipped overnight to the Norwegian Institute of Public Health in Oslo. On the day of receipt (usually within 1–2 days), plasma was aliquoted into polypropylene microtiter plates and stored at −80 °C until analyses.

Plasma folate was determined by a *Lactobacillus casei* microbiological assay [23] and plasma cobalamin (vitamin B12) by a *Lactobacillus leichmannii* microbiological assay [24]. Concurrent intake of antibiotics may interfere with microbiological assays and cause falsely reduced plasma levels of the vitamins [25], and samples with plasma folate levels <2.33 nmol/L were excluded (n = 28, i.e., the lower one percentile), leaving a total of 2797 samples to be included in the study.

Plasma levels of total homocysteine (tHcy), a marker of folate and cobalamin status, and methylmalonic acid (MMA), a marker of cobalamin status, were assayed using a GC-MS method based on methylchloroformate derivatization [26]. Plasma levels of riboflavin (vitamin B2); pyridoxal 5′-phosphate (PLP; vitamin B6); the ratio between 3-hydroxykynurenine and xanthurenic acid (HK/XA), a marker of vitamin B6 status [27]; and two markers of interferon-gamma mediated cellular immune activation, neopterin [28] and KTR (Kynurenine/Tryptophan × 1000)—the latter reflecting indoleamine-2,3-dioxygenase (IDO) activation [29]—were analyzed using a liquid chromatography-tandem mass spectrometry assay [30]. All biomarkers were measured at the laboratory of Bevital AS (www.bevital.no).

2.4. Covariates

Data on maternal age at delivery, marital status, and parity were obtained from the Medical Birth Registry of Norway. Data on maternal education, smoking habits, pre-pregnancy BMI, weight increase to pregnancy week 18, and use of supplements were obtained from the self-reported baseline cohort questionnaire. Pre-pregnancy BMI (kg/m^2) was coded as <18.5, 18.5–24.9, 25.0–29.9, 30.0–34.9, and ≥35.0. Use of supplements was coded as non-user, use of folic acid or other supplement, and use of folic acid plus other supplement, based on reported intake from four weeks prior to conception up to pregnancy week 18. A B vitamin summary score was calculated as a sum of quintiles for folate, cobalamin, PLP, and riboflavin.

2.5. Statistical Analyses

Values are presented as means with standard deviation (SD) or medians with the interquartile range. Differences between groups were examined by ANOVA, Mann-Whitney U test and the Kruskal Wallis test. Differences in categorical variables were assessed with the Chi-square test. Multiple-linear regression models were used to assess the relation between pre-pregnancy BMI, use of supplements, parity, age, and inflammation with plasma B vitamin status obtained around pregnancy week 18. The odds ratio (ORs) for having a low B vitamin status (quintile 1) according to maternal factors, including the inflammation marker neopterin, was assessed by logistic regression.

To explore non-linearity, we modeled pre-pregnancy BMI versus B vitamins and metabolic markers, using one-dimensional smoothing splines in Generalized Additive Models (GAM), in a model adjusted for adjusted for use of supplements, maternal age, parity, and neopterin.

GAMs were computed using the package mgcv (version 1.4–1) in R (The R Foundation for Statistical Computing, version 2.8.1, Vienna, Austria) [31], and the SPSS/PASW statistical program version 22 (IBM Corp, Armonk, NY, USA).the company, the city, the country) was used for all other statistical analyses. Two-sided p-values < 0.05 were considered statistically significant.

3. Results

3.1. Characteristics of the Study Population According to Pre-Pregnancy BMI

Demographic characteristics according to pre-pregnancy BMI are presented in Table 1. Fifty-eight percent of the women were multipara, and had a mean number of 1.5 (SD 0.7) former children, with no difference according to BMI group ($p = 0.14$). The majority of the women were healthy, a low percentage (0.7%) had chronic hypertension and 2% had had IVF treatment. The use of multivitamin supplements differed according to BMI group, with an increasing trend for not using any supplements with higher BMI ($p < 0.001$). Regular use of alcohol was rare and 96% reported drinking alcohol never or less than once a month after becoming pregnant. A total of 231 (8%) women reported daily smoking with a mean number of seven (SD five) cigarettes per day, with no significant difference in number between the smokers in the various BMI groups ($p = 0.80$). There was an inverse relation between pre-pregnancy BMI and weight gain to pregnancy week 18 ($r = -0.24$, $p < 0.001$) and to term ($r = -0.16$, $p < 0.001$).

Table 1. Maternal characteristics according to maternal pre-pregnancy BMI, n = 2797.

	Pre-pregnancy BMI, Categories					p Value
	<18.5	18.5–24.9	25.0–29.9	30.0–34.9	≥35.0	
	n = 80 (3%)	n = 1827 (65%)	n = 587 (21%)	n = 213 (8%)	n = 90 (3%)	
Primipara, n (%)	47 (59%)	785 (43%)	231 (39%)	86 (40%)	26 (29%)	0.001 [b]
Age, years, mean (SD)	27.8 (4.9)	29.9 (4.5)	29.9 (4.6)	29.8 (4.6)	29.5 (4.8)	0.003 [a]
Education						
Primary school, n (%)	9 (12%)	39 (2%)	15 (3%)	11 (5%)	6 (7%)	
Secondary school, n (%)	30 (41%)	623 (36%)	273 (48%)	97 (47%)	48 (55%)	<0.001 [b]
University or college, n (%)	35 (47%)	1077 (62%)	286 (50%)	98 (48%)	34 (39%)	
Use of supplements anytime from four weeks before pregnancy up to pregnancy week 18	63 (79%)	1523 (83%)	470 (79%)	156 (72%)	61 (68%)	<0.001 [b]
Use of alcohol (≥1/month), n (%)	5 (0.2%)	83 (3%)	15 (0.6%)	1 (0%)	3 (0.1%)	0.009 [b]
Daily smoking, n (%)	13 (16%)	140 (8%)	47 (8%)	22 (10%)	9 (10%)	0.04 [b]
Weight increase, kg, mean (SD), (% of pre-pregnancy weight)						
to pregnancy week 18	4.5 (3.1) (9%)	3.3 (2.9) (5%)	2.4 (3.2) (3%)	1.1 (3.5) (1%)	−0.1 (4.3) (−0.1%)	<0.001 [a] <0.001 [a]
to birth	17.3 (6.3) (35%)	15.5 (5.9) (25%)	14.8 (6.7) (20%)	11.5 (7.3) (13%)	8.7 (8.9) (8%)	<0.001 [a] <0.001 [a]
Birth weight, g, mean (SD)	3343 (635)	3575 (588)	3727 (600)	3696 (648)	3758 (755)	<0.001 [a]

[a] ANOVA: A one-way variance analysis; [b] Pearson's Chi Square test. BMI: body mass index; SD: the standard deviation.

Women in the highest pre-pregnancy BMI group (BMI ≥ 35) put on less weight during pregnancy, they were more likely to be multipara, not use micronutrient supplements, and to have a lower educational level ($p < 0.01$). The lowest mean birth weight was seen in women with a pre-pregnancy BMI <18.5 (Table 1).

3.2. Plasma B Vitamin Status According to Pre-Pregnancy BMI

There was a trend towards lower levels of B vitamins and higher levels of the metabolic markers with higher pre-pregnancy BMI (Table 2, Figure 1). The best B vitamin status was seen in women with a normal pre-pregnancy BMI (18.5–24.9), as they had the highest levels of folate, PLP, and riboflavin with the lowest tHcy and HK/XA ratio (Table 2). Cobalamin decreased with increasing BMI, but this was not reflected in the MMA levels, which were inversely related to pre-pregnancy BMI.

The circulating B-vitamins were inversely related to their functional markers, as expected. tHcy was inversely related to folate ($r = -0.48, p < 0.001$), less to cobalamin ($r = -0.24, p < 0.001$), PLP ($r = -0.16, p < 0.001$), and riboflavin ($r = -0.15, p < 0.001$). MMA was inversely related to cobalamin ($r = -0.17, p < 0.001$) and HK/XA to PLP ($r = -0.29, p < 0.001$). All B vitamins were positively related to each other ($r > 0.12, p < 0.001$).

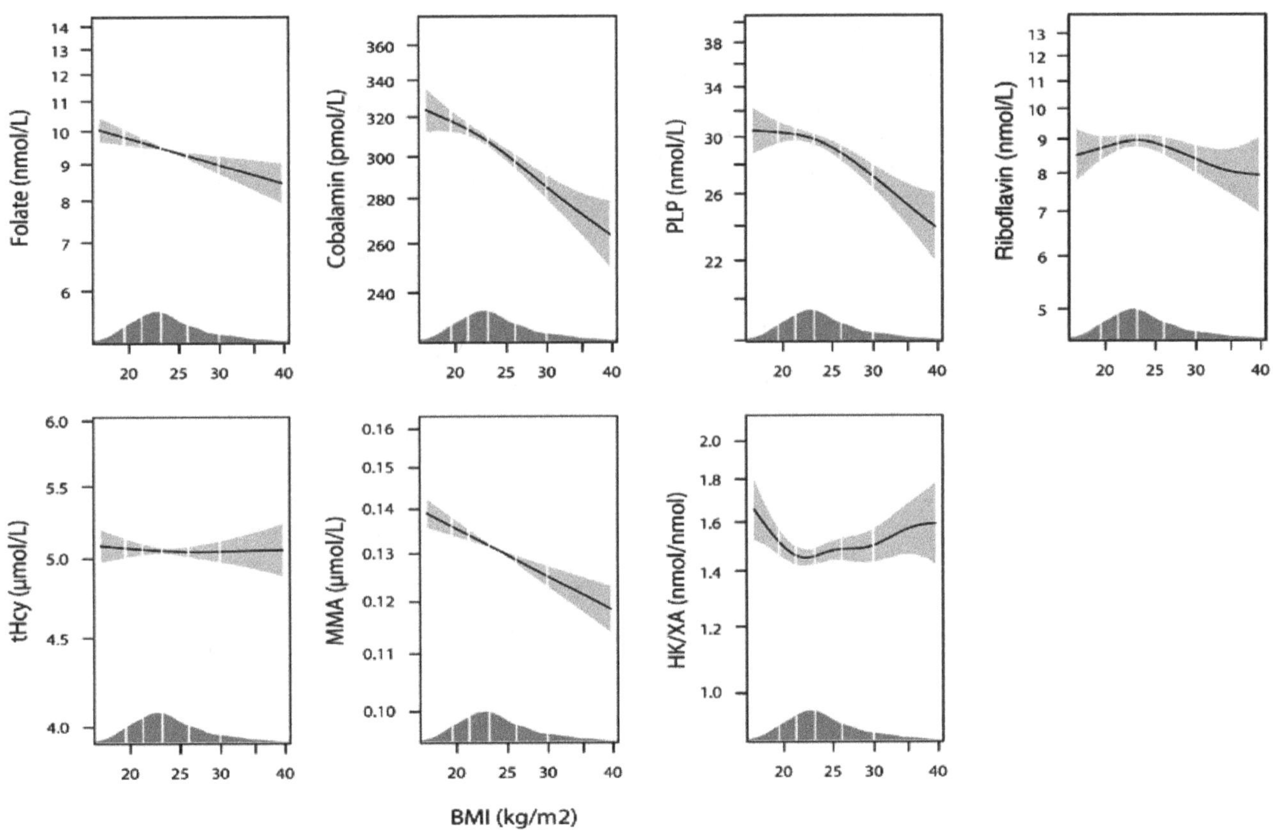

Figure 1. The association of pre-pregnancy BMI with cobalamin, folate, PLP, riboflavin, tHcy, MMA, and HK/XA by generalized additive models (GAM), adjusted for use of multisupplements, maternal age, parity, and neopterin. The solid line shows the fitted model and the shaded areas indicate 95% CIs. PLP, pyridoxal 5′phosphate; tHcy, total homocysteine; MMA, methylmalonic acid, HK/XA, 3-hydroxykynurenine/xanthurenic acid ratio.

Table 2. Maternal plasma levels of vitamins, metabolic and inflammation markers in pregnancy week 18 according to pre-pregnancy BMI, $n = 2797$.

	Pre-pregnancy BMI; Categories					p Value
	<18.5	18.5–24.9	25.0–29.9	30.0–34.9	≥35.0	
	$n = 80$	$n = 1827$	$n = 587$	$n = 213$	$n = 90$	
Plasma folate, nmol/L [a]	8.8 (6.0–15.7)	9.2 (6.3–16.0)	8.1 (5.7–12.8)	7.3 (5.1–12.2)	7.3 (5.0–12.1)	<0.001
Plasma cobalamin, pmol/L [a]	328 (243–383)	314 (254–386)	301 (240–363)	271 (220–338)	268 (204–317)	<0.001
Plasma PLP, nmol/L [a]	27.0 (21.4–39.7)	28.3 (21.8–40.7)	26.6 (20.6–35.6)	23.8 (17.4–33.7)	21.5 (17.0–30.1)	<0.001
Plasma riboflavin, nmol/L [a]	7.8 (4.8–14.4)	8.1 (5.6–13.2)	7.8 (5.2–13.9)	7.2 (5.2–11.0)	6.9 (4.4–10.1)	0.004
B vitamin status [a,b]	12.2 (3.7)	12.5 (3.6)	11.7 (3.7)	10.6 (3.7)	10.1 (3.4)	<0.001
Plasma tHcy, µmol/L [a]	5.00 (4.22–5.92)	4.91 (4.27–5.79)	4.94 (4.23–5.78)	5.04 (4.44–6.21)	5.33 (4.43–6.13)	0.03
Plasma MMA, µmol/L [a]	0.13 (0.11–0.16)	0.13 (0.11–0.16)	0.13 (0.10–0.16)	0.12 (0.10–0.15)	0.12 (0.10–0.15)	0.009
Plasma HK/XA [a]	1.6 (1.2–2.1)	1.4 (1.0–2.0)	1.5 (1.1–2.1)	1.7 (1.2–2.2)	1.8 (1.2–2.4)	<0.001
Plasma neopterine, µmol/L [a]	6.7 (6.1–8.1)	7.0 (6.1–8.1)	7.3 (6.3–8.6)	7.9 (7.0–9.1)	8.5 (7.31–9.9)	<0.001
KTR, nmol/µmol [a]	18.1 (16.0–21.5)	18.3 (16.2–20.6)	18.8 (16.8–21.2)	19.6 (17.5–22.8)	21.2 (18.5–24.0)	<0.001

[a] Median (IQR), by Kruskal Wallis test; [b] B vitamin status; summary score based on added quintiles of the 4 B vitamins, Mean (SD), by ANOVA; tHcy, total homocysteine; MMA, methylmalonic acid; HK/XA: 3-hydroxykynurenine/xanthurenic acid; KTR, kynurenine/tryptophan ratio.

3.3. *Inflammation Markers According to Pre-Pregnancy BMI*

There was a positive correlation between pre-pregnancy BMI and the inflammation markers neopterin ($r = 0.18, p < 0.001$) and KTR ($r = 0.13, p < 0.001$), as demonstrated in Figure 2. Neopterin and KTR were strongly correlated to each other ($r = 0.48, p < 0.001$).

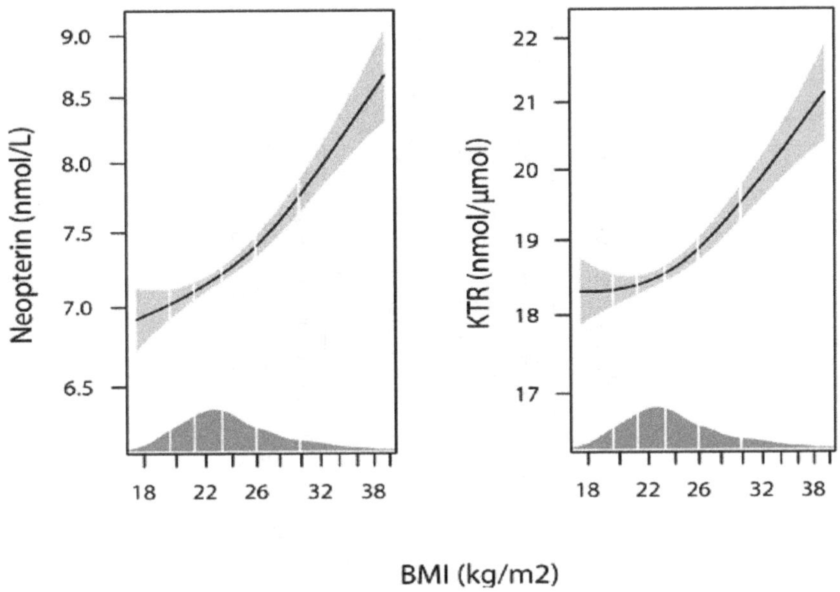

Figure 2. The association of pre-pregnancy BMI with neopterin and KTR by Generalized additive models (GAM), adjusted for use of multisupplements, maternal age, and parity. The solid line shows the fitted model and the shaded areas indicate 95% CIs. KTR, kynurenine/tryptophan ratio.

3.4. *Maternal Factors and Inflammation Markers as Determinants of Plasma B Vitamin Status in Pregnancy Week 18*

Use of supplements was the most consistent and strongest determinant for maternal B vitamin status, with significant influence on folate, cobalamin, PLP, riboflavin, tHcy, and HK/XA, in a multiple linear regression model, which additionally included pre-pregnancy BMI, age, parity, and neopterin (Table 3). In this model, pre-pregnancy BMI was a significant determinant of all vitamin markers except for riboflavin and tHcy, whereas parity was strongly negatively correlated to folate and PLP status. All parameters in the model were significantly correlated to the calculated B vitamin summary score (Table 3). Neopterin was significantly negative related to PLP, and positively to the metabolic markers tHcy, MMA, and HK/XA. Substituting neopterin with KTR in the model did not essentially change the results (data not shown). Including gestational weight gain in pregnancy week 18 as an additional factor did not change the results.

The OR for having a low calculated B vitamin summary score (quintile 1) was increased with pre-pregnancy BMI >30.0 and higher parity, and reduced with higher maternal age and use of supplements in a logistic regression model, which additionally included neopterin quartiles (Table 4). A high pre-pregnancy BMI was a predictor of low cobalamin and PLP levels, multiparity was a predictor of low folate levels, higher maternal age was associated with better folate and riboflavin status, whereas use of supplements was associated with better status of all four B vitamins. Increased inflammation, evaluated by higher neopterin levels, was only a predictor of low PLP in this model. Substituting neopterin with KTR in the model did not essentially change the results.

Table 3. Determinants of maternal plasma B vitamin status in pregnancy week 18 by multiple linear regression, $n = 2797$.

	Plasma Folate, nmol/L	Plasma Cobalamin, pmol/L	Plasma PLP, nmol/L	Plasma Riboflavin, nmol/L	Plasma tHcy, µmol/L	Plasma MMA, µmol/L	Plasma HK/XA	B Vitamin Score [a]
	B (95% CI)	B (95% CI)	B (95% CI)	B (95% CI)	B (95% CI)	B (95% CI)	B (95% CI)	B (95% CI)
Pre-pregnancy BMI [c]	−0.59 ** (−0.98, −0.20)	−16.7 ** (−22.0, −11.4)	−2.55 ** (−3.72, −1.38)	−0.60 (−1.25, 0.06)	−0.02 (−0.16, 0.12)	−0.006 ** (−0.008, −0.003)	0.11 * (0.04, 0.18)	−0.47 ** (−0.60, −0.35)
Parity [e]	−1.33 ** (−1.72, −0.95)	−3.6 (−8.8, 1.6)	−1.28 * (−2.43, −0.12)	−1.08 * (−1.73, −0.43)	−0.01 (−0.15, 0.13)	−0.001 (−0.004, 0.002)	−0.03 (−0.09, 0.04)	−0.34 ** (−0.47, −0.22)
Age [d]	2.69 ** (2.05, 3.32)	12.3 * (3.6, 20.9)	1.96 * (0.06, 3.86)	0.30 (−0.77, 1.36)	0.04 (−0.19, 0.27)	0.002 (−0.002, 0.007)	−0.12 * (−0.24, −0.01)	0.63 ** (0.43, 0.83)
Use of supplements [b]	5.14 ** (4.35, 5.94)	13.0 * (2.3, 23.7)	8.49 ** (6.12, 10.85)	1.80 * (0.48, 3.13)	−0.75 ** (−1.03, −0.47)	0.001 (−0.004, 0.007)	−0.21 * (−0.35, −0.07)	1.73 ** (1.48, 1.98)
Neopterin [f]	−0.12 (−0.35, 0.11)	−1.9 (−5.0, 1.2)	−1.00 * (−1.68, −0.31)	−0.08 (−0.47, 0.30)	0.10 * (0.02, 0.18)	0.003 ** (0.001, 0.004)	0.19 ** (0.15, 0.23)	−0.12 ** (−0.20, −0.05)

All variables were included in the model; [a] B vitamin score; added quintiles of folate, cobalamin, PLP and riboflavin; [b] No use versus use of supplements any time from four weeks before pregnancy up to pregnancy week 18; [c] Pre-pregnancy BMI, categorized; <18.5, 18.5-24.9, 25.0-29.9, 30.0-34.9, ≥35.0; [d] Age, categorized; <25 years, 25–35 years, >35 years; [e] Parity, categorized; 0, 1, 2, 3+; [f] Neopterin, quintiles; ≤5.84, 5.85–6.68, 6.69–7.50, 7.51–8.67, ≥8.68;* p value < 0.05; ** p value < 0.001. CI: indicates confidence interval.

Table 4. OR for low B vitamin status according to maternal factors, by logistic regression (n = 2797).

Independent Variables	OR (95% CI) for				
	Plasma Folate <5.45 nmol/L (Quintile 1)	Plasma Cobalamin <230 pmol/L (Quintile 1)	Plasma PLP <19.26 µmol/L (Quintile 1)	Plasma Riboflavin <4.91 µmol/L (Quintile 1)	B Vitamin Score [a] (Quintile 1)
Pre-pregnancy BMI (vs. category 2 18.5–24.9)					
<18.5	1.0 (0.5–1.8)	1.1 (0.6–1.9)	1.0 (0.5–1.8)	1.7 (1.0–2.8)	1.1 (0.7–1.9)
25.0–29.9	1.1 (0.9–1.5)	1.3 (1.0–1.6)	1.3 (1.0–1.6)	1.3 (1.0–1.7)	1.5 (1.2–1.8)
30.0–34.9	1.5 (1.0–2.1)	2.1 (1.5–2.9)	2.1 (1.6–3.0)	1.4 (1.0–2.0)	2.7 (2.0–3.7)
≥35.0	1.7 (1.0–2.8)	2.3 (1.4–3.6)	2.2 (1.4–3.5)	1.8 (1.1–3.0)	2.8 (1.7–4.3)
p trend	0.006	<0.001	<0.001	0.001	<0.001
Parity (vs. primipara)					
Para 1	1.2 (1.0–1.6)	1.1 (0.9–1.4)	1.3 (1.0–1.6)	1.3 (1.0–1.6)	1.3 (1.0–1.6)
Para 2	1.7 (1.2–2.3)	1.3 (1.0–1.7)	1.1 (0.8–1.5)	1.2 (0.9–1.6)	1.6 (1.2–2.1)
Para 3+	3.2 (2.1–4.9)	1.6 (1.0–2.4)	1.1 (0.7–1.8)	1.4 (0.9–2.2)	2.1 (1.4–3.1)
p trend	<0.001	0.02	0.36	0.11	<0.001
Maternal age (vs. ≤25 years)					
25–35	0.4 (0.3–0.6)	0.7 (0.6–1.0)	0.7 (0.7–1.0)	0.7 (0.6–1.0)	0.5 (0.4–0.7)
≥35	0.3 (0.2–0.5)	0.8 (0.5–1.2)	0.8 (0.5–1.1)	0.6 (0.4–0.9)	0.4 (0.3–0.6)
p trend	<0.001	0.11	0.11	0.004	<0.001
Use of supplements (vs. non-user)					
User	0.2 (0.2–0.2)	0.8 (0.6–1.0)	0.5 (0.4–0.6)	0.6 (0.5–0.8)	0.3 (0.3–0.4)
p trend	<0.001	0.03	<0.001	<0.001	<0.001
Neopterin (vs. ≤6.20 µmol/L, Quartile 1)					
6.21–7.17	1.1 (0.8–1.4)	1.1 (0.8–1.5)	1.1 (0.8–1.5)	0.9 (0.7–1.2)	1.0 (0.8–1.3)
7.18–8.40	1.3 (1.0–1.8)	1.0 (0.8–1.4)	1.1 (0.8–1.4)	0.9 (0.7–1.1)	1.1 (0.9–1.4)
≥8.41	1.2 (0.9–1.6)	1.2 (0.9–1.6)	1.7 (1.3–2.2)	0.9 (0.7–1.2)	1.2 (1.0–1.6)
p trend	0.11	0.24	<0.001	0.38	0.05

All variables were included in the model; [a] B vitamin score; added quintiles of folate, cobalamin, PLP and riboflavin. OR: Odds ratio.

The relations between pre-pregnancy BMI and B vitamins and metabolic markers, visualized by GAM in a model which additionally corrected for use of supplements, maternal age, parity, and neopterin, are shown in Figure 1. The association curves for folate, cobalamin, PLP, and MMA show a linear negative relation to pre-pregnancy BMI, while the relation between pre-pregnancy BMI and the other biomarkers are inverse U-shaped (riboflavin), null (tHcy), or inverse in the lower range (HK/XA).

The association curves between pre-pregnancy BMI and the inflammation markers, neopterin and KTR, visualized by GAM in a model which also corrected for use of supplements, maternal age, and parity, show a strong linear relation through the whole range of BMI values (Figure 2).

4. Discussion

4.1. Main Findings

In this study of healthy women in pregnancy week 18, use of multi supplements was the strongest maternal determinant for B vitamin status. Pre-pregnancy BMI was inversely related to folate, cobalamin, PLP, and riboflavin levels, and associated with increased markers of cellular immune activation. Inflammation seemed to be an independent predictor of low PLP levels.

4.2. Strength and Limitations

All pregnant women in Norway were invited to participate in the MoBa study, but the attendance rate was only 38.5%, rendering the cohort not representative of the Norwegian population of pregnant women. The women who participated in the MoBa study are reported to be older, more frequently vitamin users, non-smokers, and primiparous [32]. Pre-pregnancy weight was self-reported around pregnancy week 18, and as obesity is an important determinant of underreporting BMI [33], self-reporting without verification is a limitation of the study.

The samples were stored at −80 °C before analyzing. The stability of plasma metabolites according to sample handling and storage conditions has been validated and the biomarkers investigated do not change significantly during storage at −80 °C [34].

C-reactive protein, CRP, an acute phase reactant and a commonly used inflammation marker, might have added additional information about low grade inflammation, but was not analyzed, which is a limitation of the study.

4.3. Interpretation

4.3.1. Effects of Pre-Pregnancy BMI on Gestational Weight Gain and Birth Weight

In a former study of the MoBa cohort including approximately 58,000 mothers, the majority (65%) reported a normal pre-pregnancy BMI (18.5–24.9), whereas 2.9% were underweight (<18.5), and 2.6% were obese (≥35) [35], which is in accordance with the findings in the present substudy.

We observed a significant inverse relation between pre-pregnancy BMI and gestational weight gain up to pregnancy week 18 and throughout pregnancy, and despite this, a higher pre-pregnancy BMI was associated with a higher birth weight, which has been reported previously [35].

4.3.2. Pregnancy Related Changes in Biochemical Parameters

Physiological changes in pregnancy, including hemodilution, altered renal function, hormonal status, and binding-protein concentrations, affect plasma B vitamin levels and the relation to their functional metabolic markers [36,37]. Folate, cobalamin, and PLP tend to decrease, whereas riboflavin is reported to show only minor changes during pregnancy [38–42]. tHcy, a marker of folate and cobalamin deficiency [43], is 30%–60% lower in pregnant compared to nonpregnant women, with the lowest levels seen in the second trimester [44]. MMA, a marker of cobalamin deficiency [45], is reported to be reduced during the first two trimesters, thereafter gradually increasing [46]. We observed a strong inverse relation between folate and tHcy, and a weaker relation between cobalamin and MMA, as observed by others [36,47,48].

The ratio HK/XA has been shown to have a strong negative correlation with plasma levels of PLP, the active form of vitamin B6, and has been proposed as a potential markers of functional vitamin B6 status [27]. The inverse relation between PLP and HK/XA has not been previously documented in pregnant women, but we observed lower PLP and higher HK/XA ratios with increasing pre-pregnancy BMI, indicating a functional vitamin B6 deficiency, particularly in women with a pre-pregnancy BMI $\geq$30.

Extensive changes in the maternal immune system are necessary for maintaining a normal pregnancy [49] and both neopterin levels and KTR are reported to increase during pregnancy [50] Neopterin levels correlate with gestational age ($r = 0.28$, $p = 0.001$) and are reported to be higher in pregnancies complicated with preterm birth and preeclampsia [51–53].

4.3.3. Maternal Predictors for B Vitamin Status

An inverse relation between pre-pregnancy BMI and folate, vitamin D, carotenoids has formerly been reported [10,11,13]. Our results have expanded this knowledge by reporting also lower levels of PLP (vitamin B6), riboflavin (vitamin B2), and cobalamin (vitamin B12) with higher pre-pregnancy BMI.

Pre-pregnancy BMI, use of multisupplements, parity, and maternal age were all related to B vitamin status. We observed a slightly U-shaped relation between pre-pregnancy BMI and B vitamin levels in pregnancy week 18, with the best status seen in women with a normal pre-pregnancy BMI (18.5–24.9), slightly lower in underweight women (BMI < 18.5) and lowest in obese women (BMI $\geq$35.0). The strongest maternal determinant for B vitamin status was use of multisupplements, and the percentage of users was higher in normal weight compared to obese women, which might explain the inverse relation between pre-pregnancy BMI and vitamin status. Use of micronutrient supplements during pregnancy has been associated with better socioeconomic status [48], known to be related to a better diet, maternal health, and pregnancy outcome [54]. Multiparity ($\geq$3) was associated with an increased risk of folate deficiency, while maternal age >25 years was associated with a better folate status. In the MoBa cohort, the 10% who had used supplements regularly from one month before pregnancy throughout the first trimester (as recommended) were more likely to be older, married, nonsmokers, with a higher income and lower parity [54]. Compared to women with a lower pre-pregnancy BMI, obese women (BMI $\geq$ 35) had not increased their weight in pregnancy week 18, when the blood samples were collected, which might contribute to their lower micronutrient status.

4.3.4. The Complex Relation between Pre-pregnancy BMI, Inflammation, and Vitamin Levels

We observed a linear relation between pre-pregnancy BMI and the markers of cellular immune activation, neopterin and KTR, as previously reported in non-pregnant adults [16]. Inflammation is reported to be associated with lower plasma levels of several micronutrients, particularly vitamin B6 and vitamin D [18–20], but the magnitude of effect varies between different micronutrients and individuals [18,55,56]. The lower PLP levels associated with inflammation have been proposed to be due to increased PLP degradation [57] and to PLP redistribution from plasma to tissues [58], and PLP have been suggested to reflect interferon-γ-mediated immune activation [59].

In this study, neopterin was inversely related to PLP and positively to HK/XA, but not to any other vitamin, in both multiple linear and logistic regression models, which included pre-pregnancy BMI and other maternal factors. The increase in the functional marker, HK/XA, suggests that low PLP does not merely refelect altered distribution, but that inflammation may be an independent risk factor for lower vitamin B6 status.

5. Conclusions

A high pre-pregnancy BMI is associated with lower levels of folate, cobalamin, PLP, and riboflavin; and increased levels of the cellular inflammation markers, neopterin, and KTR. As an optimal micronutrient status is vital for normal fetal development, the observed lower B vitamin levels may contribute to the negative pregnancy outcomes associated with maternal obesity. Assessment of B vitamin status should be encouraged in women with a high pre-pregnancy BMI when planning a pregnancy.

Acknowledgments: We are grateful to all the families in Norway who took part in this cohort study. The Norwegian Mother and Child Cohort Study is supported by the Norwegian Ministry of Health and the Ministry of Education and Research, NIH/NIEHS (contract no. NO-ES-75558), NIH/NINDS (grant no.1 UO1 NS 047537-01), and the Norwegian Research Council/FUGE (grant no. 151918/S10).

Author Contributions: (1) Designed research: A.-L.B.-M., P.M.U., P.M., C.S., and S.E.V.; (2) Conducted research: C.R., P.M., and C.S.; (3) Analyzed data: A.-L.B.-M., A.U., R.M.N., and Ø.M.; (4) Wrote the paper: A.-L.B.-M., and P.M.U.; (5) Primary responsibility for final content: A.-L.B.-M.; (5) Primary responsibility for final content: A.-L.B.-M.; (6) All authors have read and approved the final version of the manuscript: A.-L.B.-M., A.U., Ø.M., R.M.N., C.R., P.M., C.S., S.E.V., T.R.-K., and P.M.U.

Abbreviations

MoBa: the Norwegian Mother and Child Cohort; tHcy: total homocysteine; MMA: methylmalonic acid; HK: 3-hydroxykynurenine; XA: xanthurenic acid; PLP: pyridoxal 5′-phosphate; KTR: kynurenine/tryptophan ratio; IDO: indoleamine-2,3-dioxygenase.

References

1. Swinburn, B.A.; Sacks, G.; Hall, K.D.; McPherson, K.; Finegood, D.T.; Moodie, M.L.; Gortmaker, S.L. The global obesity pandemic: Shaped by global drivers and local environments. *Lancet* **2011**, *378*, 804–814. [CrossRef]
2. Catalano, P.M.; Ehrenberg, H.M. The short- and long-term implications of maternal obesity on the mother and her offspring. *Br. J. Obstet. Gynaecol.* **2006**, *113*, 1126–1133. [CrossRef] [PubMed]
3. Stothard, K.J.; Tennant, P.W.; Bell, R.; Rankin, J. Maternal overweight and obesity and the risk of congenital anomalies: A systematic review and meta-analysis. *J. Am. Med. Assoc.* **2009**, *301*, 636–650. [CrossRef] [PubMed]
4. Boney, C.M.; Verma, A.; Tucker, R.; Vohr, B.R. Metabolic syndrome in childhood: Association with birth weight, maternal obesity, and gestational diabetes mellitus. *Pediatrics* **2005**, *115*, e290–e296. [CrossRef] [PubMed]
5. Kimmons, J.E.; Blanck, H.M.; Tohill, B.C.; Zhang, J.; Khan, L.K. Associations between body mass index and the prevalence of low micronutrient levels among US adults. *MedGenMed* **2006**, *8*, 59. [PubMed]
6. Mojtabai, R. Body mass index and serum folate in childbearing age women. *Eur. J. Epidemiol.* **2004**, *19*, 1029–1036. [CrossRef] [PubMed]
7. Samuel, L.; Borrell, L.N. The effect of body mass index on optimal vitamin D status in U.S. adults: The National Health and Nutrition Examination Survey 2001–2006. *Ann. Epidemiol.* **2013**, *23*, 409–414. [CrossRef] [PubMed]
8. Nead, K.G.; Halterman, J.S.; Kaczorowski, J.M.; Auinger, P.; Weitzman, M. Overweight children and adolescents: A risk group for iron deficiency. *Pediatrics* **2004**, *114*, 104–108. [CrossRef] [PubMed]
9. Strauss, R.S. Comparison of serum concentrations of alpha-tocopherol and beta-carotene in a cross-sectional sample of obese and nonobese children (NHANES III). National Health and Nutrition Examination Survey. *J. Pediatr.* **1999**, *134*, 160–165. [CrossRef]
10. Bodnar, L.M.; Catov, J.M.; Roberts, J.M.; Simhan, H.N. Pre-pregnancy obesity predicts poor vitamin D status in mothers and their neonates. *J. Nutr.* **2007**, *137*, 2437–2442. [PubMed]
11. Kim, H.; Hwang, J.Y.; Kim, K.N.; Ha, E.H.; Park, H.; Ha, M.; Lee, K.Y.; Hong, Y.C.; Tamura, T.; Chang, N. Relationship between body-mass index and serum folate concentrations in pregnant women. *Eur. J. Clin. Nutr.* **2012**, *66*, 136–138. [CrossRef] [PubMed]
12. Tamura, T.; Goldenberg, R.L.; Johnston, K.E.; Chapman, V.R. Relationship between pre-pregnancy BMI and plasma zinc concentrations in early pregnancy. *Br. J. Nutr.* **2004**, *91*, 773–777. [CrossRef] [PubMed]

13. Tomedi, L.E.; Chang, C.C.; Newby, P.K.; Evans, R.W.; Luther, J.F.; Wisner, K.L.; Bodnar, L.M. Pre-pregnancy obesity and maternal nutritional biomarker status during pregnancy: A factor analysis. *Public Health Nutr.* **2013**, *16*, 1414–1418. [CrossRef] [PubMed]
14. Allen, L.H. Multiple micronutrients in pregnancy and lactation: An overview. *Am. J. Clin. Nutr.* **2005**, *81*, 1206S–1212S. [PubMed]
15. Gregor, M.F.; Hotamisligil, G.S. Inflammatory mechanisms in obesity. *Ann. Rev. Immunol.* **2011**, *29*, 415–445. [CrossRef] [PubMed]
16. Theofylaktopoulou, D.; Midttun, O.; Ulvik, A.; Ueland, P.M.; Tell, G.S.; Vollset, S.E.; Nygård, O.; Eussen, S.J. A community-based study on determinants of circulating markers of cellular immune activation and kynurenines: The Hordaland Health Study. *Clin. Exp. Immunol.* **2013**, *173*, 121–130. [CrossRef] [PubMed]
17. Visser, M.; Bouter, L.M.; McQuillan, G.M.; Wener, M.H.; Harris, T.B. Elevated C-reactive protein levels in overweight and obese adults. *J. Am. Med. Assoc.* **1999**, *282*, 2131–2135. [CrossRef]
18. Duncan, A.; Talwar, D.; McMillan, D.C.; Stefanowicz, F.; O'Reilly, D.S. Quantitative data on the magnitude of the systemic inflammatory response and its effect on micronutrient status based on plasma measurements. *Am. J. Clin. Nutr.* **2012**, *95*, 64–71. [CrossRef] [PubMed]
19. Gori, A.M.; Sofi, F.; Corsi, A.M.; Gazzini, A.; Sestini, I.; Lauretani, F.; Bandinelli, S.; Gensini, G.F.; Ferrucci, L.; Abbate, R. Predictors of vitamin B6 and folate concentrations in older persons: The InCHIANTI study. *Clin. Chem.* **2006**, *52*, 1318–1324. [CrossRef] [PubMed]
20. Reyman, M.; Verrijn Stuart, A.A.; van Summeren, M.; Rakhshandehroo, M.; Nuboer, R.; de Boer, F.K.; van den Ham, H.J.; Kalkhoven, E.; Prakken, B.; Schipper, H.S. Vitamin D deficiency in childhood obesity is associated with high levels of circulating inflammatory mediators, and low insulin sensitivity. *Int. J. Obes.* **2014**. [CrossRef] [PubMed]
21. Magnus, P.; Irgens, L.M.; Haug, K.; Nystad, W.; Skjaerven, R.; Stoltenberg, C. Cohort profile: The Norwegian Mother and Child Cohort Study (MoBa). *Int. J. Epidemiol.* **2006**, *35*, 1146–1150. [CrossRef] [PubMed]
22. Nilsen, R.M.; Vollset, S.E.; Monsen, A.L.; Ulvik, A.; Haugen, M.; Meltzer, H.M.; Magnus, P.; Ueland, P.M. Infant birth size is not associated with maternal intake and status of folate during the second trimester in Norwegian pregnant women. *J. Nutr.* **2010**, *140*, 572–579. [CrossRef] [PubMed]
23. O'Broin, S.; Kelleher, B. Microbiological assay on microtitre plates of folate in serum and red cells. *J. Clin. Pathol.* **1992**, *45*, 344–347. [CrossRef] [PubMed]
24. Kelleher, B.P.; Broin, S.D. Microbiological assay for vitamin B12 performed in 96-well microtitre plates. *J. Clin. Pathol.* **1991**, *44*, 592–595. [CrossRef] [PubMed]
25. Baril, L.; Carmel, R. Comparison of radioassay and microbiological assay for serum folate, with clinical assessment of discrepant results. *Clin. Chem.* **1978**, *24*, 2192–2196. [PubMed]
26. Windelberg, A.; Arseth, O.; Kvalheim, G.; Ueland, P.M. Automated assay for the determination of methylmalonic acid, total homocysteine, and related amino acids in human serum or plasma by means of methylchloroformate derivatization and gas chromatography-mass spectrometry. *Clin. Chem.* **2005**, *51*, 2103–2109. [CrossRef] [PubMed]
27. Ulvik, A.; Theofylaktopoulou, D.; Midttun, O.; Nygard, O.; Eussen, S.J.; Ueland, P.M. Substrate product ratios of enzymes in the kynurenine pathway measured in plasma as indicators of functional vitamin B-6 status. *Am. J. Clin. Nutr.* **2013**, *98*, 934–940. [CrossRef] [PubMed]
28. Fuchs, D.; Weiss, G.; Wachter, H. Neopterin, biochemistry and clinical use as a marker for cellular immune reactions. *Int. Arch. Allergy Immunol.* **1993**, *101*, 1–6. [CrossRef] [PubMed]
29. Raitala, A.; Pertovaara, M.; Karjalainen, J.; Oja, S.S.; Hurme, M. Association of interferon-gamma +874(T/A) single nucleotide polymorphism with the rate of tryptophan catabolism in healthy individuals. *Scand. J. Immunol.* **2005**, *61*, 387–390. [CrossRef] [PubMed]
30. Midttun, O.; Hustad, S.; Ueland, P.M. Quantitative profiling of biomarkers related to B-vitamin status, tryptophan metabolism and inflammation in human plasma by liquid chromatography/tandem mass spectrometry. *Rapid Commun. Mass Spectrom.* **2009**, *23*, 1371–1379. [CrossRef] [PubMed]
31. R Development Core Team. *A Language and Environment for Statistical Computing*; R Foundation for Statistical Computing: Vienna, Austria, 2006.
32. Nilsen, R.M.; Vollset, S.E.; Gjessing, H.K.; Skjaerven, R.; Melve, K.K.; Schreuder, P.; Alsaker, E.R.; Haug, K.; Daltveit, A.K.; Magnus, P. Self-selection and bias in a large prospective pregnancy cohort in Norway. *Paediatr. Perinat. Epidemiol.* **2009**, *23*, 597–608. [CrossRef] [PubMed]

33. Visscher, T.L.; Viet, A.L.; Kroesbergen, I.H.; Seidell, J.C. Underreporting of BMI in adults and its effect on obesity prevalence estimations in the period 1998 to 2001. *Obesity* **2006**, *14*, 2054–2063. [CrossRef] [PubMed]
34. Hustad, S.; Eussen, S.; Midttun, O.; Ulvik, A.; van de Kant, P.M.; Morkrid, L.; Gislefoss, R.; Ueland, P.M. Kinetic modeling of storage effects on biomarkers related to B vitamin status and one-carbon metabolism. *Clin. Chem.* **2012**, *58*, 402–410. [CrossRef] [PubMed]
35. Stamnes Koepp, U.M.; Frost Andersen, L.; Dahl-Joergensen, K.; Stigum, H.; Nass, O.; Nystad, W. Maternal pre-pregnant body mass index, maternal weight change and offspring birthweight. *Acta Obstet. Gynecol. Scand.* **2012**, *91*, 243–249. [CrossRef] [PubMed]
36. Metz, J.; McGrath, K.; Bennett, M.; Hyland, K.; Bottiglieri, T. Biochemical indices of vitamin B12 nutrition in pregnant patients with subnormal serum vitamin B12 levels. *Am. J. Hematol.* **1995**, *48*, 251–255. [CrossRef] [PubMed]
37. Bruinse, H.W.; van den Berg, H. Changes of some vitamin levels during and after normal pregnancy. *Eur. J. Obstet. Gynecol. Reprod. Biol.* **1995**, *61*, 31–37. [CrossRef]
38. Pietrzik, K.F.; Thorand, B. Folate economy in pregnancy. *Nutrition* **1997**, *13*, 975–977. [CrossRef]
39. Milman, N.; Byg, K.E.; Bergholt, T.; Eriksen, L.; Hvas, A.M. Cobalamin status during normal pregnancy and postpartum: A longitudinal study comprising 406 Danish women. *Eur. J. Haematol.* **2006**, *76*, 521–525. [CrossRef] [PubMed]
40. Shibata, K.; Tachiki, A.; Mukaeda, K.; Fukuwatari, T.; Sasaki, S.; Jinno, Y. Changes in plasma pyridoxal 5′-phosphate concentration during pregnancy stages in Japanese women. *J. Nutr. Sci. Vitaminol.* **2013**, *59*, 343–346. [CrossRef] [PubMed]
41. Cikot, R.J.; Steegers-Theunissen, R.P.; Thomas, C.M.; de Boo, T.M.; Merkus, H.M.; Steegers, E.A. Longitudinal vitamin and homocysteine levels in normal pregnancy. *Br. J. Nutr.* **2001**, *85*, 49–58. [CrossRef] [PubMed]
42. Cunningham, P.; McDermott, L. Long chain PUFA transport in human term placenta. *J. Nutr.* **2009**, *139*, 636–639. [CrossRef] [PubMed]
43. Ueland, P.M.; Refsum, H.; Schneede, J. Determinants of plasma homocysteine. In *Homocysteine and Vascular Disease*; Robinson, K., Ed.; Kluwer Academic Publishers: Dordrecht, The Netherlands, 2000; pp. 59–84.
44. Velzing-Aarts, F.V.; Holm, P.I.; Fokkema, M.R.; van der Dijs, F.P.; Ueland, P.M.; Muskiet, F.A. Plasma choline and betaine and their relation to plasma homocysteine in normal pregnancy. *Am. J. Clin. Nutr.* **2005**, *81*, 1383–1389. [PubMed]
45. Savage, D.G.; Lindenbaum, J.; Stabler, S.P.; Allen, R.H. Sensitivity of serum methylmalonic acid and total homocysteine determinations for diagnosing cobalamin and folate deficiencies. *Am. J. Med.* **1994**, *96*, 239–246. [CrossRef]
46. Greibe, E.; Andreasen, B.H.; Lildballe, D.L.; Morkbak, A.L.; Hvas, A.M.; Nexo, E. Uptake of cobalamin and markers of cobalamin status: A longitudinal study of healthy pregnant women. *Clin. Chem. Lab. Med.* **2011**, *49*, 1877–1882. [CrossRef] [PubMed]
47. Murphy, M.M.; Molloy, A.M.; Ueland, P.M.; Fernandez-Ballart, J.D.; Schneede, J.; Arija, V.; Scott, J.M. Longitudinal study of the effect of pregnancy on maternal and fetal cobalamin status in healthy women and their offspring. *J. Nutr.* **2007**, *137*, 1863–1867. [PubMed]
48. Bjorke-Monsen, A.L.; Roth, C.; Magnus, P.; Midttun, O.; Nilsen, R.M.; Reichborn-Kjennerud, T.; Stoltenberg, C.; Susser, E.; Vollset, S.E.; Ueland, P.M. Maternal B vitamin status in pregnancy week 18 according to reported use of folic acid supplements. *Mol. Nutr. Food Res.* **2013**, *57*, 645–652. [CrossRef] [PubMed]
49. Marques, A.H.; Bjorke-Monsen, A.L.; Teixeira, A.L.; Silverman, M.N. Maternal stress, nutrition and physical activity: Impact on immune function, CNS development and psychopathology. *Brain Res.* 2015. [CrossRef] [PubMed]
50. Schrocksnadel, K.; Widner, B.; Bergant, A.; Neurauter, G.; Schrocksnadel, H.; Fuchs, D. Tryptophan degradation during and after gestation. *Adv. Exp. Med. Biol.* **2003**, *527*, 77–83. [PubMed]
51. Fuith, L.C.; Fuchs, D.; Hausen, A.; Hetzel, H.; Reibnegger, G.; Werner, E.R.; Wachter, H. Neopterin, a marker of cell-mediated immune activation in human pregnancy. *Int. J. Fertil.* **1991**, *36*, 372–375. [PubMed]
52. Von Versen-Hoeynck, F.M.; Hubel, C.A.; Gallaher, M.J.; Gammill, H.S.; Powers, R.W. Plasma levels of inflammatory markers neopterin, sialic acid, and C-reactive protein in pregnancy and preeclampsia. *Am. J. Hypertens.* **2009**, *22*, 687–692. [CrossRef] [PubMed]

53. Navolan, D.B.; Vladareanu, S.; Lahdou, I.; Ciohat, I.; Kleist, C.; Grigoras, D.; Vladareanu, R.; Terness, P.; Sas, I. Early pregnancy serum neopterin concentrations predict spontaneous preterm birth in asymptomatic pregnant women. *J. Perinat. Med.* **2016**. [CrossRef] [PubMed]
54. Nilsen, R.M.; Vollset, S.E.; Gjessing, H.K.; Magnus, P.; Meltzer, H.M.; Haugen, M.; Ueland, P.M. Patterns and predictors of folic acid supplement use among pregnant women: The Norwegian Mother and Child Cohort Study. *Am. J. Clin. Nutr.* **2006**, *84*, 1134–1141. [PubMed]
55. Theofylaktopoulou, D.; Ulvik, A.; Midttun, O.; Ueland, P.M.; Vollset, S.E.; Nygard, O.; Hustad, S.; Tell, G.S.; Eussen, S.J. Vitamins B2 and B6 as determinants of kynurenines and related markers of interferon-gamma-mediated immune activation in the community-based Hordaland Health Study. *Br. J. Nutr.* **2014**, *112*, 1065–1072. [CrossRef] [PubMed]
56. Lepski, S.; Brockmeyer, J. Impact of dietary factors and food processing on food allergy. *Mol. Nutr. Food Res.* **2013**, *57*, 145–152. [CrossRef] [PubMed]
57. Ulvik, A.; Midttun, O.; Pedersen, E.R.; Eussen, S.J.; Nygard, O.; Ueland, P.M. Evidence for increased catabolism of vitamin B-6 during systemic inflammation. *Am. J. Clin. Nutr.* **2014**, *100*, 250–255. [CrossRef] [PubMed]
58. Chiang, E.P.; Smith, D.E.; Selhub, J.; Dallal, G.; Wang, Y.C.; Roubenoff, R. Inflammation causes tissue-specific depletion of vitamin B6. *Arthritis Res. Ther.* **2005**, *7*, R1254–R1262. [CrossRef] [PubMed]
59. Torsvik, I.K.; Ueland, P.M.; Markestad, T.; Midttun, O.; Monsen, A.L. Motor development related to duration of exclusive breastfeeding, B vitamin status and B12 supplementation in infants with a birth weight between 2000–3000 g, results from a randomized intervention trial. *BMC Pediatr.* **2015**, *15*, 218. [CrossRef] [PubMed]

7

Metformin Treatment and Homocysteine

Qianying Zhang [1,†], Sheyu Li [1,†], Ling Li [2], Qianrui Li [1], Kaiyun Ren [1], Xin Sun [2] and Jianwei Li [1,*]

1 Department of Endocrinology and Metabolism, West China Hospital, Sichuan University, Chengdu 610041, China; zhangqianying314@163.com (Q.Z.); lisheyu@gmail.com (S.L.); qli.cherry@hotmail.com (Q.L.); renky.sl@foxmail.com (K.R.)
2 Chinese Evidence-based Medicine Center, West China Hospital, Sichuan University, Chengdu 610041, China; ebmliling@hotmail.com (L.L.); sunx79@hotmail.com (X.S.)
* Correspondence: jerryli678@yahoo.com
† These authors contributed equally to this work.

Abstract: The aim of this systematic review is to assess whether metformin could change the concentration of serum homocysteine (Hcy) with and without simultaneous supplementation of B-group vitamins or folic acid. A literature search was conducted in PubMed, EmBase, and Cochrane Central Register of Controlled Trials (CENTRAL) to identify randomized controlled trials (RCTs) reporting the concentration of serum Hcy in metformin-treated adults. Meta-analysis was applied to assess the association between metformin and the changes of Hcy concentration. Twelve publications were included in this study. In the overall analysis, metformin administration was not statistically associated with the change of Hcy when compared with the control treatment (mean difference (MD), 0.40 μmol/L; 95% confidence interval (CI), −0.07~0.87 μmol/L, $p = 0.10$). In the subgroup analysis, metformin was significantly associated with an increased concentration of Hcy in the absence of exogenous supplementation of folic acid or B-group vitamins (MD, 2.02 μmol/L; 95% CI, 1.37~2.67 μmol/L, $p < 0.00001$), but with a decreased concentration of serum Hcy in the presence of these exogenous supplementations (MD, −0.74 μmol/L; 95% CI, −1.19~−0.30 μmol/L, $p = 0.001$). Therefore, although the overall effect of metformin on the concentration of serum Hcy was neutral, our results suggested that metformin could increase the concentration of Hcy when exogenous B-group vitamins or folic acid supplementation was not given.

Keywords: metformin; homocysteine; vitamin B_{12}; folic acid; systematic review; meta-analysis

---

1. Introduction

Metformin, a first-line drug for type 2 diabetes mellitus (T2DM) recommended by most guidelines of diabetes, is also widely used in patients with polycystic ovary syndrome (PCOS), pre-diabetes, and other diseases involving insulin resistance [1,2]. However, Vitamin B_{12} deficiency was noted to be a potential disadvantage of metformin by the latest American Diabetes Association (ADA) guidelines [1]. A previous meta-analysis demonstrated that metformin treatment was associated with a decreased concentration of serum Vitamin B_{12} in a dose-dependent manner [3].

Homocysteine (Hcy) is a key component in the one-carbon pathway of methionine metabolism, which plays a dominant role in DNA methylation. The accumulation of Hcy, known as hyperhomocysteinemia (HHcy), is often resulted from Vitamin B_{12} deficiency [4], and is associated with an increased risk of cardiovascular diseases, cognitive impairment, cancer, chronic renal failure and other chronic diseases [4–11]. However, no consensus was reached on whether metformin could induce Hcy elevation. This systematic review aimed to assess the association between metformin administration and the changes of serum Hcy concentration with and without simultaneous supplementation of B-group vitamins or folic acid.

2. Materials and Methods

2.1. Literature Search and Study Selection

This systematic review was conducted and reported according to the Cochrane Handbook for Systematic Reviews of Interventions and the Preferred Reporting Items for Systematic Reviews and Meta-Analysis (PRISMA) statement. Literature search was conducted systematically in PubMed, EmBase, and Cochrane Central Register of Controlled Trials (CENTRAL) until January, 2016 by two authors (Q.Z. and S.L.). 'Metformin' and 'homocysteine' were used as keywords in the literature search. The references of original studies were also screened to ensure that potentially eligible publications were included. A detailed search strategy was presented in Supplementary Materials Figure S1.

We included studies which met the following criteria: (1) metformin was given as intervention while non-biguanide agents as control; (2) reporting serum Hcy concentrations as one of the outcomes; (3) designed as randomized controlled trials (RCTs). Studies with inadequate outcome data of interest, published in non-English languages, and duplicated reports were excluded. Two authors (Q.Z. and S.L.) reviewed all searched papers independently. Disagreements were settled by consensus between the two reviewers or by discussion with a third author (J.L.). The detailed inclusion and exclusion criteria were presented in Supplementary Materials Table S1.

2.2. Data Extraction and Quality Assessment

Data were obtained by two authors (Q.Z. and S.L.) independently from each included study using a predefined form. Disagreements were resolved by discussion with a third author (J.L.). The following information was extracted: title, date of publication time, author names, participant characteristics, intervention strategy, treatment received before study, background treatment (used in both groups together with the intervention), study outcomes, and method for Hcy assay. The risk of bias for each included RCT was assessed using the Cochrane Handbook for Systematic Reviews of Interventions [12].

2.3. Statistical Methods

A meta-analysis was conducted to assess the association between metformin and the changes of Hcy concentration. Considering the significant clinical heterogeneity, a random effects model was used. Subgroup analyses were conducted based on pre-defined parameters: gender, disease type, dosage of metformin, background treatment, pre-study treatment, control medication, duration of follow-up, and test method of Hcy. Pooled mean differences (MDs) and their 95% confidence intervals (CIs) were used for all continuous data. All absolute values and changes of serum Hcy concentration were unified and recorded as μmol/L. Funnel graph was also presented to evaluate the publication bias. Review Manager (RevMan 5.3 from the Cochrane Collaboration, Oxford, UK) was used for statistical analysis.

3. Results

3.1. Search Results

Twelve papers, involving 1311 participants, 1156 of whom completed the studies, were included in the pooled analysis after screening of 1227 articles (Figure 1). Reasons for excluding each paper during full-text screening were presented in Supplementary Materials Table S2 [13–25]. Among included studies, 11 were parallel trials and two were 2 × 2 factorial designed trials. The mean age of participants ranged from 24.8 to 61.4 years. The mean duration of follow-up ranged from 6 to 224 weeks. Detailed characteristics of included studies were presented in Tables 1 and 2. Additionally, primary and secondary outcomes of each included study and strategies of intervention were summarized in Supplementary Materials Tables S3 and S4.

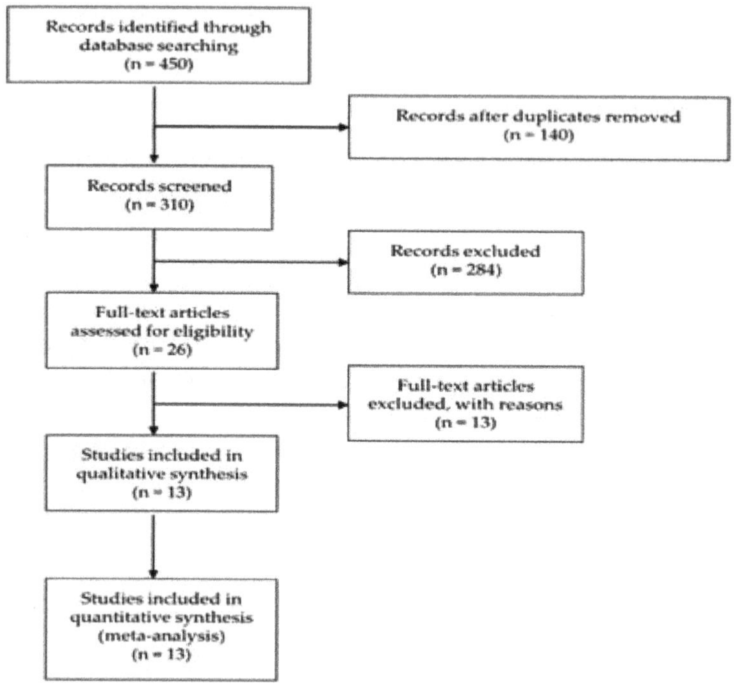

Figure 1. Flow diagram for study identification and inclusion.

Table 1. Baseline characteristics of each included study.

Study	Country	Patients, *N* (I/C)	BMI, (kg/m^2)	Age (Years)	Participants	Women (%)
Carlsen 1997 [26]	Norway	29/30	NA	53	CHD without diabetes	All men
Carlsen 2007a [27]	Norway and Turkey	31/32	NA	NA	PCOS, infertile	All women
Carlsen 2007b [27]	Norway and Turkey	16/18	NA	NA	PCOS, pregnant	All women
de Jager 2010 * [28] Wulffele 2003 * [15]	The Netherlands	131/146	30	61.4	Insulin-treated T2DM	75.5
Kilic 2011a [29]	Turkey	24/25	29.6	28.9	PCOS with IGT, BMI > 25 kg/m^2	All women
Kilic 2011b [29]	Turkey	23/24	22.4	26.5	PCOS with IGT, BMI < 25 kg/m^2	All women
Kilicdag 2005 [30]	Turkey	15/15	27.7	24.8	PCOS	All women
Sahin 2007 [31]	Turkey	74/36	28.9	58.6	Newly diagnosed T2DM	58.2
Schachter 2007a [32]	Israel	28/23	NA	NA	PCOS with IR	All women
Schachter 2007b [32]	Israel	27/24	NA	NA	PCOS with IR	All women
Derosa 2003 [33]	Italy	49/53	25.0	53.6	Drug naïve T2DM	50.0
Ghazeeri 2015 [34]	Lebanon	18/19	NA	25.8	PCOS	All women
Derosa 2004 [35]	Italy	75/73	27.9	NA	Newly diagnosed T2DM	51.2
Erem 2014 [36]	Turkey	19/19	32.4	52.4	Newly diagnosed T2DM	71.1
Hassan 2015 [37]	Egypt	30/30	27.3	NA	Newly diagnosed T2DM	All men

I/C, intervention/control group; BMI, body mass index; CHD, coronary heart disease; PCOS, polycystic ovary syndrome; T2DM, type 2 diabetes mellitus; IGT, impaired glucose tolerance; NA, not available; IR, insulin resistance. * These two analyses were short-term and long-term outcomes of the same trial, respectively. The long-term follow-up data (de Jager, 2010 [28]) were included in the quantitative analysis.

Table 2. Study characteristics of each included study.

Study ID	Intervention	Control	Primary Treatment	Washout Period	Background Treatment	Follow-up	Assay Method of Hcy	B_{12} Supplement	Folic Acid Supplement
Carlsen 1997 [26]	Metformin (2000 mg/day) [1]	Blank	Coronary artery bypass surgery or angioplasty	Lifestyle intervention and lovastatin, 40 mg daily	Lovastatin, 40 mg daily	40 weeks	HPLC	No	No
Carlsen 2007a [2] [27]	Metformin (2000 mg/day)	Placebo	NS	No	Lifestyle intervention, folic acid 0.4 mg/day and a daily multivitamin tablet	16 weeks	HPLC	1 μg/day	0.4 mg/day
Carlsen 2007b [2] [27]	Metformin (1700 mg/day)	Placebo	NS	No	Lifestyle intervention, folate 1 mg/day and a daily multi-vitamin tablet	16 weeks	HPLC	1 μg/day	1 mg/day
de Jager 2010 [28]/ Wulffele 2003 [3] [15]	Metformin (2550 mg/day) [4]	Placebo	Insulin	Insulin (12 weeks)	Insulin	224 weeks	Chromsystems kit	No	No
Kilic 2011a [5] [29]	Metformin (1700 mg/day)	Oral contraceptive	NS	No	B-group vitamins	24 weeks	CLI	2000 mg/day	No
Kilic 2011b [5] [29]	Metformin (1700 mg/day)	Oral contraceptive	NS	No	B-group vitamins	24 weeks	CLI	2000 mg/day	No
Kilicdag 2005 [30]	Metformin (1700 mg/day)	Rosiglitazone (4 mg/day)	NS	No	No	12 weeks	FPI	No	No
Sahin 2007 [31]	Metformin (1700 mg/day)	Blank	Lifestyle intervention	Lifestyle intervention (4 weeks)	Lifestyle intervention	6 weeks	CLI	No	No
Schachter 2007a [6] [32]	Metformin (1700 mg/day)	Blank	NS	No	Infertility treatment and folic acid 0.4 mg daily	Three cycles of treatment [7]	FPI	No	0.4 mg/day
Schachter 2007b [6] [32]	Metformin (1700 mg/day)	Blank	NS	No	Infertility treatment and B-group vitamins	Three cycles of treatment [7]	FPI	0.5 mg/day	0.4 mg/day
Derosa 2003 [33]	Metformin (1500–2500 mg/day) [8]	Repaglinide (2–4 mg/day) [8]	NS	Placebo	Lifestyle intervention	60 weeks	HPLC	No	No

Table 2. *Cont.*

Study ID	Intervention	Control	Primary Treatment	Washout Period	Background Treatment	Follow-up	Assay Method of Hcy	B_{12} Supplement	Folic Acid Supplement
Ghazeeri 2015 [34]	Metformin (1700 mg/day)	placebo	NS	3 months of rosuvastatin (10 mg/day)	Rosuvastatin (10 mg/day)	24 weeks	NA	No	No
Derosa 2004 [35]	Metformin (1000–3000 mg/day) [9]	Glimepiride (1–4 mg/day) [9]	NS	No	Lifestyle intervention	56 weeks	HPLC and fluorescence detection	No	No
Erem 2014 [36]	Metformin (2000 mg/day)	Pioglitazone (15–45 mg/day) [10]	No	No	Lifestyle intervention	12 months	ELISA	No	No
Hassan 2015 [37]	Metformin (1000 mg/day)	moderately calorie-restricted diet and an active lifestyle	No	No	No	3 months	enzyme-linked immunoassay and an automated fluorescence polarization analyzer	No	No

HPLC, High pressure liquid chromatography; NS, Not significant; CLI, Chemiluminescence immunoassay; FPI, Fluorescence polarization immunoassay. [1] The average daily intake of metformin was 1707 mg at week 4, 1759 mg at week 12, and 1741 mg at week 40; [2] This article included two independent RCTs; [3] These two analyses were short-term and long-term outcomes of the same trial, respectively. The long-term follow-up data (de Jager, 2010 [28]) were included in the quantitative analysis; [4] Each patient in this group was given his or her maximally tolerated daily dose (one, two, or three tablets of 850 mg) during the trial. The actual mean dose in the metformin-treated group was 2050 mg/day; [5,6] These are 2 × 2 factorial designed trials with four treatment arms in each trial; [7] This study did not report the exact duration of follow-up; [8] The average daily intake of metformin was 2000 mg, and that of repaglinide was 3 mg; [9] The average daily intake of metformin was 2500 mg, and that of glimepiride was 3 mg; [10] Each patient in this group was given his or her maximally tolerated daily dose during the trial (15 mg/day in six patients, 30 mg/day in twelve patients, and 45 mg/day in one patient).

3.2. Quality Assessment

The risk of bias of the included studies was demonstrated in Supplementary Materials Figures S2 and S3. The procedures of random sequence generation in seven studies [26,27,31,33,35–37], of allocation concealment in nine studies [26–28,31,33–37], and of blinding of participants and personnel in five studies [30,32–34,36] were not clearly described. Selective reporting risk was unclear in one study [32]. One study was at high risk of bias in allocation concealment [32], and one study provided incomplete outcome data [32]. Quality assessment of each included study was shown in Supplementary Materials Table S5.

Potential publication bias was suspected from the funnel graph analyses, which was presented in Supplementary Materials Figure S4.

3.3. Metformin and Homocysteine

The results of the overall analysis showed that metformin did not have a statistically significant effect on the concentration of Hcy when compared with the control treatment (MD, 0.40 μmol/L; 95% CI, −0.07~0.87 μmol/L, $p = 0.10$; Figure 2). Subgroup analyses according to whether the patients received folic acid or B-group vitamins supplementation showed that administration of metformin was associated with a decreased concentration of serum Hcy in the patients receiving regular folic acid or B-group vitamins (MD, −0.74 μmol/L; 95% CI, −1.19~−0.30 μmol/L, $p = 0.001$), while with an elevated concentration of serum Hcy in the patients without any supplementation (MD, 2.02 μmol/L; 95% CI, 1.37~2.67 μmol/L, $p < 0.00001$).

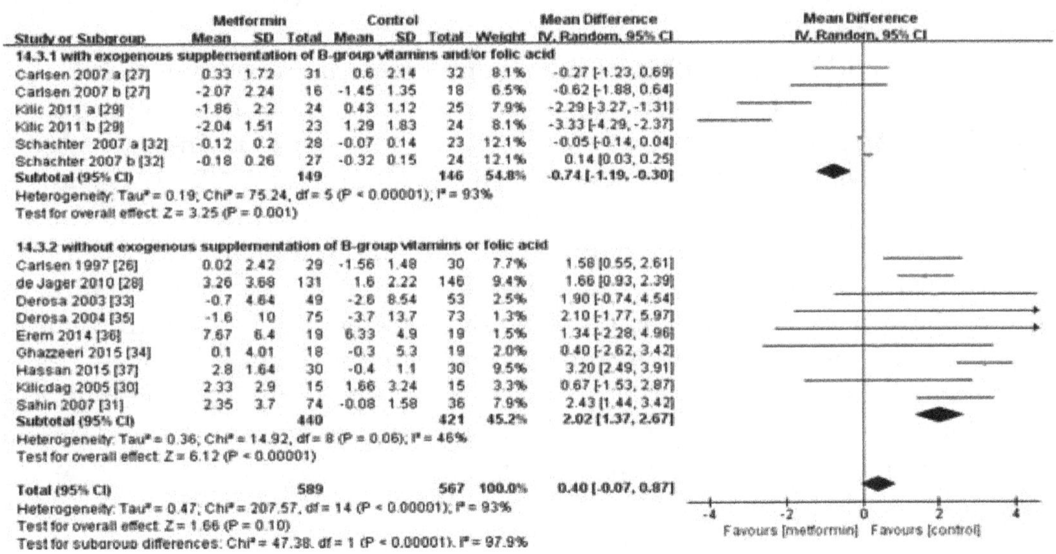

Figure 2. Overall analysis on Hcy concentration and subgroup analysis on Hcy concentration of patients with or without folic acid or B-group vitamins supplementation. The changes from baseline (Mean ± SD) between the two groups were compared. SD, standard deviation; CI, confidence interval; IV, inverse variance.

Subgroup analyses were conducted according to gender, disease type, dosage of metformin, background treatment, pre-study treatment, control treatment, duration of follow-up, change of Vitamin B_{12} concentration, and assay method of Hcy. Detailed results were presented in Supplementary Materials Table S6. It was demonstrated that the administration of metformin was associated with a significant reduction of serum Hcy among young female patients with PCOS. In addition, subgroup analysis based on the dosage of metformin showed that higher dosages of metformin (≥2000 mg daily) were associated with an elevation of serum Hcy, when compared with dosages less than 2000 mg daily (MD, 1.07 μmol/L; 95% CI, −0.17~2.30 μmol/L, $p = 0.09$).

3.4. Adverse Events

Five studies reported that more patients in the metformin group suffered gastrointestinal side effects when compared with those in the control [27,28,30,33,35]. Also, five papers did not provide any information about adverse events [26,29,31,32,34]. No death was reported. Details were shown in Supplementary Materials Table S7.

4. Discussion

Our study did not find significant association between metformin treatment and the change of serum Hcy concentration in the overall population. However, the subgroup analyses noted that metformin administration was associated with elevation of Hcy in the patients without supplementation of folic acid or B-group vitamins, which indicated that metformin might induce HHcy in the absence of exogenous folic acid or B-group vitamins supplementation.

Hcy is a sulfur amino acid with a free sulfhydryl group as the final metabolite of methionine and Vitamin B_{12} serves as a cofactor in the degeneration of Hcy to methionine. The insufficiency in Vitamin B_{12} results in the accumulation of Hcy, which is known as HHcy. HHcy is a well-established risk factor for cardiovascular diseases, cognitive impairment, and chronic renal failure [4–9], moreover, Hcy has been found to be an independent predictor of all-cause and vascular mortality [38,39]. Metformin has been demonstrated to be associated with reduction of serum Vitamin B_{12} concentration [3,40]. It has been shown that metformin could induce Vitamin B_{12} malabsorption by enhancing bacterial overgrowth, altering bacterial flora in enteric canal, and binding to the Vitamin B_{12}-intrinsic factor (IF). This malabsorption ultimately leads to a reduction of serum Vitamin B_{12} [41–45]. Hence, some researchers were calling attention to the monitoring of Vitamin B_{12} concentration in the diabetic patients treated with metformin, and suggested Vitamin B_{12} supplementation could be considered in patients with Vitamin B_{12} deficiency [3,46,47], although some authors still doubt the clinical significance of this reduction [48,49]. A recent clinical trial suggested that the metformin-associated reduction of the serum Vitamin B_{12} was due to the increased transportation and utility of Vitamin B_{12} by cells stimulated by metformin [50]. One of our subgroup analyses showed that metformin raised serum Hcy in the patients without folic acid or Vitamin B_{12} supplementation, but reduced Hcy when folic acid or Vitamin B_{12} was supplemented, indicating that metformin-associated Vitamin B_{12} reduction might be responsible for Hcy elevation, and exogenous folic acid and Vitamin B_{12} may rescue the methionine metabolic disturbance in metformin-treated patients. Considering Hcy as an important biomarker of a series of diseases and the few adverse effects of folic acid and Vitamin B_{12}, exogenous supplementation of these two vitamins could be necessary for metformin-treated patients, which is consistent with the recommendation of regular Vitamin B_{12} supplementation in the current American Association of Clinical Endocrinologists (AACE) guideline [51]. However, this recommendation had not yet been supported by well-designed randomized trials.

Our subgroup analyses also demonstrated that, the administration of metformin might cause a significant reduction of serum Hcy in young women with PCOS. However, it must be noted that, most of the young women enrolled received exogenous folic acid or B-group vitamins supplementation, and hence the observed Hcy reduction might be partially caused by the effects of exogenous folic acid or B-group vitamins. Meanwhile, estrogen, progestin, and age may also have some effects on the concentration of Hcy [5,8]. Experimental studies are required to further explain this difference.

The increase of serum Hcy concentration in the metformin-treated patients was confirmed by a series of observational studies [16–18,20,25,52–56]. These studies indicated that metformin was associated with an elevated concentration of serum Hcy compared with control treatment. Moreover, in Yilmaz's trial [20], where all the included patients were young women with PCOS but without Vitamin B_{12} or folic acid supplementation, Hcy was found to be elevated, while Vitamin B_{12} was reduced in the metformin-treated patients. In addition, Carlsen and colleagues [27] noticed that Hcy was reduced in pregnant women but not in infertile women. No explanation has been established currently, but further investigations on the pseudo reduction of Vitamin B_{12} during pregnancy and the effect of estrogen and progestin on the concentration of Hcy might help us better understand the underlying mechanism. In Carlsen's and Kilic's trials [27,29], all participants received exogenous folic acid or B-group vitamins and, interestingly, metformin-treated patients had a lower concentration of Hcy compared with controls. A possible explanation was that exogenous folic acid or B-group vitamins might counteract the reduction of the Vitamin B_{12} absorption caused by metformin [46]. In Schachter's trial [32], no matter whether the patients were treated with metformin or not, the reduction of Hcy in the patients receiving both Vitamin B_{12} and folic acid was greater than that in the patients receiving folic acid only (metformin-treated: −0.18 versus −0.12 μmol/L; metformin-untreated: −0.32 versus −0.07 μmol/L). It indicated that Vitamin B_{12} was critical in reducing serum Hcy, which could be explained by the vital role of Vitamin B_{12} in the metabolism of methionine [5].

Our study has several limitations. Firstly, the heterogeneity among the included studies was significant. Although subgroup analyses were conducted to explore possible sources of heterogeneity, factors such as weight, age, gender, and race might still influence the results of our study. Particularly, the dosage and the follow-up duration of included studies varied largely, although subgroup analyses did not find significant effects of these factors on the results. Secondly, in our subgroup analysis concerning exogenous B-group vitamins or folic acid supplementation, most patients receiving exogenous B-group vitamins or folic acid were diagnosed with PCOS or infertility, which could induce some potential biases. Further studies are required to demonstrate the interaction between metformin and B-group vitamins in patients with PCOS or infertility. Thirdly, long-term outcomes such as mortality and cardiovascular events were not studied in our analysis. Finally, the strength of the pooled results was restricted by the generally high risk of bias of included studies.

5. Conclusions

Although there is no significant change of the concentration serum Hcy between metformin-treated and non-biguanide-treated patients in the overall pooled analysis, our subgroup analysis suggested that metformin may induce an elevation of serum Hcy concentration in the absence of B-group vitamins or folic acid supplementation. Nevertheless, given the supplementation of B-group vitamins or folic acid, metformin could even be associated with reduced concentration of serum Hcy. Since HHcy is a risk factor for a series of adverse clinical outcomes, supplementation of B-group vitamins or folic acid might be necessary in metformin-treated patients, regardless of the background diseases. However, further investigations are still required to demonstrate the effects and long-term outcomes of Vitamin B_{12} or folic acid supplementation in the metformin-treated patients.

Supplementary Materials:

Table S1: Detailed inclusion and exclusion criteria of each included studies in the meta-analysis, Table S2: Rationale for excluding studies after full-text screening, Table S3: Primary and secondary outcomes of each included study, Table S4: Intervention strategy of each included study, Table S5: Rationale of quality assessment for each included study, Table S6: Summary of subgroup analysis, Table S7: Adverse events, Figure S1: Risk of bias graph: review authors' judgements about each risk of bias item presented as percentages across all included studies, Figure S2: Risk of bias summary: review authors' judgements about each risk of bias item for each included study, Figure S3: Funnel plot of comparisons.

Acknowledgments: The study was supported by grants from the National Natural Science Foundation of China (Grant No. 81400811 and 21534008), the National Basic Research Program of China (2015CB942800), the Scientific Research Project of Health and Family Planning Commission of Sichuan Province (Grant No. 130029 and 150149) and the Scientific and Technical Supporting Program of Sichuan Province (Grant No. 2014FZ0048).

Author Contributions: S.L. and J.L. designed this study; Q.Z., Q.L. and K.R. extracted the data; X.S. and L.L. are both biostatisticians from the Chinese Evidence-Based Medicine Center, West China Hospital, Sichuan University, China; X.S. provided methodological guidance of this manuscript as well as reviewed the statistics; L.L. and Q.Z. performed the data analysis and statistical procedure; Q.Z. and S.L. drafted the manuscript and all authors reviewed and revised the manuscript; J.L. is responsible for the integrity of the study as a whole.

References

1. Inzucchi, S.E.; Bergenstal, R.M.; Buse, J.B.; Diamant, M.; Ferrannini, E.; Nauck, M.; Peters, A.L.; Tsapas, A.; Wender, R.; Matthews, D.R. Management of hyperglycemia in type 2 diabetes, 2015: A patient-centered approach: Update to a position statement of the american diabetes association and the european association for the study of diabetes. *Diabetes Care* **2015**, *38*, 140–149. [CrossRef] [PubMed]
2. Global Guideline for Type 2 Diabetes—2012. Available online: http://www.idf.org/new-global-guideline-type-2-diabetes-out-now-0 (accessed on 2 January 2016).
3. Liu, Q.; Li, S.; Quan, H.; Li, J. Vitamin B12 status in metformin treated patients: Systematic review. *PLoS ONE* **2014**, *9*, e100379. [CrossRef] [PubMed]
4. Solomon, L.R. Disorders of cobalamin (vitamin B12) metabolism: Emerging concepts in pathophysiology, diagnosis and treatment. *Blood Rev.* **2007**, *21*, 113–130. [CrossRef] [PubMed]
5. Selhub, J. 5-homocysteine metabolism. *Annu. Rev. Nutr.* **1999**, *19*, 217–246. [CrossRef] [PubMed]
6. Mandaviya, P.R.; Stolk, L.; Heil, S.G. Homocysteine and DNA methylation: A review of animal and human literature. *Mol. Genet. Metab.* **2014**, *113*, 243–252. [CrossRef] [PubMed]
7. Strain, J.J.; Dowey, L.; Ward, M.; Pentieva, K.; McNulty, H. B-vitamins, homocysteine metabolism and CVD. *Proc. Nutr. Soc.* **2007**, *63*, 597–603. [CrossRef]
8. Miller, J.W. Homocysteine. In *Encyclopedia of Human Nutrition*, 3rd ed.; Elsevier: Amsterdam, The Netherlands, 2013; pp. 424–430.
9. Durand, P.P.M.; Loreau, N.; Lussier-Cacan, S.; Blache, D. Impaired homocysteine metabolism and atherothrombotic disease. *Lab. Investig.* **2011**, *81*, 645–672. [CrossRef]
10. Debreceni, B.; Debreceni, L. The role of homocysteine-lowering B-vitamins in the primary prevention of cardiovascular disease. *Cardiovasc. Ther.* **2014**, *32*, 130–138. [CrossRef] [PubMed]
11. Yang, B.; Fan, S.; Zhi, X.; Wang, Y.; Wang, Y.; Zheng, Q.; Sun, G. Prevalence of hyperhomocysteinemia in China: A systematic review and meta-analysis. *Nutrients* **2015**, *7*, 74–90. [CrossRef] [PubMed]
12. Cochrane Handbook for Systematic Reviews of Interventions. Available online: http://handbook.cochrane.org/ (accessed on 25 December 2015).
13. Gatford, K.L.; Houda, C.M.; Lu, Z.X.; Coat, S.; Baghurst, P.A.; Owens, J.A.; Sikaris, K.; Rowan, J.A.; Hague, W.M. Vitamin B12 and homocysteine status during pregnancy in the metformin in gestational diabetes trial: Responses to maternal metformin compared with insulin treatment. *Diabetes Obes. Metab.* **2013**, *15*, 660–667. [CrossRef] [PubMed]
14. Sullivan, D.; Forder, P.; Simes, J.; Whiting, M.; Kritharides, L.; Merrifield, A.; Donoghoe, M.; Colman, P.G.; Graham, N.; Haapamaki, H.; et al. Associations between the use of metformin, sulphonylureas, or diet alone and cardiovascular outcomes in 6005 people with type 2 diabetes in the field study. *Diabetes Res. Clin. Pract.* **2011**, *94*, 284–290. [CrossRef] [PubMed]
15. Wulffele, M.G.; Kooy, A.; Lehert, P.; Bets, D.; Ogterop, J.C.; Borger van der Burg, B.; Donker, A.J.; Stehouwer, C.D. Effects of short-term treatment with metformin on serum concentrations of homocysteine, folate and vitamin B12 in type 2 diabetes mellitus: A randomized, placebo-controlled trial. *J. Intern. Med.* **2003**, *254*, 455–463. [CrossRef] [PubMed]
16. Ham, A.C.; Enneman, A.W.; van Dijk, S.C.; Oliai Araghi, S.; Swart, K.M.; Sohl, E.; van Wijngaarden, J.P.; van der Zwaluw, N.L.; Brouwer-Brolsma, E.M.; Dhonukshe-Rutten, R.A.; et al. Associations between medication use and homocysteine levels in an older population, and potential mediation by vitamin B12 and folate: Data from the B-PROOF study. *Drugs Aging* **2014**, *31*, 611–621. [CrossRef] [PubMed]
17. Sahin, Y.; Unluhizarci, K.; Yilmazsoy, A.; Yikilmaz, A.; Aygen, E.; Kelestimur, F. The effects of metformin on metabolic and cardiovascular risk factors in nonobese women with polycystic ovary syndrome. *Clin. Endocrinol.* **2007**, *67*, 904–908. [CrossRef] [PubMed]
18. Rajagopal, G.; Reddy, A.P.; Venkata Harinarayan, C.; Suresh, V.; Bitla, A.; Rao, S.P.V.L.N.; Sachan, A. Effect of lifestyle modification and metformin therapy on emerging cardiovascular risk factors in overweight indian women with polycystic ovary syndrome. *Metab. Syndr. Relat. Disord.* **2012**, *10*, 273–279. [CrossRef] [PubMed]

19. Russo, G.T.; Giandalia, A.; Romeo, E.L.; Marotta, M.; Alibrandi, A.; de Francesco, C.; Horvath, K.V.; Asztalos, B.; Cucinotta, D. Lipid and non-lipid cardiovascular risk factors in postmenopausal type 2 diabetic women with and without coronary heart disease. *J. Endocrinol. Investig.* **2014**, *37*, 261–268. [CrossRef] [PubMed]
20. Yilmaz, M.; Bukan, N.; Ayvaz, G.; Karakoc, A.; Toruner, F.; Cakir, N.; Arslan, M. The effects of rosiglitazone and metformin on oxidative stress and homocysteine levels in lean patients with polycystic ovary syndrome. *Hum. Reprod.* **2005**, *20*, 3333–3340. [CrossRef] [PubMed]
21. Anderson, J.; Pena, A.S.; Sullivan, T.; Gent, R.; D'Arcy, B.; Olds, T.; Coppin, B.; Couper, J. Does metformin improve vascular health in children with type 1 diabetes? Protocol for a one year, double blind, randomised, placebo controlled trial. *BMC Pediatr.* **2013**, *13*, 108. [CrossRef] [PubMed]
22. Wulffele, M.G.; Kooy, A.; Lehert, P.; Bets, D.; Donker, A.J.; Stehouwer, C.D. Does metformin decrease blood pressure in patients with type 2 diabetes intensively treated with insulin? *Diabet. Med.* **2005**, *22*, 907–913. [CrossRef] [PubMed]
23. Luque-Ramirez, M.; Mendieta-Azcona, C.; del Rey Sanchez, J.M.; Maties, M.; Escobar-Morreale, H.F. Effects of an antiandrogenic oral contraceptive pill compared with metformin on blood coagulation tests and endothelial function in women with the polycystic ovary syndrome: Influence of obesity and smoking. *Eur. J. Endocrinol.* **2009**, *160*, 469–480. [CrossRef] [PubMed]
24. Luque-Ramirez, M.; Alvarez-Blasco, F.; Uriol Rivera, M.G.; Escobar-Morreale, H.F. Serum uric acid concentration as non-classic cardiovascular risk factor in women with polycystic ovary syndrome: Effect of treatment with ethinyl-estradiol plus cyproterone acetate versus metformin. *Hum. Reprod.* **2008**, *23*, 1594–1601. [CrossRef] [PubMed]
25. Gharakhani, M.; Neghab, N.; Farimani, M. Is reducing ovarian volume in polycystic ovarian syndrome patients after administration of metformin associated with improving cardiovascular risk factors? *Int. J. Fertil. Steril.* **2011**, *5*, 90–95. [PubMed]
26. Carlsen, S.M.; Folling, I.; Grill, V.; Bjerve, K.S.; Schneede, J.; Refsum, H. Metformin increases total serum homocysteine levels in non-diabetic male patients with coronary heart disease. *Scand. J. Clin. Lab. Investig.* **1997**, *57*, 521–527. [CrossRef]
27. Carlsen, S.M.; Kjotrod, S.; Vanky, E.; Romundstad, P. Homocysteine levels are unaffected by metformin treatment in both nonpregnant and pregnant women with polycystic ovary syndrome. *Acta Obstet. Gynecol. Scand.* **2007**, *86*, 145–150. [CrossRef] [PubMed]
28. De Jager, J.; Kooy, A.; Lehert, P.; Wulffele, M.G.; van der Kolk, J.; Bets, D.; Verburg, J.; Donker, A.J.; Stehouwer, C.D. Long term treatment with metformin in patients with type 2 diabetes and risk of vitamin B-12 deficiency: Randomised placebo controlled trial. *BMJ* **2010**, *340*, c2181. [CrossRef] [PubMed]
29. Kilic, S.; Yilmaz, N.; Zulfikaroglu, E.; Erdogan, G.; Aydin, M.; Batioglu, S. Inflammatory-metabolic parameters in obese and nonobese normoandrogenemic polycystic ovary syndrome during metformin and oral contraceptive treatment. *Gynecol. Endocrinol.* **2011**, *27*, 622–629. [CrossRef] [PubMed]
30. Kilicdag, E.B.; Bagis, T.; Zeyneloglu, H.B.; Tarim, E.; Aslan, E.; Haydardedeoglu, B.; Erkanli, S. Homocysteine levels in women with polycystic ovary syndrome treated with metformin versus rosiglitazone: A randomized study. *Hum. Reprod.* **2005**, *20*, 894–899. [CrossRef] [PubMed]
31. Sahin, M.; Tutuncu, N.B.; Ertugrul, D.; Tanaci, N.; Guvener, N.D. Effects of metformin or rosiglitazone on serum concentrations of homocysteine, folate, and vitamin B12 in patients with type 2 diabetes mellitus. *J. Diabetes Complicat.* **2007**, *21*, 118–123. [CrossRef] [PubMed]
32. Schachter, M.; Raziel, A.; Strassburger, D.; Rotem, C.; Ron-El, R.; Friedler, S. Prospective, randomized trial of metformin and vitamins for the reduction of plasma homocysteine in insulin-resistant polycystic ovary syndrome. *Fertil. Steril.* **2007**, *88*, 227–230. [CrossRef] [PubMed]
33. Derosa, G.; Mugellini, A.; Ciccarelli, L.; Crescenzi, G.; Fogari, R. Comparison of glycaemic control and cardiovascular risk profile in patients with type 2 diabetes during treatment with either repaglinide or metformin. *Diabetes Res. Clin. Pract.* **2003**, *60*, 161–169. [CrossRef]
34. Ghazeeri, G.; Abbas, H.A.; Skaff, B.; Harajly, S.; Awwad, J. Inadequacy of initiating rosuvastatin then metformin on biochemical profile of polycystic ovarian syndrome patients. *J. Endocrinol. Investig.* **2015**, *38*, 643–651. [CrossRef] [PubMed]
35. Derosa, G.; Franzetti, I.; Gadaleta, G.; Ciccarelli, L.; Fogari, R. Metabolic variations with oral antidiabetic drugs in patients with type 2 diabetes: Comparison between glimepiride and metformin. *Diabetes Nutr. Metab.* **2004**, *17*, 143–150. [PubMed]

36. Erem, C.; Ozbas, H.M.; Nuhoglu, I.; Deger, O.; Civan, N.; Ersoz, H.O. Comparison of effects of gliclazide, metformin and pioglitazone monotherapies on glycemic control and cardiovascular risk factors in patients with newly diagnosed uncontrolled type 2 diabetes mellitus. *Exp. Clin. Endocrinol. Diabetes* **2014**, *122*, 295–302. [CrossRef] [PubMed]

37. Hassan, M.H.; Abd-Allah, G.M. Effects of metformin plus gliclazide versus metformin plus glimepiride on cardiovascular risk factors in patients with type 2 diabetes mellitus. *Pak. J. Pharm. Sci.* **2015**, *28*, 1723–1730. [PubMed]

38. Anderson, J.L.; Muhlestein, J.B.; Horne, B.D.; Carlquist, J.F.; Bair, T.L.; Madsen, T.E.; Pearson, R.R. Plasma homocysteine predicts mortality independently of traditional risk factors and C-reactive protein in patients with angiographically defined coronary artery disease. *Circulation* **2000**, *102*, 1227–1232. [CrossRef] [PubMed]

39. Bates, C.J.; Mansoor, M.A.; Pentieva, K.D.; Hamer, M.; Mishra, G.D. Biochemical risk indices, including plasma homocysteine, that prospectively predict mortality in older British people: The national diet and nutrition survey of people aged 65 years and over. *Br. J. Nutr.* **2010**, *104*, 893–899. [CrossRef] [PubMed]

40. Niafar, M.; Hai, F.; Porhomayon, J.; Nader, N.D. The role of metformin on vitamin B12 deficiency: A meta-analysis review. *Intern. Emerg. Med.* **2015**, *10*, 93–102. [CrossRef] [PubMed]

41. Caspary, W.F.; Creutzfeldt, W. Analysis of the inhibitory effect of biguanides on glucose absorption: Inhibition of active sugar transport. *Diabetologia* **1971**, *7*, 379–385. [CrossRef] [PubMed]

42. Caspary, W.F.; Zavada, I.; Reimold, W.; Deuticke, U.; Emrich, D.; Willms, B. Alteration of bile acid metabolism and vitamin-B12-absorption in diabetics on biguanides. *Diabetologia* **1977**, *13*, 187–193. [CrossRef] [PubMed]

43. Scarpello, J.H.; Greaves, M.; Sladen, G.E. Small intestinal transit in diabetics. *Br. Med. J.* **1976**, *2*, 1225–1226. [CrossRef] [PubMed]

44. Schafer, G. Some new aspects on the interaction of hypoglycemia-producing biguanides with biological membranes. *Biochem. Pharmacol.* **1976**, *25*, 2015–2024. [CrossRef]

45. Carmel, R.; Rosenberg, A.H.; Lau, K.S.; Streiff, R.R.; Herbert, V. Vitamin B12 uptake by human small bowel homogenate and its enhancement by intrinsic factor. *Gastroenterology* **1969**, *56*, 548–555. [PubMed]

46. Mashavi, M.; Hanah, R.; Boaz, M.; Gavish, D.; Matas, Z.; Fux, A.; Shargorodsky, M. Effect of homocysteine-lowering therapy on arterial elasticity and metabolic parameters in metformin-treated diabetic patients. *Atherosclerosis* **2008**, *199*, 362–367. [CrossRef] [PubMed]

47. Mazokopakis, E.E.; Starakis, I.K. Recommendations for diagnosis and management of metformin-induced vitamin B12 (Cbl) deficiency. *Diabetes Res. Clin. Pract.* **2012**, *97*, 359–367. [CrossRef] [PubMed]

48. Filioussi, K.; Bonovas, S.; Katsaros, T. Should we screen diabetic patients using biguanides for megaloblastic anaemia? *Aust. Fam. Phys.* **2003**, *32*, 383–384.

49. Moore, E.M.; Mander, A.G.; Ames, D.; Kotowicz, M.A.; Carne, R.P.; Brodaty, H.; Woodward, M.; Boundy, K.; Ellis, K.A.; Bush, A.I.; et al. Increased risk of cognitive impairment in patients with diabetes is associated with metformin. *Diabetes Care* **2013**, *36*, 2981–2987. [CrossRef] [PubMed]

50. Obeid, R.; Jung, J.; Falk, J.; Herrmann, W.; Geisel, J.; Friesenhahn-Ochs, B.; Lammert, F.; Fassbender, K.; Kostopoulos, P. Serum vitamin B12 not reflecting vitamin B12 status in patients with type 2 diabetes. *Biochimie* **2013**, *95*, 1056–1061. [CrossRef] [PubMed]

51. Garber, A.J.; Abrahamson, M.J.; Barzilay, J.I.; Blonde, L.; Bloomgarden, Z.T.; Bush, M.A.; Dagogo-Jack, S.; Davidson, M.B.; Einhorn, D.; Garvey, W.T.; et al. American association of clinical endocrinologists' comprehensive diabetes management algorithm 2013 consensus statement. *Endocr. Pract.* **2013**, *19*, 536–557. [CrossRef] [PubMed]

52. Yegnanarayan, R.; Suryavanshi, M.; Singh, M.; Desai, S. A comparative study of the glycemic control of various antidiabetic agents and the role of homocysteine in the therapy of type 2 diabetes mellitus. *J. Diabetes Complicat.* **2008**, *22*, 104–111. [CrossRef] [PubMed]

53. Hoogeveen, E.K.; Kostense, P.J.; Jakobs, C.; Bouter, L.M.; Heine, R.J.; Stehouwer, C.D. Does metformin increase the serum total homocysteine level in non-insulin-dependent diabetes mellitus? *J. Intern. Med.* **1997**, *242*, 389–394. [CrossRef] [PubMed]

54. Krysiak, R.; Gilowski, W.; Okopien, B. The effect of testosterone on cardiovascular risk factors in men with type 2 diabetes and late-onset hypogonadism treated with metformin or glimepiride. *Pharmacol. Rep.* **2016**, *68*, 75–79. [CrossRef] [PubMed]
55. Sato, Y.; Ouchi, K.; Funase, Y.; Yamauchi, K.; Aizawa, T. Relationship between metformin use, vitamin B12 deficiency, hyperhomocysteinemia and vascular complications in patients with type 2 diabetes. *Endocr. J.* **2013**, *60*, 1275–1280. [CrossRef] [PubMed]
56. Wile, D.J.; Toth, C. Association of metformin, elevated homocysteine, and methylmalonic acid levels and clinically worsened diabetic peripheral neuropathy. *Diabetes Care* **2010**, *33*, 156–161. [CrossRef] [PubMed]

8

South Asian Ethnicity is Related to the Highest Risk of Vitamin B12 Deficiency in Pregnant Canadian Women

Marta Jeruszka-Bielak [1,†,§], Carly Isman [1,§], Theresa H. Schroder [1,2], Wangyang Li [1,‡], Tim J. Green [1,3] and Yvonne Lamers [1,2,*]

1 Food Nutrition and Health Program, Faculty of Land and Food Systems, The University of British Columbia, Vancouver, BC V6T 1Z4, Canada; marta_jeruszka_bielak@sggw.pl (M.J.-B.); carly.isman@gmail.com (C.I.); schrod10@mail.ubc.ca (T.H.S.); tina@medweight.ca (W.L.); Tim.Green@sahmri.com (T.J.G.)

2 BC Children's Hospital Research Institute, Vancouver, BC V5Z 4H4, Canada

3 South Australian Health Medical Research Institute, Adelaide 5000, Australia

* Correspondence: yvonne.lamers@ubc.ca

† Current address: Department of Human Nutrition, Warsaw University of Life Sciences—SGGW, 02-776 Warsaw, Poland.

‡ Current address: Medical Weight Management Centre, Coquitlam, BC V3K 7A8, Canada.

§ Shared first-authorship.

Abstract: Vitamin B12 (B12) adequacy during pregnancy is crucial for maternal health and optimal fetal development; however, suboptimal B12 status has been reported in pregnant Canadian women. Methylmalonic acid (MMA) is a sensitive indicator of B12 status. Since few studies have measured MMA during pregnancy in Canadian women, the objective of this study was to evaluate B12 status in pregnant women living in Metro Vancouver, using both plasma total B12 and MMA. We recruited a convenience sample of 320 pregnant women between 20 and 35 gestational weeks from local healthcare facilities. Plasma total B12 concentrations indicative of deficiency (<148 pmol/L) and suboptimal B12 status (148–220 pmol/L) were found in 18% and 33% of the women, respectively. Normal plasma MMA concentration (<210 nmol/L) was observed in 82% of all women. Gestational age was a strong predictor of plasma total B12 and MMA concentration, and South Asian ethnicity of B-12 deficiency and MMA concentrations. Overall, there was a high discrepancy between the prevalence of B12 inadequacy depending on the biomarker used. Independently, however, South Asian women were at particular risk for B12 deficiency, likely due to lower animal source food intake. Further study of this vulnerable group and performance testing of B12 biomarkers is warranted.

Keywords: pregnancy; cobalamin; vitamin B12; low vitamin B12 status; deficiency; methylmalonic acid; MMA; ethnicity; South Asian; predictor

1. Introduction

Maternal vitamin B12 (B12) adequacy is important for fetal growth and neurodevelopment, and for maternal and infant health. Low maternal B12 status has been associated with preterm birth [1], intra-uterine growth restriction [2], congenital heart defects [3], neural tube defects (NTDs) [4], and impaired cardiometabolic health in the offspring [5,6]. Maternal B12 status is a key determinant of infant B12 status [7,8]. Poor infant B12 status can have irreversible long-term consequences, including poor intellectual and cognitive performance later in childhood [9].

In the Canadian Health Measures Survey (Cycle 1; 2007–2009), suboptimal B12 status (serum total B12 =148–220 pmol/L) and B12 deficiency (serum total B12 <148 pmol/L) were found in 20% and 6% of adult women of all ages, respectively [10]. We previously reported a 20% prevalence of suboptimal

B12 status and 14% B12 deficiency in a convenience sample of 206 reproductive-aged women of South Asian and European ethnicity living in Metro Vancouver, with a non-significant trend for a higher prevalence of B12 deficiency in South Asian women [11]. Results of two recent prospective cohort studies of pregnant Canadian women revealed a high prevalence of low B12 status in pregnancy, with deficiency as high as 38% at delivery [12,13].

B12 deficiency is also known to be particularly high in South Asian women, with 40%–90% of women of childbearing age in India having low serum total B12 concentration and/or elevated MMA concentration [6,14,15]. This high prevalence is attributed to dietary patterns associated with little intake—low frequency and small portion sizes—of animal source foods [6]. South Asian women of childbearing age who immigrate to high-income countries are at higher risk of B12 deficiency compared to those of European descent [11,16]. The prevalence of B12 deficiency in South Asian pregnant women living in Canada has not been reported.

Biochemical B12 status can be assessed using direct indicators such as total B12 and holotranscobalamin, and functional biomarkers such as methylmalonic acid (MMA) and total homocysteine. Due to problems with the sensitivity and specificity of single measurements, the combined use of one direct and one functional biomarker has been recommended [17]; however, the majority of studies investigating B12 status have only measured total B12, including a previous study of pregnant women in Vancouver [13].

Our objective was to determine B12 status and the prevalence of B12 deficiency, using combined plasma total B12 and MMA concentrations, in a sample of healthy pregnant women in Metro Vancouver. We also aimed to identify dietary, demographic, and lifestyle factors associated with B12 status.

2. Materials and Methods

2.1. Study Population

This cross-sectional study was conducted in Metro Vancouver, British Columbia, Canada, between February 2009 and February 2010 [18]. Using convenience sampling, 340 pregnant women were recruited from BC Women's Hospital and Health Centre, Douglas College prenatal programs, and various Vancouver Coastal Health Community Health Centres. Recruitment was conducted actively by health professionals such as nurses and dietitians at these locations, as well as passively by brochures left at clinics and advertisements in local newspapers. Women were eligible to participate if they were between the 20th and 35th week of gestation, and having a singleton pregnancy. Women were excluded from participating if they had any co-morbid conditions such as gestational diabetes, cardiac or renal disease, HIV/AIDS, chronic hypertension, or autoimmune disease. The study was approved by the University of British Columbia Children's and Women's Research Ethics Board (#H08-01447). Participants provided written informed consent prior to the study.

2.2. Demographic, Lifestyle, Dietary, and Anthropometric Variables

Data were collected at a healthcare centre during a one-time interview lasting approximately 30–60 min. Participants completed a questionnaire on demographics and lifestyle factors to collect the following information: age, week of gestation, supplement use, smoking status, self-identified ethnicity, income, and highest educational level attained. We categorized women's ethnicity into European, Chinese Asian, South Asian, and "Other" ethnicities including participants of Korean, Japanese, Southeast Asian, African, Latin American, West Asian, and Arabian descent. Data for highest education level were trichotomized into the following categories: less than high school—no schooling or some elementary or completed elementary or some high school; high school degree—completed high school or some trade/vocational training or some university; university or trade school—completed trade/vocational training or completed university. Information on usual consumption of meat, fish, egg, and dairy products was collected using a qualitative questionnaire (yes/no). Participants were asked to provide their pre-pregnancy weight, and height was measured by a research assistant in order to calculate BMI.

2.3. Biochemical Analysis

Participants were asked to provide a non-fasting blood sample, from which plasma was extracted and subsequently stored at −80 °C until further analysis. Plasma samples were analyzed for B12 biomarkers unless they were haemolysed (defined by visual assessment). Plasma total B12 concentrations were measured using Microparticle Enzyme Immunoassay technology (Abbott Laboratories, Abbott Park, IL, USA). Inter-assay variation (CV %) for the medium quality control was 3.7%. Plasma MMA concentrations were quantified using liquid chromatography–tandem mass spectrometry (LC–MS/MS) (LC: Agilent Technologies, Santa Clara, CA, USA; MS/MS: SCIEX, Framingham, MA, USA) [19]. The intra- and inter-assay variations (CV %) of the method were 0.8% and 3.0%, respectively. The use of non-fasting blood samples for determining B12 status does not pose challenges in results interpretation because the indicators plasma total B12 and MMA do not underlie postprandial changes [20,21].

2.4. Statistical Analysis

To date, there are no established pregnancy-specific cutoffs for B12 biomarkers. Vitamin B12 status was categorized using the non-pregnant adult cutoffs for plasma total B12: B12 deficiency: <148 pmol/L; suboptimal B12 status: 148–220 pmol/L; B12 adequacy: >220 pmol/L. Plasma MMA concentrations were categorized as follows: <210 nmol/L, B12 replete; 210–370 nmol/L, mildly elevated MMA concentration; >370 nmol/L functional B12 deficiency [22,23].

Because plasma total B12 and MMA concentrations were skewed, non-parametric tests were applied and results are presented as medians and interquartile ranges (IQR). The impact of categorical health and lifestyle variables on total B12 concentrations was assessed using the Mann-Whitney *U* test or the Kruskal-Wallis test. The distribution of B12 deficiency, suboptimal status, and adequacy in relation to qualitative characteristics was examined with chi-squared tests using Bonferroni adjustment. Spearman's Rank correlation was used to examine the association between the biomarkers. Multiple linear and logistic regression analyses were applied to identify predictors of plasma total B12 and MMA concentrations, and predictors of B12 deficiency (dichotomized; defined as plasma total B12 <148 pmol/L) and mildly elevated MMA concentration (dichotomized; defined as plasma MMA >210 nmol/L [22]), respectively. Residuals were examined for heteroskedasticity and normality. No obvious heteroskedasticity was observed, and there were only minor deviations of the residuals from normality, which was mitigated by the large sample. Therefore, no transformation of the plasma total B12 and MMA concentrations was performed. Backwards model selection based on Akaike's Information Criterion (AIC) was used to construct the best-fit model to predict plasma total B12 or MMA concentration, B12 deficiency, or elevated MMA concentration. Prior to entry into the models, collinearity of the potential predictor variables was assessed. Statistical significance was defined as $p < 0.05$. Statistical analyses were conducted using Stata 12.1 (StataCorp LLC, College Station, TX, USA) for Windows 10 (Microsoft Corp., Redmond, WA, USA).

3. Results

3.1. Participant Characteristics

Biomarker results were obtained from 320 pregnant women; the characteristics of these participants have been previously reported [18]. Briefly, the median age was 31 years (range 16–47 years) and 63% of the participants were >30 years. Median gestational age was 30 weeks and over two-thirds of the participants were in their third trimester of pregnancy (≥27 gestational weeks). Women had a median pre-pregnancy BMI of 22.5 kg/m^2; 73% were classified as normal weight, 20% as overweight and 7% as obese. Almost half of the participants were of European descent (47%), 19% Chinese, 8% South Asians, and the remaining 26% of "other" ethnicities. The majority of women (57%) had a university degree and 6% reported to have used tobacco during pregnancy.

3.2. Plasma Total B12 and MMA Concentration

The median (IQR) plasma total B12 concentration was 215 (160, 283) pmol/L (Table 1). Plasma concentrations indicative of B12 deficiency were found in 18% of women and 33% had suboptimal B12 status (Table 1). The highest prevalence of B12 deficiency, 61.5%, was observed in women of South Asian ethnicity. Over 90% of the participants reported taking B12-containing supplements. Usual consumption of fish, meat, eggs, and dairy products was reported by 74%, 83%, 95% and 99% of the women, respectively. Plasma total B12 concentrations were higher in B12 supplement users and women with higher education. Women of South Asian ethnicity had lower plasma total B12 concentration (Table 1).

Table 1. Plasma total B12 concentration (pmol/L) and prevalence of B12 deficiency, suboptimal B12 status and B12 adequacy, stratified by demographic, anthropometric, lifestyle and dietary characteristics.

	n	Median (Interquartile Range) *	Prevalence, n (%)			
			<148 pmol/L	148–220 pmol/L	>220 pmol/L	p Value $
All participants	320	215 (160, 283)	58 (18)	106 (33)	156 (49)	
Age (years)						
<30	120	185 ^{a} (145, 245)	31 (26)	41 (34)	48 (40)	0.001 #
≥30	200	230 ^{b} (182, 298)	27 (14)	53 (26)	120 (60)	
Gestational age (weeks)						
<27	106	229 (176, 298)	16 (15)	28 (26)	62 (59)	NS
≥27	214	210 (154, 275)	42 (20)	66 (31)	106 (49)	
Pre-pregnancy body mass index (kg/m^2)						
<25	235	222 (166, 291)	39 (17)	67 (28)	129 (55)	NS
25–29.9	64	204 (151, 263)	15 (23)	19 (30)	30 (47)	
≥30	21	189 (159, 243)	4 (19)	8 (38)	9 (43)	
Ethnicity						
European	150	203 ^{a} (160, 277)	24 (16)	61 (41)	65 (43)	<0.001 #
Chinese	60	256 ^{b} (202, 311)	4 (7)	14 (23)	42 (70)	
South Asian	26	132 ^{c} (105, 231)	16 (61.5)	3 (11.5)	7 (27)	
Other	84	220 ^{a,b} (171, 269)	14 (17)	28 (33)	42 (50)	
Education						
Less than high school	21	172 ‡ (161, 209)	3 (14)	13 (62)	5 (24)	0.004 #
High school degree	77	206 (147, 264)	20 (26)	21 (27)	36 (47)	
University or trade school	221	228 ‡ (171, 287)	35 (16)	60 (27)	126 (57)	
Family income per year ($)						
<40,000	36	184 (151, 230)	7 (19)	16 (44)	13 (36)	NS
40,000 to <80,000	52	223 (171, 280)	9 (17)	14 (27)	29 (56)	
80,000 to <120,000	57	231 (160, 302)	10 (17)	17 (30)	30 (53)	
≥120,000	55	211 (176, 280)	8 (14)	18 (33)	29 (53)	
Unknown	72	225 (164, 306)	13 (18)	16 (22)	43 (60)	
Not answered	48	208 (152, 271)	11 (23)	13 (27)	24 (50)	
Smoking of tobacco during pregnancy						
Yes	18	200 (160, 237)	3 (17)	9 (50)	6 (33)	NS
No	302	219 (160, 284)	55 (18)	85 (28)	162 (54)	
Use of B12-containing supplements						
Yes	297	222 ^{a} (162, 284)	50 (17)	85 (29)	162 (54)	0.002 #
No	23	173 ^{b} (140, 221)	8 (35)	9 (39)	6 (26)	
Fish consumption						
Yes	238	223 (160, 287)	42 (18)	73 (31)	123 (52)	NS
No	82	204 (153, 258)	16 (20)	33 (40)	33 (40)	
Meat consumption						
Yes	267	216 (160, 280)	49 (18)	80 (30)	138 (52)	NS
No	18	204 (145, 302)	5 (28)	4 (22)	9 (50)	

NS, non-significant ($p > 0.05$), * Estimates within a column subgroup not sharing a common superscript letter are significantly different; Mann-Whitney U test or Kruskal-Wallis test (all $p < 0.001$) with Dunn's test for pairwise comparison ($p < 0.05$); ‡ $p = 0.065$. $ Chi-squared test to determine if the number of participants across categories of B12 status is random; # significant after Bonferroni correction, i.e., $p < 0.05/(n \text{ of tests}) = 0.05/10 = 0.005$.

The median (IQR) plasma MMA concentration was 140 (110, 187) nmol/L. The majority of pregnant women (82%) had plasma MMA concentrations indicative of B12 adequacy (<210 nmol/L; [22]), and six women (1.9%) had functional B12 deficiency (defined as having elevated MMA concentrations of >370 nmol/L; [23]). Overt B12 deficiency (defined as plasma total B12 <148 pmol/L and concurrent plasma MMA >370 nmol/L) was present in five out of the 320 women (1.6% of the study population), with three women of South Asian ethnicity. The remaining women with plasma B12 concentrations indicative of B12 deficiency had either normal (n = 31) or marginally elevated (n = 22) MMA concentrations.

There was a significant negative correlation between plasma total B12 and MMA concentrations ($\rho = -0.38$, $p < 0.0001$). Women with plasma MMA concentrations <210 nmol/L had significantly higher plasma total B12 concentrations (median 229; IQR 176, 297 pmol/L) compared to women with mildly elevated (median 157; IQR 114, 212 pmol/L) and elevated MMA concentration (median 132; IQR 107, 209 pmol/L) ($p < 0.0001$).

Plasma MMA concentrations were significantly higher in pregnant women of South Asian descent (median 223; IQR 131, 288 nmol/L) compared to European (median 144; IQR 115, 180 nmol/L), Chinese Asian (median 135; IQR 103, 190 nmol/L), and other ethnic groups (median 137; IQR 104, 174 nmol/L) ($p = 0.004$). Plasma MMA concentrations were significantly higher in third-trimester (median 146; IQR 117, 199) compared to second-trimester (median 128; IQR 96, 168) pregnant women ($p < 0.001$). There was no difference in plasma MMA concentrations with respect to pre-pregnancy BMI, supplement use, fish and meat intake, smoking, education, or income.

3.3. Predictors of B12 Status

There were complete data for multivariate analyses of 284 women after exclusion of 36 cases with missing data for meat intake and an additional case with missing data for education. The income variable was missing for 100 participants (~35%) and therefore not included in the modelling. Fish, egg, and meat intake were highly collinear with 205 out of 284 women reporting the consumption of all three. Similarly, there was a relationship between ethnicity and fish consumption with Europeans (106/140 = 76%), "Other" (54/66 = 82%), and Chinese Asian (43/56 = 77%) reporting more fish consumption than South Asians (9/22 = 41%). No similar relationship was observed between ethnicity and meat or egg consumption; however, very few women report no egg consumption (5%) or meat consumption (6%). We thus included ethnicity but excluded fish intake from the initial full model during model selection.

For plasma total B12, backwards model selection resulted in five variables remaining in the best-fit linear regression model: age, gestational age, pre-pregnancy BMI, education, and use of B12 supplements (Table 2); and two variables remaining in the best-fit logistic regression model, ethnicity and use of B12 supplements (Table 3). For plasma MMA, backwards model selection resulted in four variables remaining in the best-fit linear regression model: gestational age, ethnicity, smoking during pregnancy, and egg consumption (Table 4); and three variables remaining in the best-fit logistic regression model, gestational age, ethnicity, and egg intake (Table 5).

Plasma total B12 concentration was positively associated with age, education, and B12 supplement use (Table 2). Conversely, there was a negative relationship between gestational age and pre-pregnancy BMI with plasma total B12 concentration. Multivariate logistic regression revealed that the odds of being B12 deficient were about 10-times higher for those who self-identified as South Asians relative to those who identified as European (with "Other" and Chinese Asian ethnicity not statistically different from European ethnicity) (Table 3). The odds of being B12 deficient were 69% lower for those who were taking B12 supplements.

Table 2. Predictors of plasma total B12 concentration in linear regression model.

	Univariate		Multivariate	
	β Coefficient (95% Confidence Interval)	*p* Value	Adjusted β Coefficient (95% Confidence Interval)	Adjusted *p* Value
Age (years)	3.05 (0.49, 5.6)	0.02	2.07 (−0.54, 4.67)	0.12
Gestational age (weeks)	−3.12 (−5.63, −0.61)	0.02	−2.96 (−5.41, −0.51)	0.02
	Ethnicity			
European	reference	0.10		
Other	−5.74 (−38.8, 27.3)			
Chinese Asian	33.8 (−1.20, 68.8)			
South Asian	−26.7 (−77.4, 24.1)			
Pre-pregnancy body mass index (kg/m^2)	−3.75 (−6.74, −0.76)	0.01	−3.37 (−6.31, −0.42)	0.03
Smoking	−31.7 (−90.8, 27.3)	0.29		
	Education			
Less than high school	reference	0.02	reference	0.13
High school degree	46.4 (−11.3, 104)		32.3 (−24.6, 89.2)	
University or trade school	69.2 (16.3, 122)		50.8 (−2.61, 104)	
B12 supplement use	43.9 (−6.4, 94.2)	0.09	42.1 (−6.92, 91.1)	0.09
Fish intake	13.2 (−17.2, 43.5)	0.39		
Meat intake	13.1 (−41.2, 67.4)	0.63		
Egg intake	41.4 (−19.5, 102.3)	0.18		

p values are from likelihood ratio tests.

Table 3. Odds Ratios (OR) for having B12 deficiency, defined as plasma total B12 concentration <148 pmol/L, in logistic regression model.

	Univariate		Multivariate	
	OR (95% Confidence Interval)	*p* Value	Adjusted OR (95% Confidence Interval)	Adjusted *p* Value
Age (years)	0.95 (0.89, 1.00)	0.07		
Gestational age (weeks)	1.03 (0.97, 1.09)	0.28		
	Ethnicity			
European	reference	<0.0001	reference	<0.0001
Other	1.25 (0.57, 2.62)		1.41 (0.64, 3.04)	
Chinese Asian	0.39 (0.11, 1.08)		0.48 (0.13, 1.35)	
South Asian	8.90 (3.43, 24.7)		10.4 (3.90, 29.4)	
Pre-pregnancy body mass index (kg/m^2)	1.05 (0.98, 1.11)	0.17		
Smoking	1.07 (0.24, 3.51)	0.92		
	Education			
Less than high school	reference	0.18		
High school degree	2.01 (0.58, 9.44)			
University or trade school	1.07 (0.33, 4.79)			
B12 supplement use	0.34 (0.14, 0.91)	0.03	0.31 (0.11, 0.86)	0.03
Fish intake	0.96 (0.50, 1.95)	0.91		
Meat intake	0.59 (0.21, 1.90)	0.35		
Egg intake	0.29 (0.10, 0.91)	0.03		

p values are from likelihood ratio tests.

Plasma MMA concentration was positively associated with gestational age, ethnicity, and smoking. South Asian women had higher MMA concentration on average than European, with no discernible difference between the other ethnicities. Conversely, there was a negative relationship between plasma MMA and egg intake; however, because egg intake was nearly universal, this should be interpreted with caution. The odds of having plasma MMA concentration >210 nmol/L were about 5-times higher for those who self-identified as South Asian compared to those who self-identified as European (with Chinese Asian and "Other" ethnicities not statistically different from European). For every increase in one week of gestational age, the odds of having MMA >210 nmol/L were increased by about 11%.

Table 4. Predictors of plasma methylmalonic acid (MMA) concentration in linear regression model.

	Univariable		Multivariable	
	β Coefficient (95% Confidence Interval)	p Value	Adjusted β Coefficient (95% Confidence Interval)	Adjusted p Value
Age (years)	−1.16 (−3.05 to 0.74)	0.23		
Gestational age (weeks)	2.61 (0.78 to 4.45)	0.01	2.88 (1.11 to 4.65)	0.002
	Ethnicity			
European	reference	0.0007	reference	0.008
Other	−8.69 (−32.4 to 15.1)		−13.7 (−36.5 to 9.14)	
Chinese Asian	−13.8 (−39.0 to 11.3)		−11.4 (−35.7 to 13.0)	
South Asian	67.4 (30.9 to 104)		52.6 (15.8 to 89.4)	
Pre-pregnancy body mass index (kg/m^2)	0.57 (−1.64 to 2.79)	0.61		
Smoking	32.8 (−10.4 to 76.0)	0.14	40.7 (−1.05 to 82.4)	0.06
	Education			
Less than high school	reference	0.12		
High school degree	−32.1 (−74.7 to 10.5)			
University or trade school	−40.4 (−79.4 to −1.42)			
B12 supplement	−8.74 (−45.8 to 28.3)	0.64		
Fish intake	−17.8 (−40.0 to 4.39)	0.12		
Meat intake	−24.3 (−63.9 to 15.5)	0.23		
Egg intake	−101 (−145 to −58.2)	<0.0001	−72.6 (−117 to −28.2)	0.002

p values are from likelihood ratio tests.

Table 5. Odds Ratios (OR) for having plasma methylmalonic acid (MMA) concentration >210 nmol/L in logistic regression model.

	Univariable		Multivariable	
	OR (95% Confidence Interval)	p Value	Adjusted OR (95% Confidence Interval)	Adjusted p Value
Age (years)	0.97 (0.91 to 1.02)	0.25		
Gestational age (weeks)	1.10 (1.03 to 1.17)	0.002	1.11 (1.04 to 1.19)	0.001
	Ethnicity			
European	reference	0.001	reference	0.003
Other	0.70 (0.28 to 1.61)		0.59 (0.23 to 1.38)	
Chinese Asian	1.11 (0.47 to 2.45)		1.07 (0.45 to 2.41)	
South Asian	6.10 (2.37 to 16.2)		5.48 (1.95 to 15.8)	
Pre-pregnancy body mass index (kg/m^2)	1.01 (0.94 to 1.07)	0.84		
Smoking	0.66 (0.10 to 2.48)	0.57		
	Education			
Less than high school	reference	0.42		
High school degree	1.20 (0.37 to 4.69)			
University or trade school	0.75 (0.26 to 2.77)			
B12 supplement	0.54 (0.21 to 1.59)	0.25		
Fish intake	0.74 (0.39 to 1.46)	0.38		
Meat intake	0.43 (0.16 to 1.29)	0.12		
Egg intake	0.21 (0.07 to 0.63)	0.006	0.36 (0.10 to 1.28)	0.11

p values are from likelihood ratio tests.

4. Discussion

Vitamin B12 sufficiency in pregnancy is essential for maternal and fetal wellbeing. Assessment of B12 status of pregnant women living on the west coast of Canada using both plasma total B12 and MMA has not previously been conducted. In light of this, we measured plasma total B12 and MMA in 320 pregnant women living in Vancouver, British Columbia. We found that 33% of the women had suboptimal B12 status and 18% were B12 deficient using total B12 as sole indicator. Overt B12 deficiency, defined as plasma total B12 <148 pmol/L and concurrent plasma MMA >370 nmol/L, was uncommon and found in only 1.6% of the study population. We observed lower total B12 and higher plasma MMA concentrations in South Asian women compared to other ethnicities, and determined that the odds of being B12 deficient and having elevated MMA concentration were about 10-times and 5-times higher, respectively, for those who self-identified as South Asians relative to those who identified as European. The odds of being B12 deficient were 69% lower for those who were taking B12 supplements.

Comparing the results of studies investigating B12 status among different populations presents a number of challenges. Firstly, a wide variety of markers are used to measure B12 status, including serum/plasma total B12, MMA, total homocysteine, holotranscobalamin and total transcobalamin, and haptocorrin [24,25]. Secondly, different laboratory methods are used even for the same biomarker; for example, total B12 can be measured using microbiological [26] or immunoassays [10]. Thirdly, different cutoffs have been applied to define deficiency (e.g., for serum total B12 <125 pmol/L [27], <148 pmol/L [10,28], or even <180 pmol/L [29]). The cutoff for MMA, 210 nmol/L, was the reference value (95th percentile) of B12-replete adults with normal renal function (determined by serum creatinine) in the NHANES [22]. MMA concentrations >370 nmol/L is the "generally agreed on cutoff for elevated plasma MMA" [22] and was derived from the reference value (97.5th percentile) of healthy adults aged 40–68 years [30]. To date, there are no established cutoffs for B12 status during pregnancy for any of the B12 biomarkers. Accordingly, study findings should be compared with caution.

Two recent Canadian studies have reported the prevalence of B12 deficiency in pregnancy, with varying results. In the PREFORM study in Toronto ($n = 368$), the prevalence of suboptimal B12 status (serum total B12 <210 pmol/L) was 35% at 12–16 gestational weeks and 43% at delivery, and the prevalence of B12 deficiency (serum total B12 <148 pmol/L) was 17% and 38%, respectively [12]. In Vancouver, the prevalence of suboptimal B12 status and B12 deficiency was 21% and 10% in 264 women at 16 gestational weeks, and 35% and 23% in 220 women at delivery, respectively [13]; plasma MMA concentration was not measured in the study by Wu et al. [13]. In the PREFORM study, plasma MMA concentration was measured and the prevalence of functional B12 deficiency (defined as MMA >271 nmol/L) was two percent in early pregnancy and five percent at delivery [12]. In the present study, 26 (eight percent) of second- and third-trimester pregnant women had plasma MMA concentration >270 nmol/L. Notwithstanding the variable findings and the need for performance testing of B12 biomarkers during pregnancy, the prevalences of low total B12 concentration in pregnant Canadian women are high and highlight the importance of measuring B12 status early in pregnancy in order to develop interventions and prevent adverse maternal and fetal health outcomes.

In the present study, plasma MMA concentrations were positively associated with gestational age in these women. Differences in plasma total B12 concentrations were less pronounced and negatively correlated to gestational age. Because median MMA concentrations of women in their second (128 nmol/L) and third trimester (146 nmol/L) were well within the normal range (i.e., <210 nmol/L), the relationship we found between gestational age and MMA concentration does not appear to be clinically significant. Our findings are consistent with those of Murphy et al. [31], who reported increases in plasma MMA between the first and third trimester. In a longitudinal study in 406 Danish pregnant women, the prevalence of plasma total B12 concentrations <150 pmol/L (i.e., B12 deficiency) also increased over pregnancy, from 15% at 18 weeks of gestation, to almost 43% at 39 weeks of gestation [32]. Another prospective longitudinal study of pregnancy indicated that the prevalence of B12 deficiency increased between the second and third trimester from 8% ($n = 3$) to 35% ($n = 12$) in healthy pregnant women with B12 intake >RDA (2.6 μg/day) [28] supporting the need for pregnancy-specific cutoffs. The decrease in plasma total B12 during pregnancy could result from increased metabolic rate, active B12 transport across the placenta, and hemodilution. This suggestion is supported by the finding that plasma total B12 concentrations significantly increase postpartum, without supplementation [32,33]. Altering cutoffs for B12 biomarker concentrations in pregnant women will require extensive research to ensure the prevention of adverse health outcomes.

In our study, women who did not take supplements had double the risk of B12 deficiency compared to those who took B12-containing supplements (Table 3). Plasma total B12 concentration substantially differed between supplement users and non-users (Table 1); however, supplement use was not a significant predictor of plasma total B12 concentration (Table 2), which might be explained by the low number (n = 23/320; 7%) of women not using supplements. The prevalence of supplement use in pregnant Canadian women was reported to be very high with 89% of women using supplements in late pregnancy [34]. The B12 content in prenatal supplements in Canada greatly varies from 2 µg/day to 12 µg/day; the majority (62%) of supplement users in this study reported to use prenatal supplements with a dosage of 2.6 µg/day. Supplement use however was neither a predictor of plasma MMA concentrations nor associated with a lower risk for having elevated MMA. This finding might indicate that the majority of the women in this study were B12 replete, as reflected by their MMA concentration, and supplemental B12 only affected circulating total B12. This would support the hypothesis and B12 absorption findings by Greibe et al. [33] that the decrease in circulating total B12 concentration throughout gestation does not reflect B12 deficiency but 'normal' pregnancy-related changes in total B12 that do not impair intracellular B12 status.

An important finding of our study is that the majority of South Asian pregnant women in our cohort had suboptimal B12 status (11.5%) or were B12 deficient (61.5%). Moreover, three out of five women with overt B12 deficiency were of South Asian ethnicity. Our findings are comparable to those of a recent study on pregnant women from urban South India reporting that 51% had plasma total B12 <150 pmol/L and 76% had elevated MMA concentrations (defined as plasma MMA >260 nmol/L; compared to 46% in the current study) [15]. Of those women, 42% had impaired B12 status (i.e., total B12 <150 pmol and MMA >260 nmol/L). The study found that not consuming yogurt or fish and being primiparous were predictors of poor B12 status [15]. Cultural and religious practices that promote vegetarianism inherent to certain Indian communities around the world place these groups at greater risk of B12 deficiency during pregnancy. In a study conducted in the US, Indian women had significantly lower median serum total B12 concentrations than did "other ethnicity" (combining whites, blacks, non-Indian Asians and Latin Americans) and 24% were B12 deficient (<180 pmol/L) [29]. A randomized controlled trial of B12 supplementation in South Asian immigrant women living in New Zealand reported that 48% of the cohort (n = 62) had serum total B12 <222 pmol/L [16]. Supplementation with 6 µg of cyanocobalamin per day for six months increased serum total B12 by 30% [16].

In contrast to South Asian immigrant women, our study showed that Asian pregnant women (mostly Chinese, Southeast Asian, Japanese, Korean, and Filipino) had the highest total B12 concentrations, and the lowest prevalence of B12 inadequacy. The risk of being B12 deficient was 50% lower in Asians than in women of European descent. Similar results have been observed in an elderly population, where Asian-Americans (Chinese, Korean, Vietnamese, Japanese, or Filipino origin) had significantly higher plasma total B12 concentrations compared to European whites [35].

Without collecting quantitative data on food product consumption, we do not know what the overall B12 intake was. In our study, meat or fish consumption did not have a significant effect on plasma total B12 concentrations. Egg and dairy intake was reported by 95% and 99%, respectively, of all women. Vogiatzoglou et al. [26] found that higher consumption of dairy products (especially milk) and fish increased plasma total B12 concentrations, but meat and eggs did not. Intake of fish, but not other animal source foods, decreased the risk of having inadequate B12 status in South Indian pregnant women [15]. Of the South Asians in the current study 59% reported eating no fish, 27% no meat, and 27% no eggs. Ninety-five percent of South Asian women used B12-containing prenatal vitamin supplements compared to 89% and 100% of European and Chinese Asian women, respectively. We hypothesize that low dietary B12 intake likely contributed to the poor B12 status observed in the South Asian women.

In our study, pre-pregnancy BMI was negatively correlated with plasma total B12 ($\rho = -0.184$; $p = 0.001$) but did not significantly influence the median values of either marker or the prevalence of B12 deficiency. We observed that B12-replete pregnant women had a tendency to have a lower median BMI value. Pre-pregnancy BMI was the strongest independent predictor of plasma total B12 concentration, as was gestational age. First-trimester BMI was inversely associated with third-trimester serum total B12 concentration in a retrospective case-control study of 344 UK pregnant women who were not taking B12-containing supplements [36]. The BMI at 28 weeks of gestation was an independent predictor of circulating total B12 concentrations in UK pregnant women [37]. The Canadian Health Measures Survey 2007–2009 showed that the prevalence of B12 adequacy was lower in Canadian adults with obesity compared to normal weight and overweight adults of all age groups [10]. Being obese may alter B12 absorption, excretion or metabolism, but whether the relationship is casual [38] requires further investigation.

The strength of our research is the measurement of two biomarkers for B12 status assessment as per recommendation by an expert panel [17]. We however acknowledge the limitations of our study that include the convenience sampling and the lack of a sensitive dietary assessment tool to quantify dietary B12 intake. We also acknowledge the lack of hematological indicators, such as hemoglobin, mean corpuscular volume, or blood cell count, to investigate whether overt B12 deficiency, as observed in five women in this study, was associated with clinical outcomes. The original study did not include the measurement of hematological indicators and the retrospective analysis was not feasible for reasons of biospecimen requirements. We thus cannot conclude whether the overt B12 deficiency was of clinical concern. Women with overt B12 deficiency did not differ from the other 315 women in age (30.6 years versus 31.4 years, $p = 0.74$) or BMI (24.5 kg/m^2 versus 22.5 kg/m^2, $p = 0.42$); but reported lower intake of fish (40% versus 75%), meat (67% versus 94%), and egg (80% versus 95%). Nutritional status can be influenced by genetic modifiers of molecules involved in the digestion, absorption or metabolism of nutrients. Genetic variants related to B12 metabolism might explain some of the variation in our findings with respect to elevated MMA [39] and low total B12 concentration [40,41]; however, because we lack the women's consent for genotyping in this study, we were unable to investigate this.

The assessment of B12 status is challenged by the sensitivity and specificity limitations of individual biomarkers; we therefore followed the recommendations to using at least one direct and one functional indicator of B12 status [17] while respecting available sample volume and budget. We measured total B12, the most commonly used biomarker and direct indicator, and MMA, the more specific functional indicator of B12 deficiency compared to total homocysteine. The additional measurement of total homocysteine might not have allowed further insight to the B12 status of these women; in Canada, a folate-replete nation, elevated total homocysteine concentrations (defined as >13 μmol/L [22,42]) was observed in five percent of the general population [10] but not in pregnant Canadian women [12]. While MMA is considered the more specific indicator of B12 status, we acknowledge that MMA is influenced by renal function [43] and we lack the measurement of creatinine to control for renal function in the interpretation of elevated MMA concentration. Due to budget limits, we also did not include the measurement of folate that has an interdependent metabolic role with B12. The access to both total B12 and folate data would have allowed us to investigate the interaction of folate and B12 on biochemical outcomes. High folate status with low plasma total B12 concentration has been associated with higher MMA concentration in older adults [44–46], however not in younger adults [46]. The interaction of high folate and low B12 status on biochemical outcomes in pregnant women warrants further investigation.

5. Conclusions

Protecting women of reproductive age from B12 deficiency is important to the health of mothers and their offspring. Our study showed that a sample of pregnant women in Vancouver, Canada, had a high prevalence of low circulating total B12 concentrations, with 18% being classified as B12 deficient. However, overt B12 deficiency was present in only 1.6% of the sample. The observed discrepancy in the prevalence of B12 adequacy depending on the biomarker and cutoff used emphasizes the need for pregnancy-specific cutoffs and performance testing of B12 biomarkers during pregnancy. Independent of the biomarker used, individually or combined, South Asian pregnant women were at particular risk for B12 deficiency compared to other ethnic groups, and further study of this vulnerable group is required.

Acknowledgments: The authors thank Arianne Albert from the Women's Health Research Institute for statistical support. This research was supported by funding from the "Food, Nutrition and Health Vitamin Research Fund", Faculty of Land and Food Systems, UBC. M.J.-B. acknowledges funding from the UBC Dekaban Scholarship. Y.L. acknowledges funding from the Canadian Institutes for Health Research/Canada Research Chair Program.

Author Contributions: M.J.-B. performed data analysis, contributed to data interpretation and the drafting of this report. C.I. run the plasma MMA analyses and wrote the first draft of the report. T.H.S. contributed to sample analyses, data interpretation, and report writing. W.L. and T.J.G. designed and conducted the original study. Y.L. designed this secondary study and led the sample and data analysis, data interpretation, and report writing. All authors read and approved the final manuscript.

References

1. Ronnenberg, A.G.; Goldman, M.B.; Chen, D.; Aitken, I.W.; Willett, W.C.; Selhub, J.; Xu, X. Preconception homocysteine and B vitamin status and birth outcomes in Chinese women. *Am. J. Clin. Nutr.* **2002**, *76*, 1385–1391. [PubMed]
2. Muthayya, S.; Kurpad, A.V.; Duggan, C.P.; Bosch, R.J.; Dwarkanath, P.; Mhaskar, A.; Mhaskar, R.; Thomas, A.; Vaz, M.; Bhat, S.; et al. Low maternal vitamin B12 status is associated with intrauterine growth retardation in urban South Indians. *Eur. J. Clin. Nutr.* **2006**, *60*, 791–801. [CrossRef] [PubMed]
3. Verkleij-Hagoort, A.C.; van Driel, L.M.; Lindemans, J.; Isaacs, A.; Steegers, E.A.; Helbing, W.A.; Uitterlinden, A.G.; Steegers-Theunissen, R.P. Genetic and lifestyle factors related to the periconception vitamin B12 status and congenital heart defects: A Dutch case-control study. *Mol. Genet. Metab.* **2008**, *94*, 112–119. [CrossRef] [PubMed]
4. Molloy, A.M.; Kirke, P.N.; Troendle, J.F.; Burke, H.; Sutton, M.; Brody, L.C.; Scott, J.M.; Mills, J.L. Maternal vitamin B12 status and risk of neural tube defects in a population with high neural tube defect prevalence and no folic acid fortification. *Pediatrics* **2009**, *123*, 917–923. [CrossRef] [PubMed]
5. Stewart, C.P.; Christian, P.; Schulze, K.J.; Arguello, M.; LeClerq, S.C.; Khatry, S.K.; West, K.P., Jr. Low maternal vitamin B-12 status is associated with offspring insulin resistance regardless of antenatal micronutrient supplementation in rural Nepal. *J. Nutr.* **2011**, *141*, 1912–1917. [CrossRef] [PubMed]
6. Yajnik, C.S.; Deshpande, S.S.; Jackson, A.A.; Refsum, H.; Rao, S.; Fisher, D.J.; Bhat, D.S.; Naik, S.S.; Coyaji, K.J.; Joglekar, C.V.; et al. Vitamin B12 and folate concentrations during pregnancy and insulin resistance in the offspring: The Pune maternal nutrition study. *Diabetologia* **2008**, *51*, 29–38. [CrossRef] [PubMed]
7. Hay, G.; Clausen, T.; Whitelaw, A.; Trygg, K.; Johnston, C.; Henriksen, T.; Refsum, H. Maternal folate and cobalamin status predicts vitamin status in newborns and 6-month-old infants. *J. Nutr.* **2010**, *140*, 557–564. [CrossRef] [PubMed]
8. Duggan, C.; Srinivasan, K.; Thomas, T.; Samuel, T.; Rajendran, R.; Muthayya, S.; Finkelstein, J.L.; Lukose, A.; Fawzi, W.; Allen, L.H.; et al. Vitamin B-12 supplementation during pregnancy and early lactation increases maternal, breast milk, and infant measures of vitamin B-12 status. *J. Nutr.* **2014**, *144*, 758–764. [CrossRef] [PubMed]
9. Strand, T.A.; Taneja, S.; Ueland, P.M.; Refsum, H.; Bahl, R.; Schneede, J.; Sommerfelt, H.; Bhandari, N. Cobalamin and folate status predicts mental development scores in North Indian children 12–18 mo of age. *Am. J. Clin. Nutr.* **2013**, *97*, 310–317. [CrossRef] [PubMed]
10. MacFarlane, A.J.; Greene-Finestone, L.S.; Shi, Y. Vitamin B-12 and homocysteine status in a folate-replete population: Results from the Canadian Health Measures Survey. *Am. J. Clin. Nutr.* **2011**, *94*, 1079–1087. [CrossRef] [PubMed]
11. Quay, T.A.W.; Schroder, T.H.; Jeruszka-Bielak, M.; Li, W.; Devlin, A.M.; Barr, S.I.; Lamers, Y. High rate of suboptimal vitamin B12 status in South Asian and European women of childbearing age in Metro Vancouver. *Appl. Physiol. Nutr. Metab.* **2015**. [CrossRef] [PubMed]
12. Visentin, C.E.; Masih, S.P.; Plumptre, L.; Schroder, T.H.; Sohn, K.J.; Ly, A.; Lausman, A.Y.; Berger, H.; Croxford, R.; Lamers, Y.; et al. Low serum vitamin B-12 concentrations are prevalent in a cohort of pregnant Canadian women. *J. Nutr.* **2016**, *146*, 1035–1042. [CrossRef] [PubMed]
13. Wu, B.T.; Innis, S.M.; Mulder, K.A.; Dyer, R.A.; King, D.J. Low plasma vitamin B-12 is associated with a lower pregnancy-associated rise in plasma free choline in Canadian pregnant women and lower postnatal growth rates in their male infants. *Am. J. Clin. Nutr.* **2013**, *98*, 1209–1217. [CrossRef] [PubMed]
14. Krishnaveni, G.V.; Hill, J.C.; Veena, S.R.; Bhat, D.S.; Wills, A.K.; Karat, C.L.; Yajnik, C.S.; Fall, C.H. Low

plasma vitamin B12 in pregnancy is associated with gestational 'diabesity' and later diabetes. *Diabetologia* **2009**, *52*, 2350–2358. [PubMed]

15. Samuel, T.M.; Duggan, C.; Thomas, T.; Bosch, R.; Rajendran, R.; Virtanen, S.M.; Srinivasan, K.; Kurpad, A.V. Vitamin B(12) intake and status in early pregnancy among urban South Indian women. *Ann. Nutr. Metab.* **2013**, *62*, 113–122. [CrossRef] [PubMed]
16. Mearns, G.J.; Koziol-McLain, J.; Obolonkin, V.; Rush, E.C. Preventing vitamin B12 deficiency in South Asian women of childbearing age: A randomised controlled trial comparing an oral vitamin B12 supplement with B12 dietary advice. *Eur. J. Clin. Nutr.* **2014**, *68*, 870–875. [CrossRef] [PubMed]
17. Yetley, E.A.; Pfeiffer, C.M.; Phinney, K.W.; Bailey, R.L.; Blackmore, S.; Bock, J.L.; Brody, L.C.; Carmel, R.; Curtin, L.R.; Durazo-Arvizu, R.A.; et al. Biomarkers of vitamin B-12 status in NHANES: A roundtable summary. *Am. J. Clin. Nutr.* **2011**, *94*, 313S–321S. [CrossRef] [PubMed]
18. Li, W.; Green, T.J.; Innis, S.M.; Barr, S.I.; Whiting, S.J.; Shand, A.; von Dadelszen, P. Suboptimal vitamin D levels in pregnant women despite supplement use. *Can. J. Public Health* **2011**, *102*, 308–312. [PubMed]
19. Schroder, T.H.; Quay, T.A.; Lamers, Y. Methylmalonic acid quantified in dried blood spots provides a precise, valid, and stable measure of functional vitamin B-12 status in healthy women. *J. Nutr.* **2014**, *144*, 1658–1663. [CrossRef] [PubMed]
20. Von Castel-Roberts, K.M.; Morkbak, A.L.; Nexo, E.; Edgemon, C.A.; Maneval, D.R.; Shuster, J.J.; Valentine, J.F.; Kauwell, G.P.; Bailey, L.B. Holo-transcobalamin is an indicator of vitamin B-12 absorption in healthy adults with adequate vitamin B-12 status. *Am. J. Clin. Nutr.* **2007**, *85*, 1057–1061. [PubMed]
21. Rasmussen, K. Studies on methylmalonic acid in humans. I. Concentrations in serum and urinary excretion in normal subjects after feeding and during fasting, and after loading with protein, fat, sugar, isoleucine, and valine. *Clin. Chem.* **1989**, *35*, 2271–2276. [PubMed]
22. Pfeiffer, C.M.; Caudill, S.P.; Gunter, E.W.; Osterloh, J.; Sampson, E.J. Biochemical indicators of B vitamin status in the US population after folic acid fortification: Results from the National Health and Nutrition Examination Survey 1999–2000. *Am. J. Clin. Nutr.* **2005**, *82*, 442–450. [PubMed]
23. Holleland, G.; Schneede, J.; Ueland, P.M.; Lund, P.K.; Refsum, H.; Sandberg, S. Cobalamin deficiency in general practice. Assessment of the diagnostic utility and cost-benefit analysis of methylmalonic acid determination in relation to current diagnostic strategies. *Clin. Chem.* **1999**, *45*, 189–198. [PubMed]
24. Obeid, R.; Morkbak, A.L.; Munz, W.; Nexo, E.; Herrmann, W. The cobalamin-binding proteins transcobalamin and haptocorrin in maternal and cord blood sera at birth. *Clin. Chem.* **2006**, *52*, 263–269. [CrossRef] [PubMed]
25. Morkbak, A.L.; Hvas, A.M.; Milman, N.; Nexo, E. Holotranscobalamin remains unchanged during pregnancy. Longitudinal changes of cobalamins and their binding proteins during pregnancy and postpartum. *Haematologica* **2007**, *92*, 1711–1712. [CrossRef] [PubMed]
26. Vogiatzoglou, A.; Smith, A.D.; Nurk, E.; Berstad, P.; Drevon, C.A.; Ueland, P.M.; Vollset, S.E.; Tell, G.S.; Refsum, H. Dietary sources of vitamin B-12 and their association with plasma vitamin B-12 concentrations in the general population: The Hordaland Homocysteine Study. *Am. J. Clin. Nutr.* **2009**, *89*, 1078–1087. [CrossRef] [PubMed]
27. Ray, J.G.; Goodman, J.; O'Mahoney, P.R.; Mamdani, M.M.; Jiang, D. High rate of maternal vitamin B12 deficiency nearly a decade after canadian folic acid flour fortification. *QJM* **2008**, *101*, 475–477. [CrossRef] [PubMed]
28. Koebnick, C.; Heins, U.A.; Dagnelie, P.C.; Wickramasinghe, S.N.; Ratnayaka, I.D.; Hothorn, T.; Pfahlberg, A.B.; Hoffmann, I.; Lindemans, J.; Leitzmann, C. Longitudinal concentrations of vitamin B(12) and vitamin B(12)-binding proteins during uncomplicated pregnancy. *Clin. Chem.* **2002**, *48*, 928–933. [PubMed]
29. Carmel, R.; Mallidi, P.V.; Vinarskiy, S.; Brar, S.; Frouhar, Z. Hyperhomocysteinemia and cobalamin deficiency in young Asian Indians in the United States. *Am. J. Hematol.* **2002**, *70*, 107–114. [CrossRef] [PubMed]
30. Rasmussen, K.; Moller, J.; Ostergaard, K.; Kristensen, M.O.; Jensen, J. Methylmalonic acid concentrations in serum of normal subjects: Biological variability and effect of oral L-isoleucine loads before and after intramuscular administration of cobalamin. *Clin. Chem.* **1990**, *36*, 1295–1299. [PubMed]
31. Murphy, M.M.; Molloy, A.M.; Ueland, P.M.; Fernandez-Ballart, J.D.; Schneede, J.; Arija, V.; Scott, J.M. Longitudinal study of the effect of pregnancy on maternal and fetal cobalamin status in healthy women and their offspring. *J. Nutr.* **2007**, *137*, 1863–1867. [PubMed]
32. Milman, N.; Byg, K.E.; Bergholt, T.; Eriksen, L.; Hvas, A.M. Cobalamin status during normal pregnancy and postpartum: A longitudinal study comprising 406 Danish women. *Eur. J. Haematol.* **2006**, *76*, 521–525. [CrossRef] [PubMed]

33. Greibe, E.; Andreasen, B.H.; Lildballe, D.L.; Morkbak, A.L.; Hvas, A.M.; Nexo, E. Uptake of cobalamin and markers of cobalamin status: A longitudinal study of healthy pregnant women. *Clin. Chem. Lab. Med.* **2011**, *49*, 1877–1882. [CrossRef] [PubMed]
34. Masih, S.P.; Plumptre, L.; Ly, A.; Berger, H.; Lausman, A.Y.; Croxford, R.; Kim, Y.I.; O'Connor, D.L. Pregnant Canadian women achieve recommended intakes of one-carbon nutrients through prenatal supplementation but the supplement composition, including choline, requires reconsideration. *J. Nutr.* **2015**, *145*, 1824–1834. [CrossRef] [PubMed]
35. Carmel, R.; Green, R.; Jacobsen, D.W.; Rasmussen, K.; Florea, M.; Azen, C. Serum cobalamin, homocysteine, and methylmalonic acid concentrations in a multiethnic elderly population: Ethnic and sex differences in cobalamin and metabolite abnormalities. *Am. J. Clin. Nutr.* **1999**, *70*, 904–910. [PubMed]
36. Sukumar, N.; Venkataraman, H.; Wilson, S.; Goljan, I.; Selvamoni, S.; Patel, V.; Saravanan, P. Vitamin B12 status among pregnant women in the UK and its association with obesity and gestational diabetes. *Nutrients* **2016**, *8*, 768. [CrossRef] [PubMed]
37. Knight, B.A.; Shields, B.M.; Brook, A.; Hill, A.; Bhat, D.S.; Hattersley, A.T.; Yajnik, C.S. Lower circulating B12 is associated with higher obesity and insulin resistance during pregnancy in a non-diabetic White British population. *PLoS ONE* **2015**, *10*, e0135268.
38. Allin, K.H.; Friedrich, N.; Pietzner, M.; Grarup, N.; Thuesen, B.H.; Linneberg, A.; Pisinger, C.; Hansen, T.; Pedersen, O.; Sandholt, C.H. Genetic determinants of serum vitamin B12 and their relation to body mass index. *Eur. J. Epidemiol.* **2016**. [CrossRef] [PubMed]
39. Molloy, A.M.; Pangilinan, F.; Mills, J.L.; Shane, B.; O'Neill, M.B.; McGaughey, D.M.; Velkova, A.; Abaan, H.O.; Ueland, P.M.; McNulty, H.; et al. A common polymorphism in HIBCH influences methylmalonic acid concentrations in blood independently of cobalamin. *Am. J. Hum. Genet.* **2016**, *98*, 869–882. [CrossRef] [PubMed]
40. Thuesen, B.H.; Husemoen, L.L.; Ovesen, L.; Jorgensen, T.; Fenger, M.; Linneberg, A. Lifestyle and genetic determinants of folate and vitamin B12 levels in a general adult population. *Br. J. Nutr.* **2010**, *103*, 1195–1204. [CrossRef] [PubMed]
41. Tanwar, V.S.; Chand, M.P.; Kumar, J.; Garg, G.; Seth, S.; Karthikeyan, G.; Sengupta, S. Common variant in FUT2 gene is associated with levels of vitamin B(12) in Indian population. *Gene* **2013**, *515*, 224–228. [CrossRef] [PubMed]
42. Bailey, R.L.; Carmel, R.; Green, R.; Pfeiffer, C.M.; Cogswell, M.E.; Osterloh, J.D.; Sempos, C.T.; Yetley, E.A. Monitoring of vitamin B-12 nutritional status in the United States by using plasma methylmalonic acid and serum vitamin B-12. *Am. J. Clin. Nutr.* **2011**, *94*, 552–561. [CrossRef] [PubMed]
43. Vogiatzoglou, A.; Oulhaj, A.; Smith, A.D.; Nurk, E.; Drevon, C.A.; Ueland, P.M.; Vollset, S.E.; Tell, G.S.; Refsum, H. Determinants of plasma methylmalonic acid in a large population: Implications for assessment of vitamin B12 status. *Clin. Chem.* **2009**, *55*, 2198–2206. [CrossRef] [PubMed]
44. Selhub, J.; Morris, M.S.; Jacques, P.F. In vitamin B12 deficiency, higher serum folate is associated with increased total homocysteine and methylmalonic acid concentrations. *Proc. Natl. Acad. Sci. USA* **2007**, *104*, 19995–20000. [CrossRef] [PubMed]
45. Miller, J.W.; Garrod, M.G.; Allen, L.H.; Haan, M.N.; Green, R. Metabolic evidence of vitamin B-12 deficiency, including high homocysteine and methylmalonic acid and low holotranscobalamin, is more pronounced in older adults with elevated plasma folate. *Am. J. Clin. Nutr.* **2009**, *90*, 1586–1592. [CrossRef] [PubMed]
46. Solomon, L.R. Advanced age as a risk factor for folate-associated functional cobalamin deficiency. *J. Am. Geriatr. Soc.* **2013**, *61*, 577–582. [CrossRef] [PubMed]

9

Methionine and Choline Supply during the Periparturient Period Alter Plasma Amino Acid and One-Carbon Metabolism Profiles to Various Extents: Potential Role in Hepatic Metabolism and Antioxidant Status

Zheng Zhou [1], Mario Vailati-Riboni [1], Daniel N. Luchini [2] and Juan J. Loor [1,*]

[1] Mammalian NutriPhysioGenomics, Department of Animal Sciences and Division of Nutritional Sciences, University of Illinois, Urbana, IL 61801, USA; zzhou32@illinois.edu (Z.Z.); vailati2@illinois.edu (M.V.-R.)
[2] Adisseo North America, Alpharetta, GA 30022, USA; daniel.luchini@adisseo.com
[*] Correspondence: jloor@illinois.edu

Abstract: The objective of this study was to profile plasma amino acids (AA) and derivatives of their metabolism during the periparturient period in response to supplemental rumen-protected methionine (MET) or rumen-protected choline (CHOL). Forty cows were fed from −21 through 30 days around parturition in a 2 × 2 factorial design a diet containing MET or CHOL. MET supply led to greater circulating methionine and proportion of methionine in the essential AA pool, total AA, and total sulfur-containing compounds. Lysine in total AA also was greater in these cows, indicating a better overall AA profile. Sulfur-containing compounds (cystathionine, cystine, homocystine, and taurine) were greater in MET-fed cows, indicating an enriched sulfur-containing compound pool due to enhanced transsulfuration activity. Circulating essential AA and total AA concentrations were greater in cows supplied MET due to greater lysine, arginine, tryptophan, threonine, proline, asparagine, alanine, and citrulline. In contrast, CHOL supply had no effect on essential AA or total AA, and only tryptophan and cystine were greater. Plasma 3-methylhistidine concentration was lower in response to CHOL supply, suggesting less tissue protein mobilization in these cows. Overall, the data revealed that enhanced periparturient supply of MET has positive effects on plasma AA profiles and overall antioxidant status.

Keywords: amino acids; lactation; methyl donors; periparturient dairy cow

---

1. Introduction

Around parturition, the increased demand for nutrients to sustain fetal growth and lactation coupled with depressed dry matter intake (DMI) impose tremendous metabolic stress on dairy cows. Consequently, health problems and compromised production performance likely occur not only due to negative energy balance-induced increases in circulating free fatty acids, but a negative amino acid (AA) balance [1–3]. For instance, increased mobilization of tissue protein is often observed due to inadequate availability of AA substrates for gluconeogenesis as well as synthesis of protein in liver and mammary gland [4]. In fact, a moderate net loss of carcass protein was observed even in animals fed to predicted metabolizable protein requirements around parturition [1,5], indicating suboptimal profiles of AA may be the limiting factor for their utilization during this period. In line with this assumption, supplementing rumen-protected limiting AA has achieved various benefits in terms of lactation performance and health status of periparturient dairy cows [6–9].

Methionine (Met) is an essential sulfur-containing AA associated with various key physiologic events. Previous research has underscored the importance of Met as a limiting AA for milk protein synthesis in many diets [10,11]. Apart from its apparent key role in mammary gland and liver protein synthesis, Met also serves as substrate for sulfur-containing antioxidants, namely glutathione (GSH) and taurine [12]. In addition, as a key component of one-carbon metabolism, hundreds of methylation reactions acquire methyl groups from Met via *S*-adenosyl methionine (SAM) [13]. Furthermore, as a gluconeogenic AA, a portion of Met may be taken up by liver to sustain the abrupt increase in demand for glucose at the onset of lactation. In line with the various biologic processes relying on Met, its deficiency has often been reported in cows around parturition [3]. In fact, circulating Met concentration decreased markedly through parturition and were not restored to prepartum levels until 28 days postpartum [3].

An unfavorable circulating AA profile around parturition likely occurs due to (1) increased production of positive acute-phase proteins (APP) and immune-related proteins induced by oxidative stress and inflammation; (2) enhanced carcass protein mobilization to provide AA for gluconeogenesis; and/or (3) limited uptake of other AA and increased N excretion due to lack of Met. Recent research with periparturient dairy cows has demonstrated benefits to overall health and production performance in response to MET supplementation [7,9,14]. However, knowledge about how plasma AA and downstream products of their metabolism respond to periparturient MET supplementation is lacking.

Although choline (CHOL) is not an AA, it may regulate AA metabolism by altering AA requirements, especially Met, around parturition. For instance, Met can be regenerated when homocysteine receives a methyl group from CHOL through betaine [15–17], suggesting that CHOL supplementation can potentially reduce Met requirements around parturition. In addition, accumulation of fat in liver has been speculated to induce inflammation and oxidative stress in ruminant liver, which almost certainly would lead to increased AA requirements for production of positive APP and other immune function-related proteins [17]. As a precursor for hepatic very low-density lipoprotein (VLDL) assembly, CHOL has a crucial role in the export of triacylglycerol to prevent fatty liver by promoting phosphatidylcholine synthesis via the Kennedy pathway instead of sequential methylation using Met derived SAM, which may also spare a portion of Met around parturition.

Few studies have attempted to characterize the profile of circulating AA and their derivatives around parturition in dairy cows [3,18–20]. To our knowledge, this is the first study profiling AA and their derivatives in response to MET or CHOL supplementation around parturition. Considering that periparturient MET supplementation resulted in greater feed intake, increased milk yield, and better overall cow health while CHOL cows did not achieve similar benefits [9] (although others have reported increased milk production with CHOL [21,22]), our hypothesis was that MET and CHOL supplementation results in different alterations in AA metabolism-associated events which ultimately contribute to their distinct roles in the overall health and production efficiency of the animal.

2. Materials and Methods

2.1. Experimental Design and Treatments

All procedures for this study (protocol no. 13023) were approved by the Institutional Animal Care and Use Committee (IACUC) of the University of Illinois. Details of the experimental design have been described previously [9,23]. Briefly, the experiment was conducted as a randomized, complete, unbalanced, block design with 2 × 2 factorial arrangement of MET (Smartamine M, Adisseo NA, Alpharetta, GA, USA) and CHOL (ReaShure, Balchem Inc., New Hampton, NY, USA) level (with or without). Cows within each block were balanced for parity, previous lactation milk yield, and BCS before the close-up diet groups were assigned. A total of 81 cows were used. Treatments were control (CON, $n = 20$), with no MET or CHOL supplementation; Smartamine (SMA, $n = 21$), CON plus MET at a rate of 0.08% of DM; Reashure (REA, $n = 20$), CON + CHOL at 60 g/days; or Smartamine and Reashure (MIX, n = 20), CON + MET + CHOL. Dosage of MET was based on Osorio et al. [6], whereas CHOL was supplemented following the manufacturer's recommendations. Met as a % of metabolizable protein (MP) and the Lys:Met ratio for close-up diets were estimated to be 1.9% and 3.6:1 Lys:Met for CON, 2.4% and 2.8:1 Lys:Met for SMA, 1.9% and 3.6:1 Lys:Met for REA, and 2.4% and 2.8:1 Lys:Met for MIX. Met as a % of MP and the Lys:Met ratio for lactation diets were estimated to be 1.8% and 3.5:1 Lys:Met for CON, 2.3% and 2.7:1 Lys:Met for SMA, 1.8% and 3.5:1 Lys:Met for REA, and 2.3% and 2.7:1 Lys:Met for MIX. Per IACUC conclusions, a subset of 40 multiparous cows (10 cows/treatment) was deemed sufficient to achieve statistical power. Thus, these cows were selected randomly and used for this portion of the study. All cows received the same far-off diet from −50 to −22 days before expected parturition, the close-up diet from −21 days to expected parturition, and the lactation diet from parturition through 30 days in milk (DIM). The MET and CHOL supplements were both top-dressed from −21 ± 2 to 30 DIM once daily at the AM feeding using approximately 50 g of ground corn as carrier for all treatments. On average, cows received MET and/or CHOL supplementation for 23.1 ± 1.0 days prepartum. Supplementation of SMA (0.08% DM of TMR offered) was calculated daily for each cow. Smartamine M was supplied as small beads containing a minimum of 75% DL-Methionine (DL-Met), physically protected by a pH sensitive coating, which is considered to have a Met bioavailability of 80% [24]; therefore, per 10 g of SMA, the cows received 6 g of metabolizable Met. The REA supplement is reported to contain 28.8% choline chloride and is protected by microencapsulation. In terms of bioavailability, work from a graduate thesis using (methyl,^{2}H3)-CHOL and (methyl,^{2}H3)-Met indicated, based on differences in Met methyl flux rates, that the product has CHOL bioavailability of 72% [25]; therefore, per 60 g of REA, cows in our study would have received 12.4 g of metabolizable choline chloride. In contrast, a recent in vivo study evaluating bioavailability of REA detected low portal flux of free choline (13%) relative to abomasal delivery of choline [26], thus, indicating that only 2.3 g of free choline would have been available post-ruminally. Although assessing bioavailability of SMA and REA was beyond the scope of our study, it is important to note that the approaches for estimating "bioavailability" of CHOL in these studies was different. For instance, the work of de Veth et al. [26] did not consider the portion of CHOL partly oxidized to betaine, partly phosphorylated, and partly incorporated into lyso- and phosphatidylcholine within the enterocyte and prior to entering portal circulation. Thus, despite the low concentration of free choline any betaine generated during metabolism within enterocytes could have contributed methyl groups for remethylation of homocysteine to Met in the liver. Clearly, further studies would have to be conducted to define better CHOL needs of periparturient cows and the efficacy of available CHOL products in delivering metabolizable CHOL and its derivatives. To our knowledge, neither SMA nor REA have specific characteristics that may affect palatability of diets.

2.2. Animal Management

Dry cows were housed in a ventilated enclosed barn during the dry period and fed individually once daily at 06:30 am using an individual gate system (American Calan Inc., Northwood, NH, USA). After parturition, cows were housed in a tie-stall barn and were fed a common lactation diet once daily. Feed offered was adjusted daily to achieve ~10% refusals.

2.3. Blood Sample Collection and Analyses of Plasma AA and Their Derivatives

Blood was sampled from the coccygeal vein at −30 and −10 days relative to expected parturition date and at 4, 14 and 28 days relative to actual parturition date before the AM feeding. On average, prepartum samples were harvested at −30.8 ± 1.4 days and −10.9 ± 1.3 days relative to actual calving date. Samples were collected into evacuated tubes (BD Vacutainer; BD and Co., Franklin Lakes, NJ, USA) containing lithium heparin for isolation of plasma.

Plasma was used to analyze the concentrations of free arginine (Arg), histidine (His), isoleucine (Ile), leucine (Leu), lysine (Lys), methionine (Met), phenylalanine (Phe), threonine (Thr), tryptophan (Trp), valine (Val), asparagine (Asn), aspartate (Asp), alanine (Ala), glutamate (Glu), glutamine (Gln), glycine (Gly), proline (Pro), serine (Ser), tyrosine (Tyr), citrulline (Cit), carnosine, ornithine (Orn), sarcosine (Sar), cystathionine, cystine, homocystine, taurine, α-aminoadipic acid, α-aminobutyric acid, β-alanine, γ-aminobutyric acid (GABA), hydroxylysine, hydroxyproline, phosphoserine, 1-methyl histidine, and 3-methyl histidine at the University of Missouri Agriculture Experiment Station Chemical Laboratories (Columbia, MO, USA) using high performance liquid chromatography [27,28]. Plasma total GSH was measured using a commercial kit (Cat. No. NWH-GSH01; Northwest Life Science Specialties LLC, Vancouver, WA, USA). The essential amino acid (EAA) pool included Arg + His + Ile + Leu + Lys + Met + Phe + Thr + Trp + Val; the NEAA pool included Asn + Asp + Ala + Gln + Glu + Gly + Pro + Ser + Tyr; total AA was the sum of EAA and non-essential amino acid (NEAA); the total sulfur-containing compounds (TSC) included Met + cystine + cystathionine + homocysteine + taurine + GSH.

2.4. Liver Sample Collection and Quantitative RT-PCR (qPCR)

Liver was sampled via puncture biopsy [29] from cows under local anesthesia at approximately 08:00 am on days −10, 7, 20, and 30 days relative to parturition. Liver was frozen immediately in liquid nitrogen and stored until analysis. The qPCR was performed in liver samples as described previously [7].

2.5. Statistical Analysis

Data were analyzed using PROC MIXED of SAS (SAS Institute Inc., Cary, NC, USA) according to the following model:

$$Y_{ijklm} = \mu + b_i + M_j + C_k + MC_{jk} + T_l + TM_{jl} + TC_{kl} + TMC_{jkl} + A_{m:ijk} + \varepsilon_{ijklm}$$

where Y_{ijklm} is the dependent, continuous variable; μ is the overall mean; b_i is the random effect of the ith block; M_j is the fixed effect of MET (j = with or without); C_k is the fixed effect of CHOL (k = with or without); T_l is the fixed effect of time (day or week) of the experiment; A_m is the random effect of the mth animal (cow); ε_{ijklm} is the residual error. The covariate of parity (2nd vs. 3rd lactation and above) and concentrations obtained at −30 days for various AA and derivatives were maintained in the model for all variables when significant ($p < 0.05$). Plasma AA and derivatives and hepatic gene expression were analyzed at various time points that were not equally spaced. Therefore, the first order ante-dependence covariance structure 1 (ANTE(1)) was used for repeated measures. Variables were assessed for normality of distribution using the Shapiro-Wilk test. When the normality assumption was rejected, data were log-transformed before statistical analysis. Back transformed data are reported in tables and figures for ease of interpretation. Data reported are least square means for each time point and least square means separation between treatments and time points were performed using the PDIFF statement. Statistical differences were declared significant at $p < 0.05$ and tendencies at $p < 0.10$.

3. Results

3.1. Essential AA

Main effects of MET, CHOL, and their interactions with time for essential AA are presented in Table 1. Means for MET × CHOL are presented in Table S1. Overall, plasma concentrations of Arg, His, Lys, and Trp decreased soon after parturition (4 days). In contrast, circulating Met concentration increased at 4 days (Figure 1). As expected, MET-supplemented cows had greater plasma Met concentration at all time points ($p < 0.01$, Figure 1E) compared with cows without MET. In fact, the proportion of Met in EAA ($p < 0.01$, Figure 2A) and total AA pool (TAA) ($p < 0.01$, Figure 2C) also was greater in response to MET supplementation. In contrast, plasma Met ($p > 0.10$, Figure 1F) and Met%EAA ($p > 0.10$, Figure 2B) levels were not different in response to CHOL supplementation. A main effect of MET ($p = 0.02$) also was detected for Lys, the second most-limiting AA for milk production, mainly due to greater plasma concentrations at −10 days and 14 days (M × D $p < 0.05$, Figure 1C). Similarly, plasma Arg concentration also was greater ($p = 0.02$) in MET cows owing to greater concentrations at −10 days and 14 days (M × D $p < 0.05$, Figure 1A), but not at 4 days postpartum. Although greater Thr was detected in MET cows at −10 days (M × D $p < 0.05$, Figure 1G), Thr concentrations were not greater at other time points measured postpartum in MET-supplemented cows, hence, overall only a tendency ($p = 0.09$) was detected in these cows. In addition to greater ($p < 0.01$) Trp in MET cows, a main effect of CHOL also was detected for Trp ($p = 0.04$, Figure 1I,J). Despite the lack of main effects of MET for plasma His, Phe and total branched-chain amino acids (BCAA = sum of Val, Leu, and Ile) concentrations, the EAA tended to be greater ($p = 0.06$) in response to MET mainly owing to greater EAA concentration prepartum (M × D $p < 0.05$, Figure 1K).

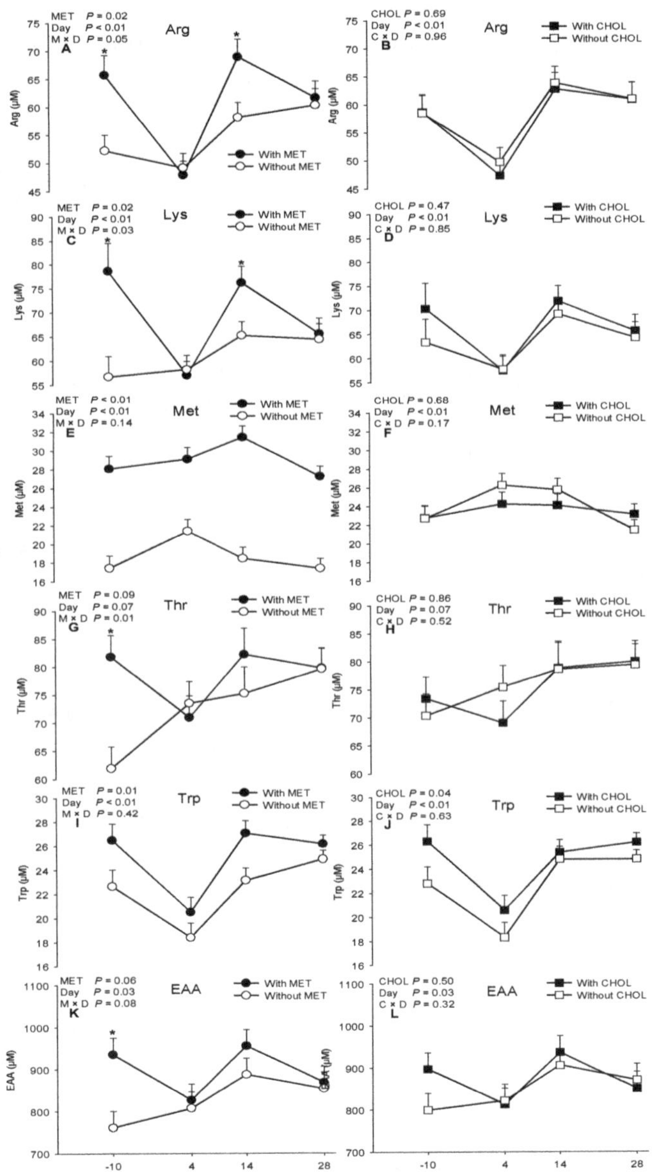

Figure 1. Effects of supplementing multiparous Holstein cows during the periparturient period (−21 through 30 days around parturition) with rumen-protected methionine (MET; Smartamine M, Adisseo NA, Alpharetta, GA, USA) or rumen-protected choline (CHOL; ReaShure, Balchem Inc., New Hampton, NY, USA) on circulating concentrations of arginine, lysing, methionine, threonine, tryptophan, and total essential AA (EAA). Values are means, with standard errors represented by vertical bars.

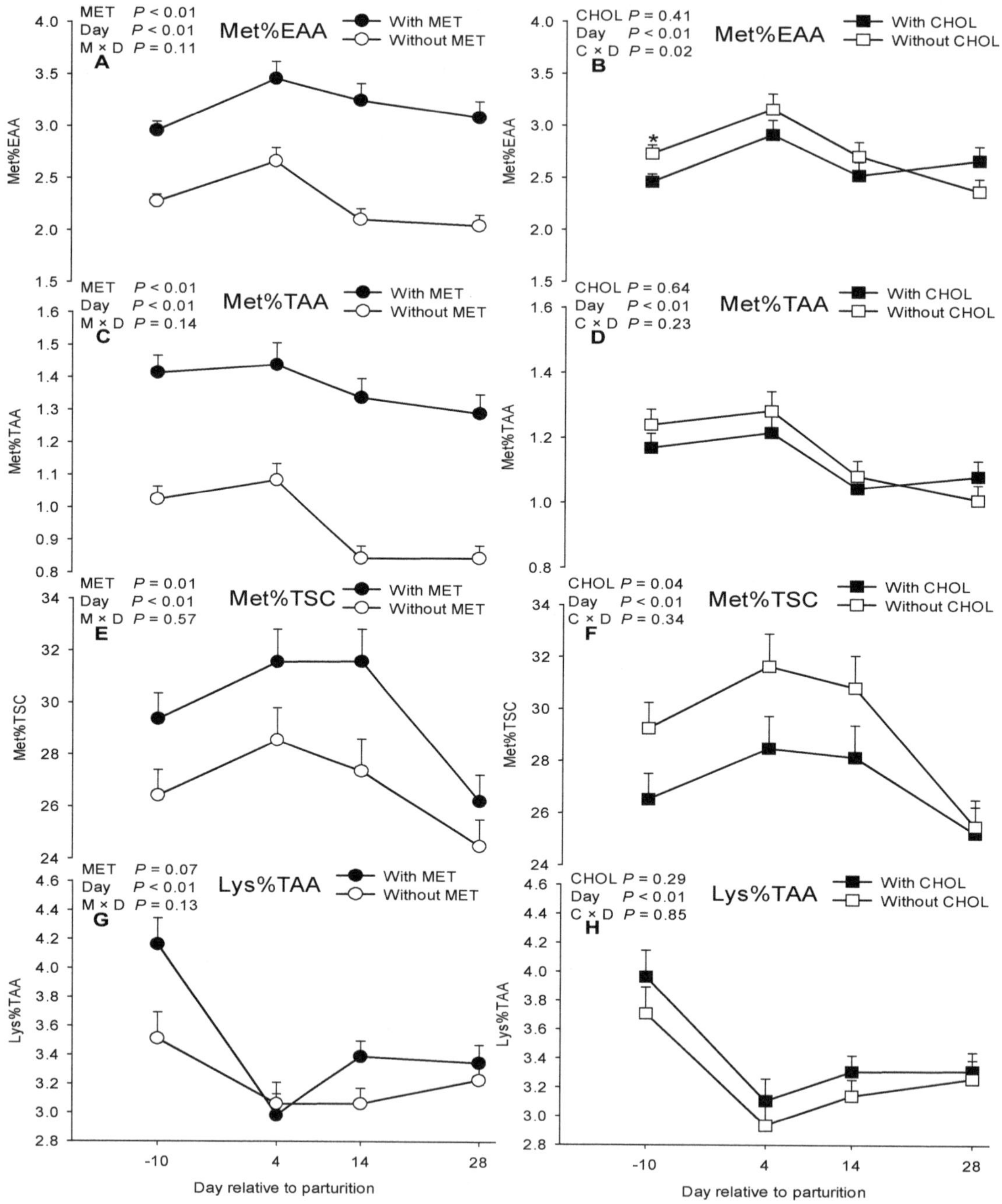

Figure 2. Effects of supplementing multiparous Holstein cows during the periparturient period (−21 through 30 days around parturition) with rumen-protected methionine (MET; Smartamine M, Adisseo NA) or rumen-protected choline (CHOL; ReaShure, Balchem Inc.) on proportions of circulating Met in essential amino acids (Met%EAA), total amino acids (Met%TAA), total sulfur-containing compounds (Met%TSC), and proportion of Lys in TAA (Lys%TAA). Values are means, with standard errors represented by vertical bars.

Table 1. Plasma proteinogenic AA concentrations during the periparturient period in cows supplemented with or without rumen-protected MET and CHOL.

	MET		CHOL			Day				p-Value [2]				
AA (μM)	Without	With	Without	With	SEM [1]	−10	4	14	28	MET [3]	CHOL [4]	Time	M × T [5]	C × T [6]
Essential AA														
Arginine	54.75	60.43	57.99	57.05	1.75	58.58^{ab}	48.47^{c}	63.29^{a}	60.92^{ab}	0.02	0.69	<0.01	0.05	0.96
Histidine	52.38	54.55	54.04	52.87	1.18	57.28^{a}	53.53^{b}	52.30^{b}	50.92^{b}	0.19	0.49	<0.01	0.13	0.17
Isoleucine	95.58	103.61	100.64	98.40	4.42	98.18	95.54	106.87	97.83	0.19	0.72	0.18	0.07	0.36
Leucine	153.31	161.79	152.70	162.43	6.69	151.35^{b}	153.51^{b}	173.18^{a}	152.92^{b}	0.35	0.31	0.03	0.27	0.31
Lysine	60.99	68.74	63.47	66.06	2.45	66.75^{ab}	57.56^{c}	70.47^{a}	64.91^{b}	0.02	0.47	<0.01	0.03	0.85
Methionine	18.65	28.95	24.04	23.55	0.83	22.75^{c}	25.25^{a}	24.92^{ab}	22.27^{c}	<0.01	0.68	<0.01	0.14	0.17
Phenylalanine	46.64	47.09	45.88	47.86	1.02	45.00^{b}	47.64^{b}	51.16^{a}	43.97^{b}	0.75	0.17	<0.01	0.26	0.92
Threonine	72.55	78.67	75.93	75.30	2.50	71.87	72.22	78.70	79.66	0.09	0.86	0.07	0.01	0.52
Tryptophan	22.26	25.04	22.68	24.61	0.64	24.56^{ab}	19.44^{c}	25.08^{a}	25.50^{a}	<0.01	0.04	<0.01	0.42	0.63
Valine	226.77	244.54	229.16	241.99	9.32	230.11	223.02	249.41	240.25	0.17	0.33	0.08	0.26	0.31
BCAA [7]	476.69	510.97	483.71	503.55	19.87	480.67	473.17	530.28	491.93	0.21	0.48	0.08	0.19	0.27
EAA	827.12	896.20	849.22	874.1	25.54	848.26^{bc}	816.78^{bc}	921.2^{a}	860.39^{ab}	0.06	0.50	0.03	0.08	0.32
Met%EAA	2.26	3.18	2.73	2.64	0.09	2.59^{b}	3.04^{a}	2.62^{b}	2.52^{b}	<0.01	0.41	<0.01	0.11	0.23
Non-essential AA														
Alanine	187.39	206.37	198.37	195.39	5.55	188.83^{b}	175.45^{c}	211.30^{a}	211.95^{a}	0.02	0.71	<0.01	0.05	0.32
Asparagine	34.90	39.63	37.78	36.61	1.48	27.82^{c}	34.08^{b}	45.67^{a}	44.19^{a}	0.02	0.56	<0.01	0.22	0.42
Aspartate	4.21	4.79	4.24	4.76	0.21	4.91^{a}	3.78^{b}	4.80^{a}	4.57^{a}	0.04	0.07	<0.01	0.59	0.14
Glutamate	35.93	38.34	36.44	37.81	1.04	44.24^{a}	32.17^{d}	37.84^{b}	35.24^{c}	0.10	0.36	<0.01	0.54	0.38
Glutamine	246.22	259.53	257.92	247.82	6.18	278.17^{a}	252.84^{b}	242.52^{b}	237.96^{b}	0.15	0.25	<0.01	0.21	0.29
Glycine *	426.83	406.23	427.39	405.67	15.10	236.99^{c}	456.97^{b}	536.19^{a}	435.98^{b}	0.35	0.31	<0.01	0.92	0.22
Proline	72.30	78.24	74.03	76.50	2.02	59.19^{c}	67.52^{b}	90.21^{a}	84.15^{a}	0.04	0.39	<0.01	0.35	0.74
Serine	86.62	88.92	88.67	86.87	2.28	73.88^{c}	90.85^{b}	100.78^{a}	85.57^{b}	0.48	0.58	<0.01	0.16	0.49
Tyrosine	40.82	43.39	40.78	43.43	1.53	42.03^{a}	36.26^{b}	46.32^{a}	43.80^{a}	0.24	0.24	<0.01	0.08	0.94
NEAA [8]	1114.59	1151.58	1153.58	1112.59	24.79	946.13^{c}	1136.83^{b}	1301.27^{a}	1177.00^{b}	0.29	0.24	<0.01	0.36	0.23
TAA [9]	1926.95	2052.97	1995.87	1982.22	41.32	1781.41^{d}	1947.89^{bc}	2215.47^{a}	2035.97^{b}	0.03	0.82	<0.01	0.10	0.53
Met%TAA	0.94	1.37	1.15	1.13	0.04	1.20^{a}	1.25^{a}	1.06^{b}	1.05^{b}	<0.01	0.64	<0.01	0.14	0.23
Lys%TAA	3.22	3.47	3.26	3.42	0.10	3.84^{a}	3.02^{c}	3.23^{bc}	3.29^{b}	0.08	0.28	<0.01	0.13	0.85

* Significant ($p < 0.05$) parity effect observed. Labeled means in a row without a common superscript letter differ ($p < 0.05$). [1] Greatest SEM; [2] MET × CHOL interaction was included in the supplemental file; [3] Overall effect of MET supplementation; [4] Overall effect of CHOL supplementation; [5] Interaction of MET × time; [6] Interaction of CHOL × time; [7] Branched-chain AA; [8] Non-essential AA; [9] Total AA.

3.2. Non-Essential AA

Main effects of MET, CHOL, and their interactions with time for non-essential proteinogenic AA are presented in Table 1. Means for MET × CHOL are presented in Table S1. Similar to EAA, plasma concentrations of Asp, Glu, Gln, and Tyr decreased soon after parturition (Figure 3). In contrast, plasma concentrations of Asn, Gly, Pro, and Ser increased at 4 days compared with −10 days. Although total NEAA did not change ($p > 0.10$) in response to MET or CHOL, TAA in MET-supplemented cows was greater ($p = 0.03$, Figure 3K) as a result of an overall tendency for greater EAA together with greater Asn, Asp, Ala, and Pro ($p < 0.05$, Figure 3A,C,E,I) as well as a tendency for greater Glu ($p = 0.10$, Figure 3G).

It is noteworthy that similarly to Arg and Lys (M × D $p < 0.05$, Figure 1A,C), plasma Ala concentrations were already greater (M × D $p < 0.05$, Figure 3A) at −10 days prepartum in MET cows. After parturition, plasma Arg, Lys, and Ala were not different regardless of MET supplementation at 4 days, but were again greater at 14 days (M × D $p < 0.05$, Figure 1A,C and Figure 3A) in MET cows. Unlike Met, only a tendency for greater ($p = 0.06$, Figure 3D) Asp was detected in response to CHOL.

3.3. Sulfur-Containing Compounds

Main effects of MET, CHOL, and their interactions with time for sulfur-containing compounds are presented in Table 2. Means for MET × CHOL are presented in Table S2. As expected, MET supplementation increased plasma concentrations of cystathionine, cystine, homocysteine, and taurine ($p < 0.05$, Figure 4A,C,E,G), which account for the greater overall plasma TSC level at all time points evaluated (M × D $p < 0.05$, Figure 4I). Similar to Ala, Arg, and Lys, greater ($p < 0.01$) cystine and cystathionine concentrations were also detected in response to MET due to greater plasma level at −10, 14, and 28 days (M × D $p < 0.05$, Figure 4A,C). In addition to increased circulating sulfur-containing compounds, MET also increased the proportion of Met in TSC ($p = 0.01$, Figure 2E). In contrast, although plasma cystine concentration was greater ($p < 0.01$, Figure 4D) in response to CHOL supplementation, a decreased proportion of Met in TSC was detected in CHOL cows around parturition ($p = 0.03$, Figure 2F).

3.4. Non-Proteinogenic AA and Derivatives

Main effects of MET, CHOL, and their interactions with time for non-proteinogenic AA and derivatives are presented in Table 2. Means for MET × CHOL are presented in Table S2. Although no main effect of MET or CHOL was detected for ornithine, greater Cit ($p < 0.01$, Figure 5I) and a tendency ($p = 0.07$, Figure 5K) for greater urea were observed in MET-supplemented cows in addition to greater Arg. Besides taurine, plasma concentrations of carnosine, another antioxidant, was also greater ($p = 0.02$, Figure 5G) in MET cows. Although no main effect of CHOL was detected for carnosine, greater (C × D $p < 0.05$, Figure 5H) concentrations were detected at −10 days and 28 days. γ-aminobutyric acid was greater both in MET- and CHOL-supplemented cows ($p < 0.05$, Figure 5E,F). The indicator of protein mobilization, 3-methylhistidine, was lower in CHOL cows ($p = 0.02$, Figure 5D). Similarly, plasma 1-methylhistidine concentration also was lower in these cows ($p = 0.04$).

3.5. Pyruvate Carboxylase and Phosphoenolpyruvate Carboxykinase 1 Expression

Main effects of MET, CHOL, and their interactions with time for expression of *pyruvate carboxylase* (*PC*) and *phosphoenolpyruvate carboxykinase 1* (*PCK1*) are presented in Table 3. Means for MET × CHOL are presented in Table S3. Main effects of MET and CHOL or interactions were not detected ($p > 0.05$) for the mRNA expression of *PC* and *PCK1*.

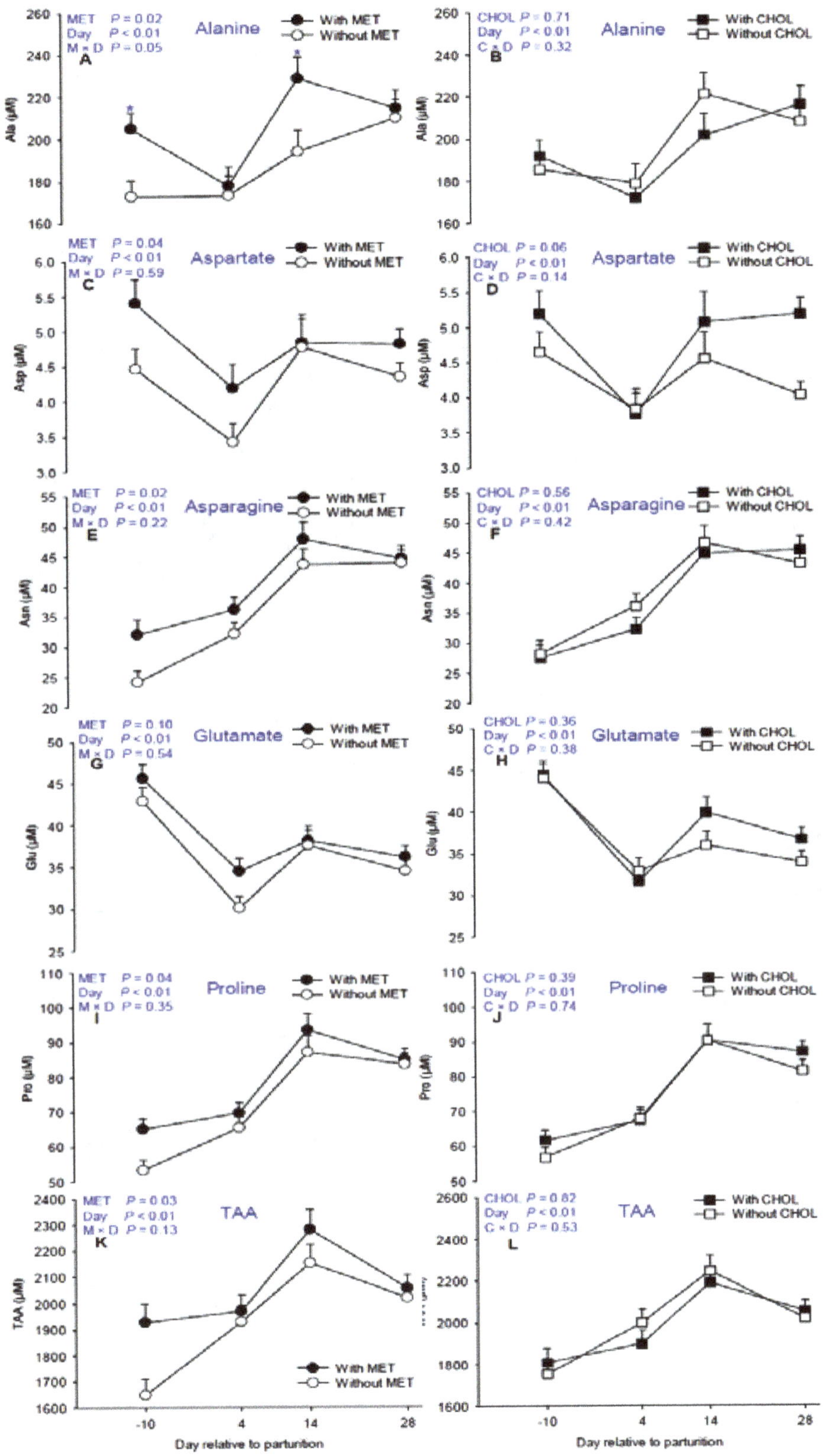

Figure 3. Effects of supplementing multiparous Holstein cows during the periparturient period (−21 through 30 days around parturition) with rumen-protected methionine (MET; Smartamine M, Adisseo NA) on circulating concentrations of free alanine, aspartate, asparagine, glutamate, proline, and total AA (TAA). Values are means, with standard errors represented by vertical bars.

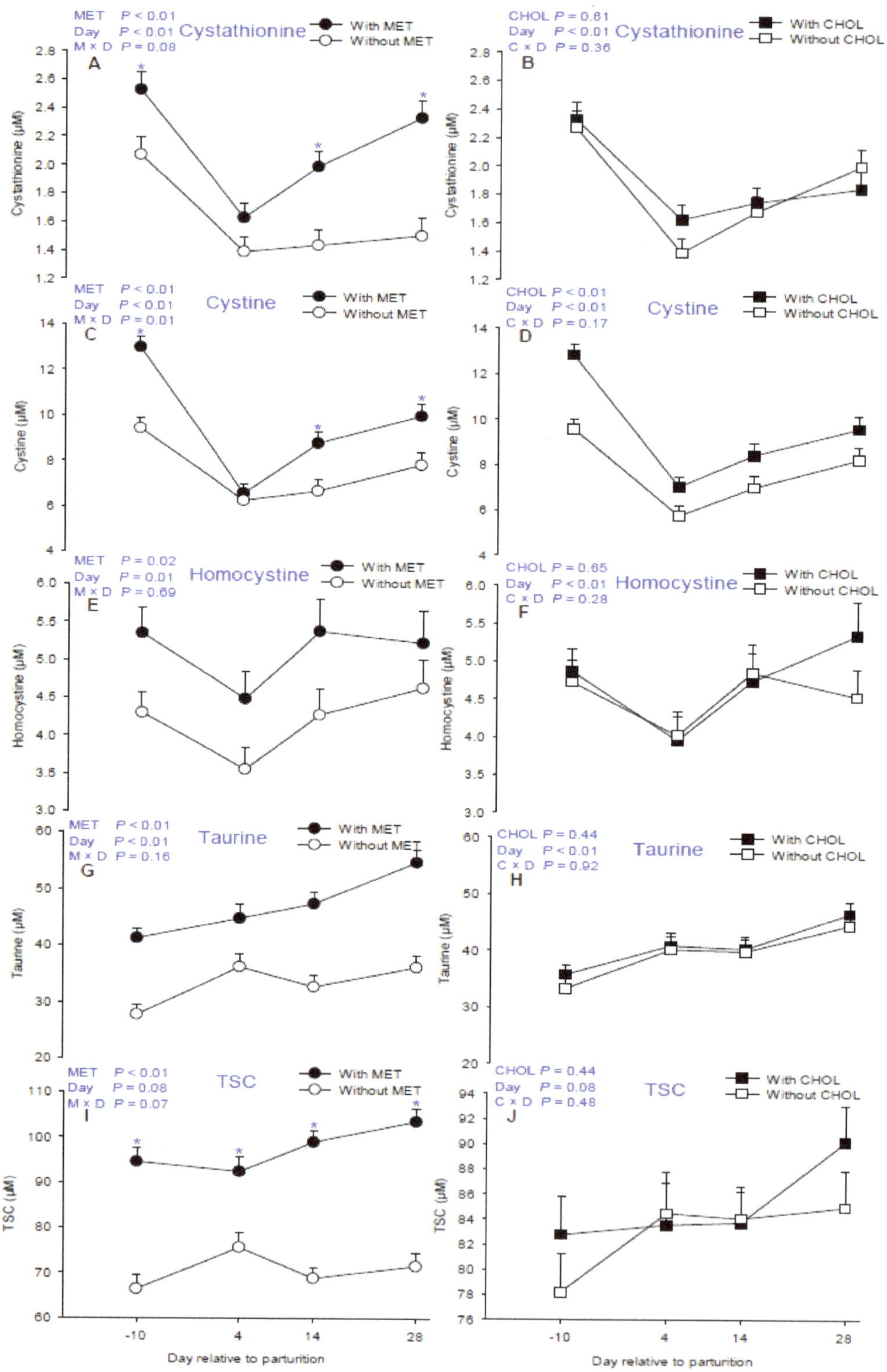

Figure 4. Effects of supplementing multiparous Holstein cows during the periparturient period (−21 through 30 days around parturition) with rumen-protected methionine (MET; Smartamine M, Adisseo NA) on circulating concentrations of cystathionine, cystine, homocysteine, taurine, and total sulfur-containing compounds (TSC). Values are means, with standard errors represented by vertical bars.

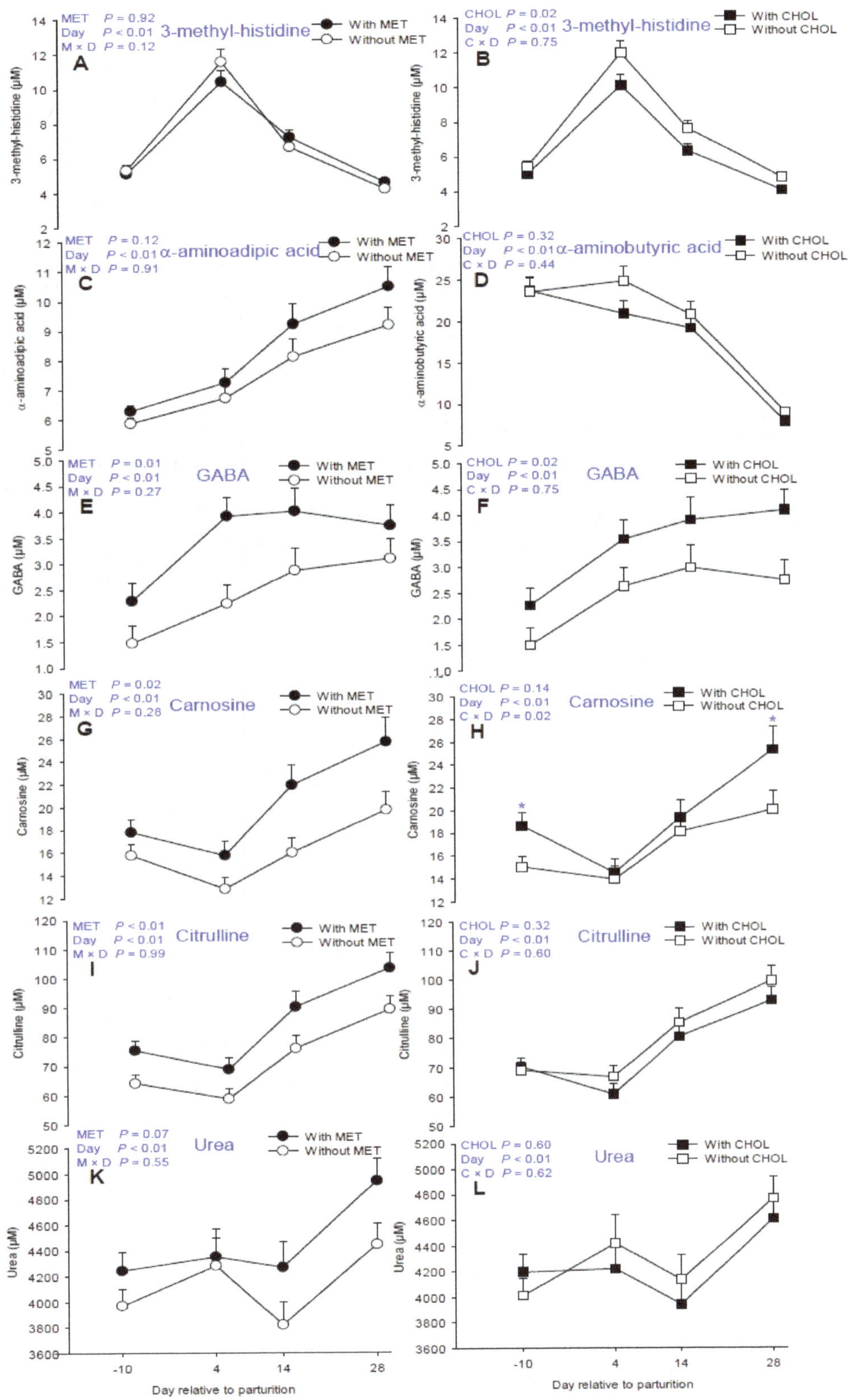

Figure 5. Effects of supplementing multiparous Holstein cows during the periparturient period (−21 through 30 days around parturition) with rumen-protected methionine (MET; Smartamine M, Adisseo NA) or rumen-protected choline (CHOL; ReaShure, Balchem Inc.) on proportions of circulating 1-methyl histidine, 3-methyl histidine, γ-amino butyric acid, carnosine, citrulline, and urea. Values are means, with standard errors represented by vertical bars.

Table 2. Plasma non-proteinogenic AA and AA derivatives concentrations during the periparturient period in cows supplemented with or without rumen-protected MET and CHOL.

	MET		CHOL			Day				*p*-Value [2]				
Parameter (μM)	**Without**	**With**	**Without**	**With**	**SEM [1]**	**−10**	**4**	**14**	**28**	**MET [3]**	**CHOL [4]**	**Time**	**M × T [5]**	**C × T [6]**
AA and derivatives [#]														
1-methyl histidine	15.36	16.56	16.79	15.15	0.57	12.82^{c}	12.58^{c}	18.38^{b}	21.85^{a}	0.12	0.04	<0.01	0.36	0.50
3-methyl histidine	6.44	6.48	6.97	5.99	0.29	5.21^{c}	11.00^{a}	6.91^{b}	4.40^{d}	0.92	0.02	<0.01	0.12	0.75
α-aminoadipic acid	7.37	8.15	8.03	7.48	0.36	6.09^{d}	6.99^{c}	8.65^{b}	9.81^{a}	0.12	0.27	<0.01	0.91	0.30
α-aminobutyric acid	15.64	19.78	18.13	17.07	0.81	8.94^{c}	23.60^{a}	22.77^{a}	19.93^{b}	<0.01	0.32	<0.01	0.61	0.44
β-alanine	9.06	8.87	8.81	9.11	0.32	8.97	8.69	9.24	8.94	0.68	0.50	0.54	0.96	0.92
γ-aminobutyric acid	2.42	3.49	2.46	3.45	0.29	1.88^{b}	3.08^{a}	3.44^{a}	3.41^{a}	0.01	0.02	<0.01	0.27	0.75
Carnosine *	15.88	19.92	16.60	19.07	1.29	16.74^{c}	14.20^{d}	18.71^{b}	22.51^{a}	0.02	0.14	<0.01	0.30	0.02
Citrulline	71.19	83.47	79.08	75.14	2.92	69.61^{c}	63.69^{c}	82.86^{b}	96.11^{a}	<0.01	0.30	<0.01	0.99	0.60
Glutathione	4.68	4.73	4.84	4.57	0.27	4.60^{b}	6.11^{a}	4.35^{bc}	3.76^{c}	0.89	0.50	<0.01	0.50	0.74
Hydroxylysine	0.32	0.28	0.30	0.29	0.04	0.33	0.29	0.33	0.25	0.37	0.79	0.21	0.61	0.70
Hydroxyproline	15.19	15.36	15.42	15.13	0.48	12.80^{c}	18.10^{a}	16.31^{b}	13.89^{c}	0.81	0.67	<0.01	0.94	0.12
Ornithine	29.14	32.00	30.48	30.60	1.35	39.37^{a}	22.11^{d}	30.04^{c}	33.25^{b}	0.13	0.95	<0.01	0.12	0.45
Phosphoserine	6.22	6.18	6.07	6.33	0.18	5.53^{c}	5.91^{bc}	6.72^{ab}	6.74^{a}	0.88	0.30	<0.01	0.71	0.91
Sarcosine	10.65	11.43	11.50	10.58	0.56	8.32^{b}	11.31^{a}	12.03^{a}	12.50^{a}	0.33	0.27	<0.01	0.76	0.37
Urea	4121.63	4442.94	4323.55	4235.16	123.89	4104.53^{bc}	4317.26^{b}	4036.81^{c}	4687.49^{a}	0.07	0.60	<0.01	0.55	0.62
Sulfur-containing compounds														
Cystathionine	1.60	2.12	1.84	1.89	0.07	2.30	1.51	1.71	1.92	<0.01	0.61	<0.01	0.08	0.36
Cystine	7.56	9.58	7.65	9.48	34.5	11.20^{a}	6.41^{d}	7.73^{c}	8.92^{b}	<0.01	0.02	<0.01	0.01	0.17
Homocystine	4.17	5.10	4.52	4.70	0.30	4.80^{a}	3.99^{b}	4.80^{a}	4.92^{a}	0.02	0.65	0.01	0.69	0.28
Taurine	33.23	47.04	39.43	40.84	1.28	34.51	40.49	40.06	45.48	<0.01	0.44	<0.01	0.16	0.92
TSC [7]	70.65	97.37	82.47	85.95	1.93	80.52	84.03	83.93	87.57	<0.01	0.44	0.08	0.07	0.48
Met%TSC	28.44	31.4	31.09	28.74	0.72	29.65^{b}	32.35^{ab}	31.15^{b}	26.51^{c}	0.01	0.03	<0.01	0.74	0.24

* Significant ($p < 0.05$) parity effect observed. Labeled means in a row without a common superscript letter differ ($p < 0.05$). [#] β-aminobutyric acid undetectable; [1] Greatest SEM; [2] MET × CHOL interaction was included in the supplemental file; [3] Overall effect of MET supplementation; [4] Overall effect of CHOL supplementation; [5] Interaction of MET × time; [6] Interaction of CHOL × time; [7] Total sulfur-containing AAs and derivatives (methionine, cystathionine, cystine, homocysteine, and taurine).

Table 3. Hepatic relative *PC*[#] and *PCK1* mRNA expression during the periparturient period in cows supplemented with or without rumen-protected MET and CHOL.

	MET		CHOL			Day				*p*-Value [2]				
Genes	**Without**	**With**	**Without**	**With**	**SEM [1]**	**−10**	**7**	**20**	**30**	**MET [3]**	**CHOL [4]**	**Time**	**M × T [5]**	**C × T [6]**
PC	2.12	2.02	2.09	2.05	0.07	1.49^{c}	2.88^{a}	2.23^{b}	1.93^{d}	0.33	0.70	<0.01	0.28	0.34
PCK1	2.27	2.43	2.39	2.31	0.10	1.57^{c}	2.62^{ab}	2.74^{a}	2.69^{ab}	0.27	0.55	<0.01	0.48	0.46

* Significant ($p < 0.05$) parity effect observed. Labeled means in a row without a common superscript letter differ ($p < 0.05$). [#] *PC* = pyruvate carboxylase; *PCK1* = Phosphoenolpyruvate carboxykinase 1; [1] Greatest SEM; [2] MET × CHOL interaction was included in the supplemental file; [3] Overall effect of MET supplementation; [4] Overall effect of CHOL supplementation; [5] Interaction of MET × time; [6] Interaction of CHOL × time.

4. Discussion

A detailed discussion of production performance and immunometabolic status of the cows has been published elsewhere [8,9,23].

4.1. Enhancing the Supply of MET Improved Plasma AA Profiles

MET and Lys in the MP are the most-limiting AA in a wide-range of diets for dairy cows due to their low concentrations in feed protein relative to their "apparent required amounts in digestible protein" [30]. During the periparturient period, the decreased feed intake coupled with increased AA requirements to sustain fetal growth and lactation lead to greater tissue protein mobilization evidenced in the present study by the highest plasma 3-methyl histidine at 4 days regardless of treatments. Although AA released from tissue mobilization can partly mitigate the demand for AA, cow body tissue protein is relatively low in Met and Lys [31]. Consequently, this physiological stage is characterized by an overall decrease in circulating AA, especially the most-limiting AA (e.g., Met and Lys). Apart from limiting milk production, according to von Liebig's hypothesis commonly described with the analogy of a water barrel with broken staves, inadequate Met availability also could potentially limit the utilization of other circulating AA [32]. Strategies to increase circulating Met are, thus, expected to improve overall circulating AA profiles and utilization during the periparturient period.

Apart from greater plasma Met, the fact that various proteinogenic circulating EAA (Arg, Lys, Met, Thr, and Trp), NEAA (Ala, Asn, Asp, Glu, Gln, and Pro) and non-proteinogenic AA (Cit) were greater in response to rumen-protected MET supplementation is an indication of a better circulating AA profile during the periparturient period. However, it cannot be ignored that MET cows had greater DMI both prepartum and postpartum [9,23]. Therefore, the DMI increase in MET-supplemented cows might have contributed to the observed increase in circulating EAA and TAA. It is noteworthy that despite concomitant increases in circulating Met, EAA and TAA, the proportion of Met in EAA and TAA (Met%EAA and Met%TAA) as well as the proportion of Lys in TAA were increased in response to MET supplementation, indicating a better AA profile at least in regards to limiting AA, i.e., Met and Lys.

Considering the overall greater milk yield, milk protein %, and milk protein yield [9,23], it is reasonable to speculate that MET supplementation contributes to better lactation performance both by increasing intake and proportion of Met and Lys in the circulating AA pool. Although CHOL can, in theory, promote in vivo synthesis of Met or indirectly spare Met by reducing the use of Met for CHOL synthesis, the lack of change in circulating AA in the present study and the fact that flux from CHOL to MET was not increased in response to CHOL supplementation in lactating goats [33] and transition dairy cows [34] do not support such hypothesis.

4.2. Utilization of Circulating AA Close to Parturition

Around parturition, the demand for AA for glucose and protein synthesis increases abruptly and results in greatly increased AA uptake from the circulation [35]. The few published reports have revealed that circulating AA concentrations in dairy cows generally reach a nadir close to parturition mainly as a result of increased demand for milk protein synthesis and gluconeogenesis coupled with insufficient dietary intake [3,18,20,36]. In agreement with these reports, regardless of treatment, we detected the lowest circulating concentrations of most AA at 4 days relative to parturition.

Although circulating concentrations of multiple AA (Ala, Arg, Lys) and derivatives (cystine, cystathionine) in MET-supplemented cows were already greater at −10 days compared with cows without MET supplementation and regained greater levels at 14 days postpartum, the circulating concentrations of all AA and derivatives at 4 days were similar regardless of MET supplementation. Whether the lack of difference in circulating concentrations of these AA at 4 days in MET cows was due to inadequate supply in the circulation (e.g., AA from intake and tissue mobilization) [37] or enhanced utilization (e.g., greater liver and mammary uptake) remains unknown. However, the fact that average DMI at day 4 remained greater (+3.33 kg/days more) in MET-supplemented cows [9,23], together with similar 3-methylhistidine in cows with or without MET supplementation, seems to support an overall greater, rather than lower, AA supply at 4 days in response to MET supplementation. In line with the increase in AA supply, MET-supplemented cows regained greater concentrations of these AA at 14 days.

In terms of AA utilization, a previous study detected the greatest liver uptake of EAA at 4 days postpartum in dairy cows [35]. Similarly, hepatic uptake of total NEAA, especially Ala, also was substantially greater in the periparturient period, underscoring that this AA acts as a precursor for glucose synthesis [35,38]. The greater (+4.10 kg/day more) milk yield in MET-supplemented cows at 4 days [9,23] could have caused an increase in uptake of these AA by mammary gland soon after parturition, hence, resulting in lower plasma AA concentration relative to −10 days. Presumably, greater mammary availability of AA accounted for the greater milk protein % [9,23].

It is also noteworthy that a reduction in net flux of carbon from volatile fatty acids across the liver and an increase in glucose release was detected early postpartum in a previous report [35], indicating that the greatest flux through citric acid cycle occurs soon after parturition. Considering the severe negative energy balance and depressed DMI soon after parturition, the increased demand for energy and glucose synthesis by the liver likely accounted for the increase in citric acid flux. Whether periparturient MET supplementation in the present study enhanced gluconeogenesis by promoting AA flux through the citric acid cycle is unknown, but does not seem to be related to regulation at the transcriptional level as evidenced by unchanged mRNA abundance of the key gluconeogenic genes *PC* and *PCK1*.

4.3. Sulfur-Containing Compound Pool and Metabolism

Met and cysteine are the two sulfur-containing AA that are incorporated into proteins. Apart from their well-known role in contributing sulfur bonds during protein synthesis, Met and cysteine are precursors for downstream functional compounds (homocysteine, cystathionine, and taurine) and, thus, are considered the principal components in vivo of the sulfur-containing compound pool [12]. The fact that circulating concentrations of all sulfur-containing compounds measured (except GSH) were greater in MET-supplemented cows during the periparturient period indicate an enriched sulfur-containing compound pool.

It is noteworthy that other than Met, all other plasma sulfur-containing compounds measured are components of the transsulfuration pathway. Considering plasma homocysteine concentrations are highly-dependent on intracellular homocysteine metabolism in liver [39], and cystathionine is a sensitive marker of changes in flux through the transsulfuration pathway [40], the greater homocysteine and cystathionine concentrations indicate increased hepatic flux through this pathway in response to MET supplementation. In addition to the involvement of sulfur-containing compounds, the fact that circulating concentrations of α-aminobutyric acid also were greater in MET-supplemented cows indicates increased flux through the transsulfuration pathway [41]. Considering the key role of Met as the most-limiting AA for milk protein synthesis, the fact that it is the major precursor for sulfur-containing compounds in the transsulfuration pathway indicates that such increase may result in depletion of Met which could potentially give rise to unfavorable lactation performance. However, despite the increased flux through the transsulfuration pathway, the sustained greater circulating concentration of Met and proportion of Met in TSC during the periparturient period indicates that sufficient Met was available in MET-supplemented cows even at 4 days. In contrast, although greater circulating cystine was detected in response to CHOL supplementation, the proportion of Met in TSC was decreased, indicating enhanced flux through the transsulfuration pathway at the expense of Met. Whether the decrease of plasma Met proportion in TSC in the CHOL-supplemented cows contributed to the lack of benefit in performance is unknown; however, it does not seem to support the hypothesis that CHOL can promote Met synthesis in vivo in periparturient dairy cows.

Around parturition, the increased demand for nutrients and energy leads to an increase in the production reactive oxygen metabolites (ROM), the accumulation of which could deplete antioxidants and give rise to oxidative stress that may cause substantial tissue damage and render cows more susceptible to various health disorders [42,43]. Because of their marked ability to scavenge ROM and free radicals, among the sulfur-containing compounds measured, taurine and GSH are considered potent intracellular antioxidants [44]. Hence, in non-ruminants, hepatic concentrations of GSH and taurine have been widely-used as oxidative stress biomarkers [45–47]. Because the liver is the main site of taurine synthesis and releases it into plasma [48], its concentration in the circulation reflects hepatic synthesis [49]. Therefore, the greater overall circulating taurine in response to MET supplementation indicates greater hepatic and extra-hepatic taurine availability and, hence, potentially less oxidative stress in these cows. However, although previous results from our group revealed greater total and reduced hepatic GSH in MET-supplemented cows [14,50], plasma GSH was barely detectable and did not respond to MET. Considering that concentration of GSH in whole blood was 200-fold higher than in plasma due to high concentration in erythrocytes, small amounts of hemolysis may lead to great variations in plasma GSH concentration [51]. Therefore, plasma GSH may not be a reliable oxidative stress biomarker for periparturient dairy cows.

4.4. AA Derivatives

AA derivatives have unique metabolic properties and, thus, many have been adopted as biomarkers for metabolic status. For instance, because 3-methylhistidine is released from the catabolism of actin and myosin in skeletal muscle and is not further metabolized in the body, it has been regarded as a reliable marker for tissue protein mobilization [52]. Assuming that renal blood flow was not altered by CHOL supplementation, the overall lower plasma 3-methylhistidine in response to CHOL supplementation during the periparturient period indicates a lower degree of muscle catabolism. Considering that CHOL supplementation did not result in greater milk yield, the lower degree of tissue mobilization could denote better production efficiency. However, the fact that CHOL supplementation did not alter energy corrected milk (ECM):DMI and fat corrected milk (FCM):DMI does not support such hypothesis. Although lower circulating 1-methylhistidine concentration also was observed in response to CHOL, the postpartum pattern of a gradual increase with time indicates that it is not a suitable indicator of muscle catabolism considering that it was at its greatest right after parturition.

The antioxidant activity of carnosine in non-ruminants has been demonstrated both in terms of reducing oxidative damage and improving the enzymatic and non-enzymatic activity of other antioxidants [53]. The fact that supplementation of carnosine in non-ruminants was able to rescue the prooxidant-antioxidant balance by restoring depleted levels of blood GSH and activities of antioxidant enzymes [54] indicates that circulating carnosine concentrations could decrease in events of oxidative stress. Although the contribution of carnosine to restoring prooxidant–antioxidant balance under physiologic (without carnosine supplementation) conditions remains unknown, the overall greater circulating carnosine together with greater circulating taurine as well as hepatic GSH reported previously [8] indicate a less pronounced oxidative stress status in response to periparturient MET supplementation.

As a neurotransmitter distributed in both neural and non-neural tissue, GABA has various physiologic functions including feed intake regulation [55]. In rats, GABA-B agonist administration increased intake by attenuating satiety signals [56]. In lactating dairy cows, increased DMI in response to rumen-protected GABA supplementation during mid-lactation has been reported [55,57]. The greater circulating GABA in response to periparturient MET supplementation along with the greater DMI [9,23] seem to suggest a role of GABA in mediating DMI regulation by MET. However, considering that CHOL supplementation failed to increase periparturient DMI, yet resulted in a similar increase in circulating GABA, seems to argue against a regulatory role of this molecule in the control of intake at least around parturition.

5. Conclusions

The greater Ala, Arg, and Lys together with cystine and cystathionine concentrations at −10 days and 14 days, but not at 4 days, in cows fed MET indicated greater utilization of these AA and derivatives at the time of most-severe negative AA balance. The enriched circulating sulfur-containing compound pool together with greater α-aminobutyric acid revealed enhanced transsulfuration pathway activity in response to MET supplementation. Despite the greater circulating cystine in CHOL cows, the lower proportion of Met in TSC indicates enhanced flux through the transsulfuration pathway at the expense of Met. Whether the decrease in the proportion of Met was due to insufficient choline supplementation remains unknown. As a precursor for Met synthesis in vivo, it is possible that increasing periparturient choline supplementation could mitigate a decrease in Met. Although plasma GSH did not differ in response to MET due to barely detectable concentrations in plasma, the greater circulating taurine and carnosine indicate less oxidative stress in MET-supplemented cows. In conclusion, the overall better health and production performance reported previously in MET cows was due, at least in part, to a better plasma AA profile and overall lower oxidative stress status. Hence, the lack of change in AA profiles could be one of the reasons preventing CHOL-fed cows from achieving comparable performance and health benefits during the periparturient period.

Supplementary Materials:

RNA Extraction and mRNA Expression Calculation, Table S1: Plasma proteinogenic AA concentrations during the transition period in cows supplemented with or without rumen-protected methionine (MET) and choline (CHOL), Table S2: Plasma non-proteinogenic AA and AA derivatives concentrations during the transition period in cows supplemented with or without rumen-protected MET and CHOL, Table S3: Hepatic relative *PC* and *PCK1* mRNA expression during the transition period in cows with or without rumen-protected MET and CHOL.

Acknowledgments: This work was supported by Adisseo Inc., NA, Alpharetta, GA, USA. Zheng Zhou was a recipient of a doctoral fellowship from China Scholarship Council, Beijing, China.

Author Contributions: J.J.L. and D.N.L. conceived and designed the experiments; Z.Z. and M.V.-R. performed the experiments; Z.Z. analyzed the data; Z.Z. wrote the paper.

References

1. Bell, A.W.; Burhans, W.S.; Overton, T.R. Protein nutrition in late pregnancy, maternal protein reserves and lactation performance in dairy cows. *Proc. Nutr. Soc.* **2000**, *59*, 119–126. [CrossRef] [PubMed]
2. Goff, J.P.; Horst, R.L. Physiological changes at parturition and their relationship to metabolic disorders. *J. Dairy Sci.* **1997**, *80*, 1260–1268. [CrossRef]
3. Zhou, Z.; Loor, J.J.; Piccioli-Cappelli, F.; Librandi, F.; Lobley, G.E.; Trevisi, E. Circulating amino acids during the peripartal period in cows with different liver functionality index. *J. Dairy Sci.* **2016**, *99*, 2257–2267. [CrossRef] [PubMed]
4. Overton, T.R. Substrate utilization for hepatic gluconeogenesis in the transition dairy cow. In Proceedings of the 1998 Cornell Nutrition Conference for Feed Manufacturers, Syracuse, NY, USA, 19 October 1998; pp. 237–246.
5. McNeill, D.M.; Slepetis, R.; Ehrhardt, R.A.; Smith, D.M.; Bell, A.W. Protein requirements of sheep in late pregnancy: Partitioning of nitrogen between gravid uterus and maternal tissues. *J. Anim. Sci.* **1997**, *75*, 809–816. [CrossRef] [PubMed]
6. Osorio, J.S.; Ji, P.; Drackley, J.K.; Luchini, D.; Loor, J.J. Supplemental smartamine m or metasmart during the transition period benefits postpartal cow performance and blood neutrophil function. *J. Dairy Sci.* **2013**, *96*, 6248–6263. [CrossRef] [PubMed]
7. Osorio, J.S.; Ji, P.; Drackley, J.K.; Luchini, D.; Loor, J.J. Smartamine M and MetaSmart supplementation during the peripartal period alter hepatic expression of gene networks in 1-carbon metabolism, inflammation, oxidative stress, and the growth hormone-insulin-like growth factor 1 axis pathways. *J. Dairy Sci.* **2014**, *97*, 7451–7464. [CrossRef] [PubMed]

8. Zhou, Z.; Bulgari, O.; Vailati-Riboni, M.; Trevisi, E.; Ballou, M.A.; Cardoso, F.C.; Luchini, D.N.; Loor, J.J. Rumen-protected methionine compared with rumen-protected choline improves immunometabolic status in dairy cows during the peripartal period. *J. Dairy Sci.* **2016**, *99*, 8956–8969. [CrossRef] [PubMed]
9. Zhou, Z.; Vailati-Riboni, M.; Trevisi, E.; Drackley, J.K.; Luchini, D.N.; Loor, J.J. Better postpartal performance in dairy cows supplemented with rumen-protected methionine compared with choline during the peripartal period. *J. Dairy Sci.* **2016**, *99*, 8716–8732. [CrossRef] [PubMed]
10. Pisulewski, P.M.; Rulquin, H.; Peyraud, J.L.; Verite, R. Lactational and systemic responses of dairy cows to postruminal infusions of increasing amounts of methionine. *J. Dairy Sci.* **1996**, *79*, 1781–1791. [CrossRef]
11. Schwab, C.G.; Bozak, C.K.; Whitehouse, N.L.; Mesbah, M.M. Amino acid limitation and flow to duodenum at four stages of lactation. 1. Sequence of lysine and methionine limitation. *J. Dairy Sci.* **1992**, *75*, 3486–3502. [CrossRef]
12. Brosnan, J.T.; Brosnan, M.E. The sulfur-containing amino acids: An overview. *J. Nutr.* **2006**, *136*, 1636S–1640S. [PubMed]
13. Ulrey, C.L.; Liu, L.; Andrews, L.G.; Tollefsbol, T.O. The impact of metabolism on DNA methylation. *Hum. Mol. Genet.* **2005**, *14*, R139–R147. [CrossRef] [PubMed]
14. Zhou, Z.; Vailati-Riboni, M.; Luchini, D.; Loor, J.J. Rumen-protected methyl donors during the transition period: Circulating plasma amino acids in response to supplemental rumen-protected methionine or choline. In Proceedings of the ASAS-ADSA-CSAS-WSASAS Joint Annual Meetings, Salt Lake City, UT, USA, 19–23 July 2016.
15. Wong, E.R.; Thompson, W. Choline oxidation and labile methyl groups in normal and choline-deficient rat liver. *Biochim. Biophys. Acta* **1972**, *260*, 259–271. [CrossRef]
16. Li, Z.; Vance, D.E. Phosphatidylcholine and choline homeostasis. *J. Lipid Res.* **2008**, *49*, 1187–1194. [CrossRef] [PubMed]
17. Pinotti, L.; Baldi, A.; Dell'Orto, V. Comparative mammalian choline metabolism with emphasis on the high-yielding dairy cow. *Nutr. Res. Rev.* **2002**, *15*, 315–332. [CrossRef] [PubMed]
18. Doepel, L.; Lapierre, H.; Kennelly, J.J. Peripartum performance and metabolism of dairy cows in response to prepartum energy and protein intake. *J. Dairy Sci.* **2002**, *85*, 2315–2334. [CrossRef]
19. Meijer, G.A.L.; Vandermeulen, J.; Bakker, J.G.M.; Vanderkoelen, C.J.; Vanvuuren, A.M. Free amino-acids in plasma and muscle of high-yielding dairy-cows in early lactation. *J. Dairy Sci.* **1995**, *78*, 1131–1141. [CrossRef]
20. Verbeke, R.; Roets, E.; Peeters, G. Variations in the concentrations of free amino acids in the plasma of the dairy cow at parturition. *J. Dairy Res.* **1972**, *39*, 355–364. [CrossRef] [PubMed]
21. Sales, J.; Homolka, P.; Koukolova, V. Effect of dietary rumen-protected choline on milk production of dairy cows: A meta-analysis. *J. Dairy Sci.* **2010**, *93*, 3746–3754. [CrossRef] [PubMed]
22. Shahsavari, A.; D'Occhio, M.J.; Al Jassim, R. The role of rumen-protected choline in hepatic function and performance of transition dairy cows. *Br. J. Nutr.* **2016**, *116*, 35–44. [CrossRef] [PubMed]
23. Zhou, Z.; Vailati-Riboni, M.; Trevisi, E.; drackley, J.K.; Luchini, D.; Loor, J.J. Better postpartal performance in dairy cows supplemented with rumen-protected methionine than choline during the peripartal period. *J. Dairy Sci.* **2016**, in press.
24. Graulet, B.; Richard, C.; Robert, J.C. Methionine availability in plasma of dairy cows supplemented with methionine hydroxy analog isopropyl ester. *J. Dairy Sci.* **2005**, *88*, 3640–3649. [CrossRef]
25. Benoit, S.L.A. *Can Choline Spare Methioinine from Catabolism in Lactating Mice and Dairy Cows?* University of Maryland: College Park, MD, USA, 2009.
26. De Veth, M.J.; Artegoitia, V.M.; Campagna, S.R.; Lapierre, H.; Harte, F.; Girard, C.L. Choline absorption and evaluation of bioavailability markers when supplementing choline to lactating dairy cows. *J. Dairy Sci.* **2016**, *99*, 9732–9744. [CrossRef] [PubMed]
27. Fekkes, D. State-of-the-art of high-performance liquid chromatographic analysis of amino acids in physiological samples. *J. Chromatogr. B Biomed. Appl.* **1996**, *682*, 3–22. [CrossRef]
28. Deyl, Z.; Hyanek, J.; Horakova, M. Profiling of amino acids in body fluids and tissues by means of liquid chromatography. *J. Chromatogr.* **1986**, *379*, 177–250. [CrossRef]
29. Dann, H.M.; Morin, D.E.; Bollero, G.A.; Murphy, M.R.; Drackley, J.K. Prepartum intake, postpartum induction of ketosis, and periparturient disorders affect the metabolic status of dairy cows. *J. Dairy Sci.* **2005**, *88*, 3249–3264. [CrossRef]

30. National Research Council (NRC). *Nutrient Requirements of Dairy Cattle*, 7th ed.; The National Academies Press: Washington, DC, USA, 2001.
31. O'Connor, J.D.; Sniffen, C.J.; Fox, D.G.; Chalupa, W. A net carbohydrate and protein system for evaluating cattle diets: IV. Predicting amino acid adequacy. *J. Anim. Sci.* **1993**, *71*, 1298–1311. [PubMed]
32. Mitchell, H.H.; Block, R.J. Some relationships between the amino acid contents of proteins and their nutritive values for the rat. *J. Biol. Chem.* **1946**, *163*, 599–620. [CrossRef] [PubMed]
33. Emmanuel, B.; Kennelly, J.J. Kinetics of methionine and choline and their incorporation into plasma lipids and milk components in lactating goats. *J. Dairy Sci.* **1984**, *67*, 1912–1918. [CrossRef]
34. Zhou, Z.; Garrow, T.A.; Dong, X.; Luchini, D.N.; Loor, J.J. Hepatic activity and transcription of betaine-homocysteine methyltransferase, methionine synthase, and cystathionine synthase in periparturient dairy cows are altered to different extents by supply of methionine and choline. *J. Nutr.* **2016**, in press. [CrossRef] [PubMed]
35. Larsen, M.; Kristensen, N.B. Precursors for liver gluconeogenesis in periparturient dairy cows. *Animal* **2013**, *7*, 1640–1650. [CrossRef] [PubMed]
36. Meijer, G.A.; van der Meulen, J.; Bakker, J.G.; van der Koelen, C.J.; van Vuuren, A.M. Free amino acids in plasma and muscle of high yielding dairy cows in early lactation. *J. Dairy Sci.* **1995**, *78*, 1131–1141. [CrossRef]
37. Komaragiri, M.V.; Erdman, R.A. Factors affecting body tissue mobilization in early lactation dairy cows. 1. Effect of dietary protein on mobilization of body fat and protein. *J. Dairy Sci.* **1997**, *80*, 929–937. [CrossRef]
38. Kuhla, B.; Nurnberg, G.; Albrecht, D.; Gors, S.; Hammon, H.M.; Metges, C.C. Involvement of skeletal muscle protein, glycogen, and fat metabolism in the adaptation on early lactation of dairy cows. *J. Prot. Res.* **2011**, *10*, 4252–4262. [CrossRef] [PubMed]
39. Schalinske, K.L.; Smazal, A.L. Homocysteine imbalance: A pathological metabolic marker. *Adv. Nutr.* **2012**, *3*, 755–762. [CrossRef] [PubMed]
40. Guttormsen, A.B.; Solheim, E.; Refsum, H. Variation in plasma cystathionine and its relation to changes in plasma concentrations of homocysteine and methionine in healthy subjects during a 24-h observation period. *Am. J. Clin. Nutr.* **2004**, *79*, 76–79. [PubMed]
41. Stabler, S.P.; Sekhar, J.; Allen, R.H.; O'Neill, H.C.; White, C.W. Alpha-lipoic acid induces elevated *S*-adenosylhomocysteine and depletes *S*-adenosylmethionine. *Free Radic. Biol. Med.* **2009**, *47*, 1147–1153. [CrossRef] [PubMed]
42. Bernabucci, U.; Ronchi, B.; Lacetera, N.; Nardone, A. Influence of body condition score on relationships between metabolic status and oxidative stress in periparturient dairy cows. *J. Dairy Sci.* **2005**, *88*, 2017–2026. [CrossRef]
43. Castillo, C.; Hernandez, J.; Bravo, A.; Lopez-Alonso, M.; Pereira, V.; Benedito, J.L. Oxidative status during late pregnancy and early lactation in dairy cows. *Vet. J.* **2005**, *169*, 286–292. [CrossRef] [PubMed]
44. Young, I.S.; Woodside, J.V. Antioxidants in health and disease. *J. Clin. Pathol.* **2001**, *54*, 176–186. [CrossRef] [PubMed]
45. Romeu, M.; Nogues, R.; Marcas, L.; Sánchez-Martos, V.; Mulero, M.; Martinez-Vea, A.; Mallol, J.; Giralt, M. Evaluation of oxidative stress biomarkers in patients with chronic renal failure: A case control study. *BMC Res. Notes* **2010**, *3*, 20–26. [CrossRef] [PubMed]
46. Vetrani, C.; Costabile, G.; Di Marino, L.; Rivellese, A.A. Nutrition and oxidative stress: A systematic review of human studies. *Int. J. Food Sci. Nutr.* **2013**, *64*, 312–326. [CrossRef] [PubMed]
47. Saharan, S.; Mandal, P.K. The emerging role of glutathione in Alzheimer's disease. *J. Alzheimer's Dis.* **2014**, *40*, 519–529.
48. Garcia, R.A.; Stipanuk, M.H. The splanchnic organs, liver and kidney have unique roles in the metabolism of sulfur amino acids and their metabolites in rats. *J. Nutr.* **1992**, *122*, 1693–1701. [PubMed]
49. Hayes, K.C.; Sturman, J.A. Taurine in metabolism. *Annu. Rev. Nutr.* **1981**, *1*, 401–425. [CrossRef] [PubMed]
50. Osorio, J.S.; Trevisi, E.; Ji, P.; Drackley, J.K.; Luchini, D.; Bertoni, G.; Loor, J.J. Biomarkers of inflammation, metabolism, and oxidative stress in blood, liver, and milk reveal a better immunometabolic status in peripartal cows supplemented with smartamine M or MetaSmart. *J. Dairy Sci.* **2014**, *97*, 7437–7450. [CrossRef] [PubMed]
51. Pocius, P.A.; Clark, J.H.; Baumrucker, C.R. Glutathione in bovine blood: Possible source of amino acids for milk protein synthesis. *J. Dairy Sci.* **1981**, *64*, 1551–1554. [CrossRef]

52. Harris, C.I.; Milne, G. The urinary excretion of Nt-methyl histidine by cattle: Validation as an index of muscle protein breakdown. *Br. J. Nutr.* **1981**, *45*, 411–422. [CrossRef] [PubMed]
53. Boldyrev, A.A.; Aldini, G.; Derave, W. Physiology and pathophysiology of carnosine. *Physiol. Rev.* **2013**, *93*, 1803–1845. [CrossRef] [PubMed]
54. Aydin, A.F.; Kucukgergin, C.; Ozdemirler-Erata, G.; Kocak-Toker, N.; Uysal, M. The effect of carnosine treatment on prooxidant-antioxidant balance in liver, heart and brain tissues of male aged rats. *Biogerontology* **2010**, *11*, 103–109. [CrossRef] [PubMed]
55. Cheng, J.B.; Bu, D.P.; Wang, J.Q.; Sun, X.Z.; Pan, L.; Zhou, L.Y.; Liu, W. Effects of rumen-protected *gamma*-aminobutyric acid on performance and nutrient digestibility in heat-stressed dairy cows. *J. Dairy Sci.* **2014**, *97*, 5599–5607. [CrossRef] [PubMed]
56. Higgs, S.; Barber, D.J. Effects of baclofen on feeding behaviour examined in the runway. *Prog. Neuro-Psychopharmacol.* **2004**, *28*, 405–408. [CrossRef] [PubMed]
57. Wang, D.M.; Wang, C.; Liu, H.Y.; Liu, J.X.; Ferguson, J.D. Effects of rumen-protected *gamma*-aminobutyric acid on feed intake, lactation performance, and antioxidative status in early lactating dairy cows. *J. Dairy Sci.* **2013**, *96*, 3222–3227. [CrossRef] [PubMed]

Maternal Folate Status and the BHMT c.716G>A Polymorphism Affect the Betaine Dimethylglycine Pathway during Pregnancy

Jose M. Colomina [1,2], Pere Cavallé-Busquets [2,3], Sílvia Fernàndez-Roig [1,2], Pol Solé-Navais [1,2], Joan D. Fernandez-Ballart [1,2], Mónica Ballesteros [4], Per M. Ueland [5], Klaus Meyer [6] and Michelle M. Murphy [1,2,*]

1 Area of Preventive Medicine and Public Health, Faculty of Medicine and Health Sciences, Universitat Rovira i Virgili, IISPV, C/Sant Llorenç 21, Reus 43201, Spain; josemaria.colomina@urv.cat (J.M.C.); silviafroig@gmail.com (S.F.-R.); pol.sole@urv.cat (P.S.-N.); joan.fernandez-ballart@urv.cat (J.D.F.-B.)

2 Ciberobn Fisiopatología de la Obesidad y Nutrición (CB06/03), Instituto Carlos III, Madrid 28029, Spain; pecavalle@grupsagessa.com

3 Area of Obstetrics and Gynaecology, Hospital Universitari Sant Joan, Reus and Universitat Rovira i Virgili, Reus 43204, Spain

4 Area of Obstetrics and Gynaecology, Hospital Universitari Joan XXIII, Tarragona and Universitat Rovira i Virgili, Tarragona 43005, Spain; mobape71@yahoo.es

5 Section for Pharmacology, Department of Internal Medicine, University of Bergen, Bergen N-5020, Norway; per.ueland@ikb.uib.no

6 Bevital A/S, Laboratory building, 9th floor, Bergen N-5021, Norway; klaus.meyer@bevital.no

* Correspondence: michelle.murphy@urv.cat

Abstract: The effect of the betaine: homocysteine methyltransferase BHMT c.716G>A (G: guanosine; A: adenosine) single nucleotide polymorphism (SNP) on the BHMT pathway is unknown during pregnancy. We hypothesised that it impairs betaine to dimethylglycine conversion and that folate status modifies its effect. We studied 612 women from the Reus Tarragona Birth Cohort from $\leq$12 gestational weeks (GW) throughout pregnancy. The frequency of the variant BHMT c.716A allele was 30.8% (95% confidence interval (CI): 28.3, 33.5). In participants with normal-high plasma folate status (>13.4 nmol/L), least square geometric mean [95% CI] plasma dimethylglycine (pDMG, µmol/L) was lower in the GA (2.35 [2.23, 2.47]) versus GG (2.58 [2.46, 2.70]) genotype at $\leq$12 GW ($p < 0.05$) and in the GA (2.08 [1.97, 2.19]) and AA (1.94 [1.75, 2.16]) versus GG (2.29 [2.18, 2.40]) genotypes at 15 GW ($p < 0.05$). No differences in pDMG between genotypes were observed in participants with possible folate deficiency ($\leq$13.4 nmol/L) (p for interactions at $\leq$12 GW: 0.023 and 15 GW: 0.038). PDMG was lower in participants with the AA versus GG genotype at 34 GW (2.01 [1.79, 2.25] versus 2.44 [2.16, 2.76] and at labour, 2.51 [2.39, 2.64] versus 3.00 [2.84, 3.18], ($p < 0.01$)). Possible deficiency compared to normal-high folate status was associated with higher pDMG in multiple linear regression analysis (β coefficients [SEM] ranging from 0.07 [0.04], $p < 0.05$ to 0.20 [0.04], $p < 0.001$ in models from early and mid-late pregnancy) and the AA compared to GG genotype was associated with lower pDMG (β coefficients [SEM] ranging from −0.11 [0.06], $p = 0.055$ to −0.23 [0.06], $p < 0.001$). Conclusion: During pregnancy, the BHMT pathway is affected by folate status and by the variant BHMT c.716A allele.

Keywords: pregnancy; folate; betaine: homocysteine methyltransferase; BHMT c.716G>A; betaine; dimethylglycine

---

1. Introduction

The importance of one carbon metabolism and homocysteine regulation in foetal development and optimal pregnancy outcome is well established. Homocysteine remethylation contributes not only to homocysteine homeostasis but also to the provision of methyl groups essential for foetal development. Homocysteine is remethylated to methionine by the ubiquitous folate and cobalamin-dependent methionine synthase (MTR; EC 2.1.1.13) and by betaine:homocysteine methyltransferase (BHMT; EC 2.1.1.5) that occurs mainly in the kidney and liver [1]. The estimated consumption of homocysteine by MTR and BHMT is similar in rat liver [2] but globally the MTR reaction is thought to prevail in mammals based on the fact that BHMT activity has only been detected in some organs such as the liver and kidney [3,4] with conflicting reports regarding its presence in the brain [1,5,6]. To the best of our knowledge this information is not available in human studies to date but a study of healthy Dutch adults reported that the inverse association between folate and fasting plasma total homocysteine (tHcy) was stronger than that between betaine and tHcy, suggesting that the MTR reaction prevails under normal circumstances [7]. Some studies also provide indirect evidence for interaction between both remethylation pathways and upregulation of the BHMT pathway when folate status is low [8–12]. Serum folate was positively associated with betaine and inversely associated with dimethylglycine in a study of healthy Dutch adults [8] and serum dimethylglycine was higher in folate-deficient compared to normal status adults in a USA study [9]. Stronger negative associations between betaine and post-methionine load tHcy were observed when serum folate status was low [10] or in the absence of B vitamin supplement use [11]. We reported an apparent shift in the roles of folate and betaine in homocysteine homeostasis as folate status declines with advancing pregnancy and that low plasma folate status was associated with low plasma betaine and high dimethylglycine and a high dimethylglycine/betaine ratio [12].

BHMT c.716G>A (also known as 742G>A, rs3733890) is a common single nucleotide polymorphism (SNP) in which arginine is substituted by glutamine at position 239 [13]. Numerous human studies reported no effect of the SNP on tHcy [14–18]. However, a Norwegian study did report that plasma dimethylglycine decreased with increasing number of A alleles [17].

The BHMT c.716G>A SNP in pregnant women has been associated with increased risk of placental abruption [16]. There are conflicting reports of the effect of the SNP in the foetus on foetal development outcomes. The variant allele was associated with increased risk of grave neural tube defects (NTDs) [19–21] but reduced risk of orofacial cleft [22] and Down syndrome [23,24]. Interestingly, in Liu et al.'s study [19], the risk of NTDs associated with the variant A allele was only observed in pregnancies of women that did not take folic acid supplements.

We hypothesised that the BHMT c.716G>A polymorphism impedes the conversion of betaine to dimethylglycine during pregnancy. We tested how plasma folate status affects plasma betaine and dimethylglycine according to BHMT c.716G>A genotype throughout pregnancy.

2. Experimental Section

2.1. Participants

A total of 612 women that were recruited before November 2014 from the pregnancy phase of the Reus-Tarragona Birth Cohort (RTBC) were studied. The RTBC is an observational longitudinal study of maternal nutritional status and pregnancy that is being carried out by the Area of Preventive Medicine and Public Health, Universitat Rovira i Virgili and the Areas of Obstetrics and Gynaecology of the University Hospitals: Sant Joan, Reus and Joan XXIII, Tarragona (Spain). The study design and participant recruitment have been previously described [12]. Briefly, women attending their first antenatal visit with a viable singleton pregnancy confirmed by ultrasonography that provided a fasting blood sample at or before the 12th gestational week (GW) were eligible to participate in the study. Exclusion criteria included chronic diseases, surgical interventions affecting nutritional status or medication affecting folate or cobalamin metabolism. The study was carried out with ethical approval from the ethics committees of both participating hospitals and the research has been registered at Clinical Trials. gov: NCT01778205. All participants were informed of the nature and aims of the study and provided signed consent.

Participant age and body mass index (BMI) were recorded at the first antenatal check-up. Data regarding lifestyle, habits and supplement use from periconception throughout pregnancy was collected by the study team using questionnaires at 20 and 32 GW. Socioeconomic status of the participants was defined as low, middle or high according to the family unit income, education level and occupation of both parents [25]. Participants were classified as smokers throughout pregnancy, smokers during the first trimester and non-smokers based on first and second trimester as well as cord plasma cotinine concentrations (see biochemical determinations). Since plasma cotinine is indicative of recent smoking data from questionnaires and prenatal check-ups regarding declared smoking activity by the participants was also considered.

In line with the Spanish Obstetrics and Gynaecology Society recommendations [26], women were advised to take daily prenatal supplements containing 400 μg folic acid during the first trimester. The specific supplements recommended for this study were composed of 400 μg folic acid and 2 μg cyanocobalamin.

2.2. *Blood Sample Collection and Biochemical and Genetic Determinations*

Fasting blood samples were collected at ≤12, 15, 24–27 and 34 GW and nonfasting samples on admission to hospital with confirmed labour and from the umbilical cord. Maternal blood was drawn from the antecubital vein, and cord blood from the vein, into vacutainers containing EDTA-K_2. Samples were kept at 4 °C for a maximum of 1 h before separating plasma of which aliquots were immediately stored at −80 °C in the Institut d'Investigació Sanitària Pere Virgili biobank (Reus (Tarragona), Spain). Leukocytes were isolated from the blood cells remaining after plasma separation and DNA extracted from these using the Puregene DNA extraction kit (Gentra Systems, Minneapolis, MN, USA). Samples were transported on dry ice to Bevital (www.bevital.no, Bergen, Norway), carrying out biochemical analyses in batches comprising complete pregnancies within 18 months of collection. Plasma folate was determined by microbiological assay with *Lactobacillus casei* [27]. Plasma concentrations of choline, betaine, dimethylglycine, total homocysteine (tHcy) were measured by liquid chromatography–tandem mass spectrometry [28,29]. Plasma cotinine, which is an indicator of recent nicotine exposure, was also determined by liquid chromatography–tandem mass spectrometry [30] and plasma creatinine by modified Jaffé method (Química Clínica Aplicada SA, Amposta, Tarragona, Spain). Classification as current smoker was based on plasma cotinine >10 ng/mL at ≤12 GW (first trimester smoker) and 24–27 GW or in the cord (smoker throughout pregnancy). The maternal BHMT c.716G>A SNP was determined by Matrix-Assisted Laser Desorption/Ionization Time-Of-Flight Mass Spectrometry (MALDI-TOF/MS) as previously described [31].

2.3. *Statistical Analysis*

Previously, we reported a shift in folate status between early and mid-late pregnancy in line with the overall cessation of folic acid supplement use or change in supplement type between the first and second or third trimesters of pregnancy [12]. To account for change in plasma folate status during pregnancy, and to classify plasma folate status according to WHO criteria [32], participants were classified into possibly deficient (plasma folate ≤ 13.4 nmol/L) or normal-high (plasma folate > 13.4 nmol/L) status categories during early pregnancy (based on plasma folate at ≤12 or 15 GW) and again during mid-late pregnancy (based on plasma folate at 24–27 or 34 GW). In the event of falling into different categories at different time points within the corresponding phase of pregnancy, normal-high status was assigned during early pregnancy and the predominant status out of the 3 time points was assigned in mid-late pregnancy. In any analysis using plasma folate status, the category occurring during the corresponding phase of pregnancy was used.

Natural log transformation was applied to normalise the distribution of plasma variables as required for the application of parametric tests. Thus, geometric means (95% CI) are reported for plasma folate, betaine, choline, dimethylglycine and tHcy. In all other cases medians (25th percentile, 75th percentile) are reported and frequencies are reported as % (95% CI). Proportions were compared using the chi-square test and the same test was also used to test the Hardy Weinberg equilibrium of the observed allele frequencies.

Plasma folate, choline, betaine, dimethylglycine and dimethylglycine/betaine ratio and tHcy were compared between the different BHMT c.716G>A genotypes at each gestational period and in the cord by ANCOVA adjusting for gestational age (weeks) at the time of the blood sample, and plasma folate status (in all models except for plasma folate models). The dimethylglycine models were also adjusted for plasma betaine. Interaction between plasma folate status and BHMT c.716G>A genotype in their effects on plasma dimethylglycine, dimethylglycine/betaine ratio and tHcy was tested and if observed, stratified analysis according to folate status was performed.

Changes in plasma concentrations of folate, choline, betaine, dimethylglycine, the dimethylglycine/betaine ratio and tHcy during pregnancy were assessed using 2-factor repeated measures ANOVA (General linear model; Intrasubject factor time of pregnancy and intersubject factor BHMT c.716G>A genotype) with posthoc Bonferroni correction of p values to account for multiple comparisons. The first trimester time point was used as the reference.

Multiple linear regression analysis was used to investigate the effects of plasma folate status and of maternal BHMT c.716G>A genotype on plasma dimethylglycine at each stage of pregnancy and in the cord. The models were adjusted for plasma betaine and gestational age at corresponding time of blood sample. The usual diagnostic techniques for multiple linear regression analysis were applied (Cook's distance to identify influential cases and analysis of residuals). Interaction between plasma folate status and BHMT c.716G>A genotype was also tested. All analyses were carried out with SPSS (SPSS Inc., Chicago, IL, USA) for Windows, version 22.0.

3. Results

Participation in the study by eligible candidates and completion (defined as live birth) is illustrated in Figure 1. Of the women screened at their first prenatal check-up, 42.4% were eligible to participate in the study. Of the 624 participants that entered the study (93.8% of those eligible) first trimester data was collected from 612 and 562 went on to have live births.

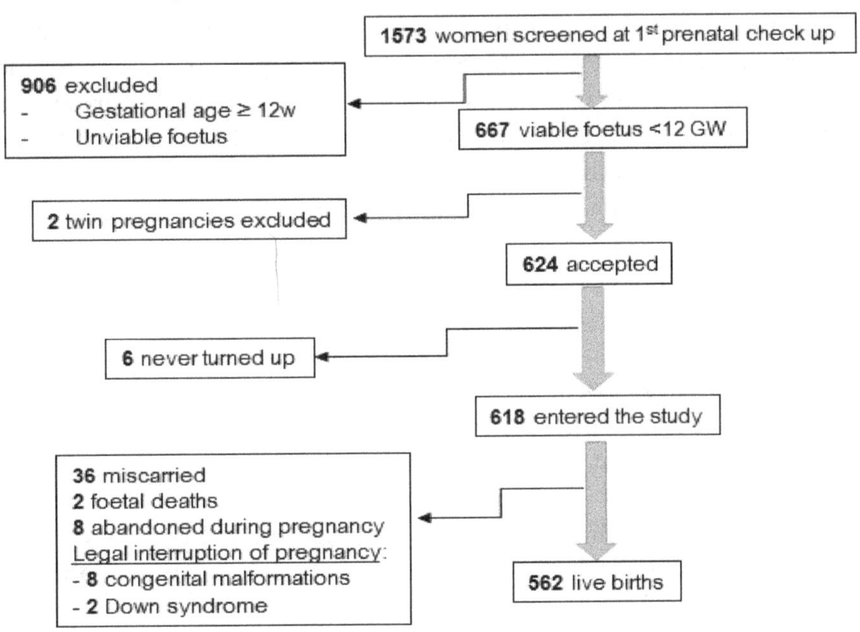

Figure 1. Flow chart of participation in the study.

Participant lifestyle, plasma folate, cobalamin, choline, tHcy and obstetrical characteristics are summarised in Table 1. This data shows that 80.9% of the women reported planning their pregnancy and 34.1% took folic acid supplements before becoming pregnant. Active smoking during the first trimester and throughout pregnancy was observed in 28.1% and in 17% of the participants respectively. The frequency of the BHMT c.716A allele was 30.8% (95% CI: 28.3, 33.5) and the genotypes were in Hardy Weinberg equilibrium (chi square for observed compared to expected genotype frequencies: 1.64).

Table 1. Participant characteristics (n = 612).

Age (Year) [1]		**32.0 (29.0, 35.0)**
Body mass index (kg/m^2) [1]		23.0 (20.9, 25.4)
Planned pregnancy [2]		80.9 (77.3, 84.0)
Previous pregnancy [2]		52.6 (48.6, 56.5)
Socioeconomic status [2,3]	High	43.6 (39.6, 47.6)
	Mid	49.6 (45.5, 53.6)
	Low	6.8 (5.1, 9.1)
Smoking during pregnancy [2]	First trimester	28.1 (24.7, 31.8)
	Throughout pregnancy	17.0 (14.2, 20.3)
Folic acid supplement use [2]	Preconception	34.1 (30.2, 38.2)
	First trimester	93.8 (91.5, 95.4)
	Mid-late pregnancy	53.9 (49.6, 58.1)
BHMT c.716G>A [2]	GG	48.9 (45.0, 52.9)
	GA	40.5 (36.6, 44.4)
	AA	10.6 (8.4, 13.3)

G: guanosine; A: adenosine. Values are [1] median (25th percentile, 75th percentile), [2] % (95% confidence interval); [3] based on total income, occupation and education level of both parents.

Plasma folate, choline, betaine and dimethylglycine concentrations, dimethylglycine/betaine ratios and tHcy at each time point of pregnancy and in the cord, according to maternal BHMT c.716G>A genotype are reported in Table 2. Plasma folate, choline, betaine or tHcy did not differ among genotypes at any time of pregnancy. Lower plasma dimethylglycine was observed in the heterozygote compared to homozygote common genotype at $\leq$12 GW and at labour. This was also true for the homozygote variant genotype during late pregnancy. A lower plasma dimethylglycine/betaine ratio was observed in the homozygote variant compared to heterozygote genotype at $\leq$12 GW and compared to the homozygote common genotype at 34 GW. This was also true for the heterozygote compared to the homozygote common genotype at 15 GW. Further adjustment of the ANCOVA models for plasma creatinine and smoking habit did not alter the results.

Plasma betaine gradually decreased in all of the genotypes throughout pregnancy. Plasma dimethylglycine fluctuated in a U shape pattern in the homozygote common and heterozygote genotypes where end of pregnancy concentrations were higher than in early pregnancy. However, in the homozygote variant genotype, plasma dimethylglycine concentrations remained lower than in early pregnancy, throughout pregnancy. The plasma dimethylglycine/betaine ratio gradually increased during pregnancy in all genotypes.

Interactions between plasma folate category and the effect of BHMT c.716G>A genotype on dimethylglycine were observed at $\leq$12 and 15 GW and on the dimethylglycine/betaine ratio at $\leq$12 GW.

A stratified analysis of plasma dimethylglycine for each genotype according to plasma folate status in early pregnancy is illustrated in Figure 2. In the normal-high category of plasma folate status, lower plasma dimethylglycine was observed in the heterozygote compared to the homozygote common genotype at both $\leq$12 and 15 GW and in the homozygote variant compared to homozygote common genotype at 15 GW.

Table 2. Plasma folate, choline, betaine, dimethylglycine and tHcy during pregnancy and in the cord according to maternal BHMT c.716G>A genotype.

	BHMT c.716G>A Genotype	≤12 GW [546] [1]	15 GW [440]	24–27 GW [500]	34 GW [485]	Labour [478]	Cord [465]
Folate (nmol/L)	GG	26.8 (24.5, 29.2)	25.6 (23.3, 28.1)	13.3 ^{a} (12.2, 14.6)	10.9 ^{a} (9.9, 12.1)	10.8 ^{a} (9.7, 11.9)	23.9 (22.2, 25.7)
	GA	25.5 (23.2, 28.0)	24.6 (22.3, 27.1)	12.9 ^{a} (11.7, 14.2)	10.7 ^{a} (9.7, 11.9)	10.8 ^{a} (9.7, 12.1)	24.2 (22.4, 26.1)
	AA	24.5 (20.2, 29.6)	25.4 (20.8, 31.1)	12.6 ^{a} (10.3, 15.3)	12.0 ^{a} (9.6, 15.1)	10.2 ^{a} (8.2, 12.9)	22.6 (19.1, 26.6)
	ANCOVA [3] *models*	NS	NS	NS	NS	NS	NS
Choline (μmo/L)	GG	7.6 (7.4, 7.9)	7.7 (7.5, 7.9)	9.1 ^{a} (8.9, 9.4)	10.3 ^{a} (10.1, 10.6)	11.7 ^{a} (11.3, 12.1)	28.1 (26.8, 29.5)
	GA	7.7 (7.4, 7.9)	7.7 (7.5, 8.0)	9.2 ^{a} (9.0, 9.5)	10.4 ^{a} (10.1, 10.7)	11.7 ^{a} (11.3, 12.2)	28.9 (27.5, 30.4)
	AA	7.6 (7.2, 8.1)	8.0 (7.5, 8.5)	9.5 ^{a} (9.0, 10.1)	10.5 ^{a} (9.9, 11.2)	11.6 ^{a} (10.7, 12.5)	29.8 (26.8, 33.1)
	ANCOVA [3] *models*	NS	NS	NS	NS	NS	NS
Betaine (μmol/L)	GG	20.9 (20.2, 21.6)	14.6 ^{a} (14.2, 15.1)	12.8 ^{a} (12.4, 13.1)	12.8 ^{a} (12.5, 13.1)	13.1 ^{a} (12.7, 13.5)	24.7 (24.0, 25.4)
	GA	21.8 (21.0, 22.6)	15.3 ^{a} (14.8, 15.8)	13.1 ^{a} (12.7, 13.4)	13.3 ^{a} (12.9, 13.7)	13.4 ^{a} (13.0, 13.8)	25.1 (24.3, 25.8)
	AA	20.2 (18.8, 21.8)	14.5 ^{a} (13.6, 15.5)	12.7 ^{a} (11.9, 13.4)	13.0 ^{a} (12.3, 13.8)	12.7 ^{a} (11.9, 13.5)	25.3 (23.8, 27.0)
	ANCOVA [3] *models*	NS	NS	NS	NS	NS	NS
Dimethylglycine (μmol/L)	GG	2.58 (2.47, 2.69)	2.29 ^{a} (2.19, 2.39)	2.22 ^{a} (2.12, 2.33)	2.51 (2.39, 2.64)	3.00 ^{a} (2.84, 3.18)	3.73 (3.55, 3.92)
	GA	2.37 (2.26, 2.48) *	2.12 ^{a} (2.02, 2.22)	2.11 ^{a} (2.00, 2.22)	2.39 (2.27, 2.52)	2.69 ^{a} (2.53, 2.86) *	3.54 (3.36, 3.73)
	AA	2.50 (2.28, 2.74)	2.08 ^{a} (1.88, 2.30)	2.02 ^{a} (1.82, 2.24)	2.01 ^{a} (1.79, 2.25) **,†	2.44 (2.16, 2.76) **	3.29 (2.95, 3.67)
	ANCOVA [4] *models*	$p = 0.026$	$p = 0.040$	NS	$p = 0.002$	$p = 0.002$	NS
	Folate genotype interaction	$p = 0.023$	$p = 0.058$	NS	NS	NS	NS
Dimethylglycine/betaine	GG	0.13 (0.12, 0.14)	0.17 ^{a} (0.16, 0.18)	0.19 ^{a} (0.18, 0.21)	0.22 ^{a} (0.20, 0.24)	0.26 ^{a} (0.23, 0.28)	0.17 (0.15, 0.18)
	GA	0.12 (0.11, 0.13)	0.15 ^{a} (0.14, 0.16) *	0.18 ^{a} (0.16, 0.19)	0.20 ^{a} (0.18, 0.22)	0.23 ^{a} (0.21, 0.26)	0.15(0.14, 0.16)
	AA	0.15 (0.13, 0.17) †	0.15 (0.13, 0.17)	0.18 ^{a} (0.15, 0.22)	0.16 (0.12, 0.20) *	0.22 ^{a} (0.17, 0.27)	0.14 (0.11, 0.16)
	ANCOVA [5] *models*	$p = 0.009$	$p = 0.018$	NS	$p = 0.020$	NS	$p = 0.044$
	Folate genotype interaction	$p = 0.038$	NS	NS	NS	NS	NS
Total homocysteine (μmol/L)	GG	5.2 (5.1, 5.4)	4.5 ^{a} (4.4, 4.7)	4.6 ^{a} (4.5, 4.8)	5.3 (5.1, 5.4)	6.2 ^{a} (6.0, 6.5)	4.8 (4.7, 5.0)
	GA	5.3 (5.1, 5.4)	4.4 ^{a} (4.3, 4.6)	4.7 ^{a} (4.5, 4.8)	5.4 (5.2, 5.6)	6.2 ^{a} (5.9, 6.4)	4.9 (4.7, 5.2)
	AA	5.3 (5.0, 5.6)	4.5 ^{a} (4.3, 4.8)	4.6 ^{a} (4.3, 4.9)	5.2 (4.9, 5.6)	6.0 ^{a} (5.6, 6.5)	4.9 (4.5, 5.3)
	ANCOVA [4] *models*	NS	NS	NS	NS	NS	NS

G: guanosine; A: adenosine; GW: gestational weeks; NS: non-significant. [1] n varies between time points due to participant loss due to complications, non-attendance of programmed blood draw or delivery elsewhere or failure to collect blood samples in the labour ward; [2] values are least square geometric means (95% confidence interval); [3] adjusting for plasma folate status and gestational age at time of blood draw; [4] adjusting for plasma folate status, plasma betaine and gestational age at time of blood draw. ANCOVA Bonferroni posthoc: * $p < 0.05$, ** $p < 0.01$ versus GG; † $p < 0.05$, versus GA; Two-factor repeated measures ANOVA versus ≤12 GW (intrasubject factor: gestational age; intersubject factor: BHMT c.716G>A genotype) followed by post hoc Bonferroni correction for multiple comparisons: ^{a} $p < 0.001$.

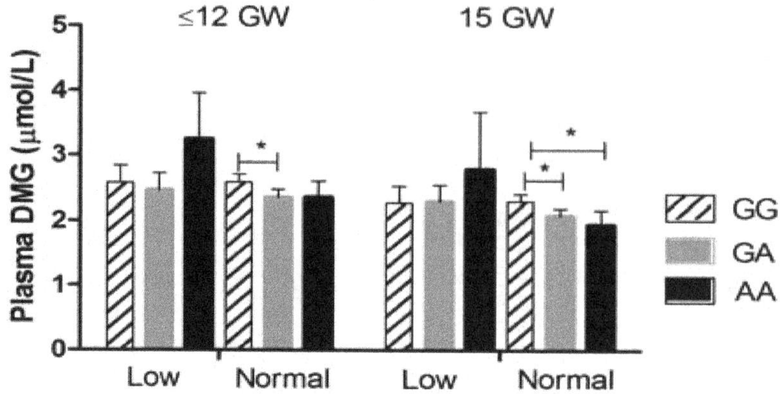

Figure 2. Plasma dimethylglycine according to BHMT c.716G>A genotype and folate status in early pregnancy. G: guanosine; A: adenosine; GW: Gestational weeks. Low: possibly deficient (plasma folate ≤ 13.4 nmol/L). Normal: normal-high (plasma folate > 13.4 nmol/L). At ≤12 GW, Low: GG (n = 57), GA (n = 48), AA (n = 14); Normal: GG (n = 231), GA (n = 193), AA (n = 47). At 15 GW, Low: GG (n = 37), GA (n = 40), AA (n = 6); Normal: GG (n = 169), GA (n = 141), AA (n = 34). The triple screening blood sample at 15 GW is optional and blood samples were available from less participants. Values are least square geometric means. Error bars represent 95% confidence interval. Comparisons between genotypes were made using ANCOVA adjusting for plasma betaine and gestational age at time of blood draw with posthoc Bonferroni correction for multiple comparisons of p values: * $p < 0.05$.

The associations between plasma folate status and BHMT c.716G>A genotype with plasma dimethylglycine throughout pregnancy and in the cord are reported in Table 3. Low compared to normal-high plasma folate status was positively associated with plasma dimethylglycine throughout pregnancy and in the cord. Compared to the homozygous common BHMT GG genotype, both variant GA and AA genotypes were associated with lower plasma dimethylglycine during early and late pregnancy. The observed associations were stronger in the case of the homozygote AA variant genotype during late pregnancy and in the cord. Further adjustment of the multiple linear regression models for plasma creatinine and smoking habit did not alter the results.

Table 3. Change in plasma dimethylglycine throughout pregnancy according to plasma folate category, and BHMT c.716G>A genotype.

		Model [1]		**Plasma Folate Category** [2]	**BHMT c.716G>A Genotype**	
		R^2	F (n)	Possibly deficient vs. normal-high	GA vs. GG	AA vs. GG
Early	≤12 GW	15.4	22.5 (592) ***	0.07 (0.04) [3],*	−0.08 (0.03) **	−0.04 (0.05)
	15 GW	12.0	12.6 (427) ***	0.07 (0.04) #	−0.08 (0.03) *	−0.11 (0.06) †
Mid-late	24–27 GW	11.6	14.3 (507) ***	0.13 (0.03) ***	−0.06 (0.04)	−0.10 (0.06)
	34 GW	18.9	23.8 (492) ***	0.20 (0.04) ***	−0.06 (0.04)	−0.23 (0.06) ***
	Labour	13.2	15.5 (477) ***	0.15 (0.04) ***	−0.11 (0.04) *	−0.21 (0.07) **
	Cord	5.0	5.7 (447) ***	0.08 (0.04) *	−0.05 (0.04) *	−0.13 (0.06) *

F: analysis of variance F-test of overall significance; G: guanosine; A: adenosine; GW: Gestational weeks. [1] Multiple linear regression analysis: dependent variable plasma dimethylglycine. Adjusted for plasma betaine and gestational age at time of blood draw; [2] Pregnancy (possibly deficient: ≤13.4 nmol/L; normal-high: >13.4 nmol/L); [3] β coefficient (standard error of the mean). * $p < 0.05$, ** $p < 0.01$, *** $p < 0.001$, † $p = 0.055$, # $p = 0.087$.

4. Discussion

4.1. Principal Findings

This study reports for the first time that the A-allele of the BHMT c.716G>A SNP is associated with lower plasma dimethylglycine during pregnancy and in the cord. Low folate status, on the other hand is associated with higher plasma dimethylglycine during mid and late pregnancy and in the cord. Folate status and genotype interacted during early pregnancy and stratification by plasma folate status category showed that the effect of the variant BHMT c.716A allele on dimethylglycine was limited to women with normal-high folate status. By late pregnancy, the variant allele's effect was independent of folate status.

4.2. Comparison with Previous Studies and Interpretation

We observed similar frequencies of the BHMT c.716G>A genotypes as previously reported in studies from Europe [14,17,33].

We interpret the lower plasma dimethylglycine concentrations observed in the presence of the variant BHMT c.716A allele to mean that the conversion of betaine to dimethylglycine is low in pregnant women carrying the A-allele. A similar observation was previously reported in a population study [17]. On the other hand, the higher plasma dimethylglycine concentrations when folate status is low, suggests BHMT upregulation when MTR activity is reduced. In early pregnancy when MTR activity was not reduced by low folate availability, the effects of lower BHMT activity in the presence of the BHMT c.716 A-allele are evident. We hypothesised that this effect would be more pronounced at mid-late pregnancy and with low folate status when the BHMT pathway is more active [12]. Our results showed decreased betaine to dimethylglycine conversion in the variant A-allele carriers, but in early pregnancy this effect was limited to women with normal-high folate status. In vitro experiments have shown that BHMT expression and activity may be modified by the molecular environment. SAM has been shown to inhibit BHMT transcription in human cells [34,35] and SAM [36] and to a lesser extent SAH [36,37] to inhibit BHMT activity in rat liver extracts. Methionine has also been shown to inhibit BHMT [38,39]. A study in MTHFR-deficient mice supplemented with very high doses of folic acid showed that despite greater betaine utilisation, likely for homocysteine remethylation, it was insufficient to maintain SAM concentrations [40]. Despite the differences in molecular environment between *in vivo* and *in vitro* studies, they shed light on potential mechanisms that may lead to our observed effects. A speculative suggestion from our data is that high folate status can lead to BHMT inhibition, with the inhibitory effect being stronger on the variant enzyme. Some studies have investigated the effect of folate on BHMT. Liver *BHMT* expression was reported to be lower in the offspring of rat dams supplemented with folic acid during pregnancy [41] but was unaffected by excessive folic acid intake in mice [40]. It has also been suggested that betaine is spared when folate status is replete [42]. It is possible that the combination of both mechanisms, replete folate status and the variant allele, lead to reduced conversion of betaine to dimethylglycine. Cessation of prenatal folic acid supplementation at the end of the first trimester was associated with a sharp reduction in folate status, and from mid pregnancy the genotype effect on dimethylglycine was independent of folate status.

No differences in plasma betaine concentrations between the different genotypes were observed. This is not surprising because a stable betaine pool is maintained even when the BHMT pathway is upregulated [9,43], possibly to spare betaine for its principal functions as an osmolyte [44] and in protein stabilisation [45].

4.3. Implications

BHMT expression and activity in foetal livers has been reported to increase with gestational age in human [5,46] and pig studies [47] which is in line with increased BHMT activity in late pregnancy that we suggest here. Interestingly, foetal liver MTR activity decreases in the third trimester [5]. This supports the idea of complementarity between the BHMT and MTR pathways in late pregnancy and our observations indirectly support this hypothesis.

Here we show that the BHMT c.716G>A polymorphism, previously associated with foetal developmental defects, affects the BHMT pathway during pregnancy. In situations of upregulation of the MTR and BHMT pathways, such as in pregnancy, the effect of the SNP on BHMT activity may become more evident. Anomalies in homocysteine remethylation affect homocysteine homeostasis as well as methyl group supply to essential epigenetic reactions. Elevated maternal homocysteine has been associated with pregnancy complications affecting both maternal and foetal health as well as foetal development [48] and with lasting developmental effects into childhood [49]. Inhibition of BHMT has been shown to cause hyperhomocysteinaemia in mice [50]. We did not observe an effect of the variant allele on homocysteine. However, the extent of the effect of the SNP on BHMT activity in humans is unknown. Pregnancy itself has a profound effect on homocysteine [51] and may mask any potential effects of the SNP. Comparison of associations between betaine and homocysteine before and after the implementation of mandatory fortification of flour with folic acid in the USA showed that the inverse correlation reported in Framingham study participants with low folate status prior to fortification, was no longer observed post-fortification [52].

Potential modification of effects of folate status by the BHMT c.716G>A SNP should be considered when contrasting/interpreting results from fortified versus non-fortified populations or supplement versus non-supplement users. In addition, the importance of the BHMT pathway in homocysteine homeostasis may be less important in folate-replete populations.

4.4. Strengths and Limitations

A strength of this study is its longitudinal design and follow up from very early pregnancy. It was carried out in the absence of mandatory fortification with folic acid and therefore the effects of prenatal folic acid supplement use were observed. Samples were processed according to specific protocols to prevent artefacts in plasma analyte concentrations caused by temperature and time before separation of blood cells [53].

When folic acid supplementation ceased there was a large drop in plasma folate as we reported previously [12]. Sample power may have been limited in analyses of the effect of the BHMT c.716AA genotype during early pregnancy. However many significant effects of this genotype on dimethylglycine were observed in mid-late pregnancy and in the cord. Another potential limitation to the study was the difference in folic acid supplement use between women. They were recommended to take prenatal supplements containing 400 μg of folic acid during the first trimester. However some took other brands of folic acid containing higher doses or extended their folic acid use beyond the first trimester. We dealt with this in our analysis by classifying the women into plasma folate status categories in early and again in mid-late pregnancy to account for the difference in status that we expected to arise due to differences in patterns of supplement use.

Although there is increasing evidence that BHMT plays an important role in one carbon metabolism many aspects regarding the mechanisms involved are unclear. Information regarding the effect of the common BHMT c.716G>A polymorphism on BHMT activity and how it is affected by variations in molecular environment is lacking.

5. Conclusions

We conclude that dimethylglycine during pregnancy is affected by both folate status and the BHMT c.716G>A polymorphism.

Acknowledgments: This work was supported by funding from Comisión Interministerial de Ciencia y Tecnología, Spain [SAF 2005-05096]; Instituto de Salud Carlos III, Fondo de Investigaciones Sanitarias (cofinanced by FEDER) [FIS: 10/00335 and FIS: 13/02500] and Centros de Investigación Biomédica en Red CB06/03; Institut d'Investigació Sanitària Pere Virgili 2010/21; Agència de Gestió d'Ajuts Universitaris i de Recerca [SGR 2009-1237] and from Italfarmaco SA, Madrid, Spain. Jose M Colomina received a Universitat Rovira i Virgili (URV) Martí Franques predoctoral research grant.

Author Contributions: J.M.C., S.F.-R., J.D.F.-B. and M.M.M. developed the hypothesis, designed the study and analysed the data. P.C.-B. and M.B. recruited the participants and carried out the pregnancy phase of the study. S.F.-R., P.S.-N. and J.M.C. collected lifestyle and dietary data from the participants and processed samples for biobanking. P.M.U. and K.M. were responsible for the biochemical and genetic determinations. All authors participated in the writing of the paper and approved the final version.

References

1. McKeever, M.P.; Weir, D.G.; Molloy, A.; Scott, J.M. Betaine-homocysteine methyltransferase: Organ distribution in man, pig and rat and subcellular distribution in the rat. *Clin. Sci.* **1991**, *81*, 551–556. [CrossRef] [PubMed]
2. Finkelstein, J.D.; Martin, J.J. Methionine metabolism in mammals. Distribution of homocysteine between competing pathways. *J. Biol. Chem.* **1984**, *259*, 9508–9513. [PubMed]
3. Finkelstein, J.D. Methionine metabolism in mammals. *J. Nutr. Biochem.* **1990**, *1*, 228–237. [CrossRef]
4. Lambert, B.D.; Titgemeyer, E.C.; Stokka, G.L.; DeBey, B.M.; Löest, C.A. Methionine supply to growing steers affects hepatic activities of methionine synthase and betaine-homocysteine methyltransferase, but not cystathionine synthase. *J. Nutr.* **2002**, *132*, 2004–2009. [PubMed]
5. Gaull, G.E.; Von Berg, W.; Räihä, N.C.; Sturman, J.A. Development of methyltransferase activities of human fetal tissues. *Pediatr. Res.* **1973**, *7*, 527–533. [PubMed]
6. Sunden, L.F.; Renduchintala, M.S.; Park, E.I.; Miklasz, S.D.; Garrow, T.A. Betaine-homocysteine methyltransferase expression in porcine and human tissues and chromosomal localization of the human gene. *Arch. Biochem. Biophys.* **1997**, *345*, 171–174. [CrossRef] [PubMed]
7. Melse-Boonstra, A.; Holm, P.I.; Ueland, P.M.; Olthof, M.; Clarke, R.; Verhoef, P. Betaine concentration as a determinant of fasting total homocysteine concentrations and the effect of folic acid supplementation on betaine concentrations. *Am. J. Clin. Nutr.* **2005**, *81*, 1378–1382. [PubMed]
8. Imbard, A.; Smulders, Y.M.; Barto, R.; Smith, D.E.C.; Kok, R.M.; Jakobs, C.; Blom, H.J. Plasma choline and betaine correlate with serum folate, plasma S-adenosyl-methionine and S-adenosyl-homocysteine in healthy volunteers. *Clin. Chem. Lab. Med.* **2013**, *51*, 683–692. [CrossRef] [PubMed]
9. Allen, R.H.; Stabler, S.P.; Lindenbaum, J. Serum betaine, *N,N*-dimethylglycine and *N*-methylglycine levels in patients with cobalamin and folate deficiency and related inborn errors of metabolism. *Metabolism* **1993**, *42*, 1448–1460. [CrossRef]
10. Holm, P.I.; Ueland, P.M.; Vollset, S.E.; Midttun, Ø.; Blom, H.J.; Keijzer, M.B.; den Heijer, M. Betaine and folate status as cooperative determinants of plasma homocysteine in humans. *Arterioscler. Thromb. Vasc. Biol.* **2005**, *25*, 379–385. [CrossRef] [PubMed]
11. Holm, P.I.; Bleie, Ø.; Ueland, P.M.; Lien, E.; Refsum, H.; Nordrehaug, J.E.; Nygård, O. Betaine as a determinant of postmethionine load total plasma homocysteine before and after B-vitamin supplementation. *Arterioscler. Thromb. Vasc. Biol.* **2004**, *24*, 301–307. [CrossRef] [PubMed]
12. Fernàndez-Roig, S.; Cavallé-Busquets, P.; Fernandez-Ballart, J.D.; Ballesteros, M.; Berrocal-Zaragoza, M.I.; Salat-Batlle, J.; Ueland, P.M.; Murphy, M.M. Low folate status enhances pregnancy changes in plasma betaine and dimethylglycine concentrations and the association between betaine and homocysteine. *Am. J. Clin. Nutr.* **2013**, *97*, 1252–1259.
13. Park, E.I.; Garrow, T. Interaction between dietary methionine and methyl donor intake on rat liver betaine-homocysteine methyltransferase gene expression and organization of the human gene. *J. Biol. Chem.* **1999**, *274*, 7816–7824. [CrossRef] [PubMed]
14. Heil, S.G.; Lievers, K.J.; Boers, G.H.; Verhoef, P.; den Heijer, M.; Trijbels, F.J.; Blom, H.J. Betaine-homocysteine methyltransferase (BHMT): Genomic sequencing and relevance to hyperhomocysteinemia and vascular disease in humans. *Mol. Genet. Metab.* **2000**, *71*, 511–519. [CrossRef] [PubMed]
15. Weisberg, I.S.; Park, E.; Ballman, K.V.; Berger, P.; Nunn, M.; Suh, D.S.; Breksa, A.P.; Garrow, T.A.; Rozen, R. Investigations of a common genetic variant in betaine-homocysteine methyltransferase (BHMT) in coronary artery disease. *Atherosclerosis* **2003**, *167*, 205–214. [CrossRef]
16. Ananth, C.V.; Elsasser, D.; Kinzler, W.L.; Peltier, M.R.; Getahun, D.; Leclerc, D.; Rozen, R.R. Polymorphisms in methionine synthase reductase and betaine-homocysteine *S*-methyltransferase genes: Risk of placental abruption. *Mol. Genet. Metab.* **2007**, *91*, 104–110. [CrossRef] [PubMed]
17. Fredriksen, A.; Meyer, K.; Ueland, P.M.; Vollset, S.E.; Grotmol, T.; Schneede, J. Large-scale population-based metabolic phenotyping of thirteen genetic polymorphisms related to one-carbon metabolism. *Hum. Mutat.* **2007**, *28*, 856–865. [CrossRef] [PubMed]
18. Liang, S.; Zhou, Y.; Wang, H.; Qian, Y.; Ma, D.; Tian, W.; Persaud-Sharma, V.; Yu, C.; Ren, Y.; Zhou, S.; et al. The effect of multiple single nucleotide polymorphisms in the folic acid pathway genes on homocysteine metabolism. *Biomed. Res. Int.* **2014**, *2014*, 560183. [CrossRef] [PubMed]

19. Liu, J.; Qi, J.; Yu, X.; Zhu, J.; Zhang, L.; Ning, Q.; Luo, X. Investigations of single nucleotide polymorphisms in folate pathway genes in Chinese families with neural tube defects. *J. Neurol. Sci.* **2014**, *337*, 61–66. [CrossRef] [PubMed]
20. Shaw, G.M.; Lu, W.; Zhu, H.; Yang, W.; Briggs, F.B.S.; Carmichael, S.L.; Barcellos, L.F.; Lammer, E.J.; Finnell, R.H. 118 SNPs of folate-related genes and risks of spina bifida and conotruncal heart defects. *BMC Med. Genet.* **2009**, *10*, 49. [CrossRef] [PubMed]
21. Boyles, A.L.; Billups, A.V.; Deak, K.L.; Siegel, D.G.; Mehltretter, L.; Slifer, S.H.; Bassuk, A.G.; Kessler, J.A.; Reed, M.C.; Nijhout, H.F.; et al. Neural tube defects and folate pathway genes: Family-based association tests of gene-gene and gene-environment interactions. *Environ. Health Perspect.* **2006**, *114*, 1547–1552. [CrossRef] [PubMed]
22. Mostowska, A.; Hozyasz, K.K.; Wojcicki, P.; Dziegelewska, M.; Jagodzinski, P.P. Associations of folate and choline metabolism gene polymorphisms with orofacial clefts. *J. Med. Genet.* **2010**, *47*, 809–815. [CrossRef] [PubMed]
23. Zampieri, B.L.; Biselli, J.M.; Goloni-Bertollo, E.M.; Vannucchi, H.; Carvalho, V.M.; Cordeiro, J.A.; Pavarino, E.C. Maternal risk for Down syndrome is modulated by genes involved in folate metabolism. *Dis. Markers* **2012**, *32*, 73–81. [CrossRef] [PubMed]
24. Amorim, M.R.; Moura, C.M.; Gomes, A.D.; Barboza, H.N.; Lopes, R.B.; Ribeiro, M.G.; Costa Lima, M.A. Betaine–homocysteine methyltransferase 742G>A polymorphism and risk of down syndrome offspring in a Brazilian population. *Mol. Biol. Rep.* **2013**, *40*, 4685–4689. [CrossRef] [PubMed]
25. Álvarez-Dardet, C.; Alonso, J.; Domingo, A.; Regidor, E. *La Medición de la Clase Social en Ciencias de la Salud*; SG Editores, SEE: Barcelona, Spain, 1995.
26. Dirección General de Salud Pública (Ministerio de Sanidad y Consumo—Gobierno de España). *Recomendaciones Sobre Suplementación con ácido Fólico para la Prevención de Defectos del Tubo Neural*; Dirección General de Salud Pública: Madrid, Spain, 2001; Volume 25.
27. Molloy, A.M.; Scott, J.M. Microbiological assay for serum, plasma, and red cell folate using cryopreserved, microtiter plate method. *Methods Enzymol.* **1997**, *281*, 43–53. [PubMed]
28. Holm, P.I.; Ueland, P.M.; Kvalheim, G.; Lien, E.A. Determination of choline, betaine, and dimethylglycine in plasma by a high-throughput method based on normal-phase chromatography-tandem mass spectrometry. *Clin. Chem.* **2003**, *49*, 286–294. [CrossRef] [PubMed]
29. Ueland, P.M.; Midttun, O.; Windelberg, A.; Svardal, A.; Skålevik, R.; Hustad, S. Quantitative profiling of folate and one-carbon metabolism in large-scale epidemiological studies by mass spectrometry. *Clin. Chem. Lab. Med.* **2007**, *45*, 1737–1745. [CrossRef] [PubMed]
30. Midttun, Ø.; Hustad, S.; Ueland, P.M. Quantitative profiling of biomarkers related to B-vitamin status, tryptophan metabolism and inflammation in human plasma by liquid chromatography/tandem mass spectrometry. *Rapid Commun. Mass Spectrom.* **2009**, *23*, 1371–1379. [CrossRef] [PubMed]
31. Meyer, K.; Fredriksen, A.; Ueland, P.M. High-level multiplex genotyping of polymorphisms involved in folate or homocysteine metabolism by matrix-assisted laser desorption/ionization mass spectrometry. *Clin. Chem.* **2004**, *50*, 391–402. [CrossRef] [PubMed]
32. World Health Organization. Serum and Red Blood Cell Folate Concentrations for Assessing Folate Status in Populations. Vitamin and Mineral Nutrition Information System. 2012. Available online: http://apps.who.int/iris/bitstream/10665/75584/1/WHO_NMH_NHD_EPG_12.1_eng.pdf (accessed on 6 September 2016).
33. Giusti, B.; Sestini, I.; Saracini, C.; Sticchi, E.; Bolli, P.; Magi, A.; Gori, A.M.; Marcucci, R.; Gensini, G.F.; Abbate, R. High-throughput multiplex single-nucleotide polymorphism (SNP) analysis in genes involved in methionine metabolism. *Biochem. Genet.* **2008**, *46*, 406–423. [CrossRef] [PubMed]
34. Castro, C.; Breksa, A.P.; Salisbury, E.; Garrow, T.A. Betaine-Homocysteine S-Methyltransferase (BHMT) Transcription Is Inhibited by S-Adenosylmethionine (ADOMET). In *Chemistry and Biology of Pteridines and Folates*; Milstien, S., Kapatos, G., Levine, R.A., Shane, B., Eds.; Springer: Bethesda, Spain, 2002; pp. 549–556.
35. Ou, X.; Yang, H.; Ramani, K.; Ara, A.I.; Chen, H.; Mato, J.M.; Lu, S.C. Inhibition of human betaine-homocysteine methyltransferase expression by S-adenosylmethionine and methylthioadenosine. *Biochem. J.* **2007**, *401*, 87–96. [CrossRef] [PubMed]
36. Finkelstein, J.D.; Martin, J.J. Inactivation of betaine-homocysteine methyltransferase by adenosylmethionine and adenosylethionine. *Biochem. Biophys. Res. Commun.* **1984**, *118*, 14–19. [CrossRef]
37. Finkelstein, J.D.; Kyle, W.E.; Harris, B.J. Methionine metabolism in mammals: Regulatory effects of S-adenosylhomocysteine. *Arch. Biochem. Biophys.* **1974**, *165*, 774–779. [CrossRef]

38. Finkelstein, J.D.; Harris, B.J.; Kyle, W.E. Methionine metabolism in mammals: Kinetic study of betaine-homocysteine methyltransferase. *Arch. Biochem. Biophys.* **1972**, *153*, 320–324. [CrossRef]
39. Szegedi, S.S.; Castro, C.C.; Koutmos, M.; Garrow, T.A. Betaine-homocysteine S-methyltransferase-2 is an S-methylmethionine-homocysteine methyltransferase. *J. Biol. Chem.* **2008**, *283*, 8939–8945. [CrossRef] [PubMed]
40. Christensen, K.E.; Mikael, L.G.; Leung, K.Y.; Lévesque, N.; Deng, L.; Wu, Q.; Malysheva, O.V.; Best, A.; Caudill, M.A.; Greene, N.D.; et al. High folic acid consumption leads to pseudo-MTHFR deficiency, altered lipid metabolism, and liver injury in mice. *Am. J. Clin. Nutr.* **2015**, *101*, 646–658. [CrossRef] [PubMed]
41. Chmurzynska, A.; Malinowska, A.M. Homocysteine homeostasis in the rat is maintained by compensatory changes in cystathionine β-synthase, betaine-homocysteine methyltransferase, and phosphatidylethanolamine N-methyltransferase gene transcription occurring in response to maternal protein and folic acid intake during pregnancy and fat intake after weaning. *Nutr. Res.* **2011**, *31*, 572–577. [PubMed]
42. Eussen, S.J.P.M.; Ueland, P.M.; Clarke, R.; Blom, H.J.; Hoefnagels, W.H.L.; van Staveren, W.; de Groot, L.C.P.G.M. The association of betaine, homocysteine and related metabolites with cognitive function in Dutch elderly people. *Br. J. Nutr.* **2007**, *98*, 960–968. [CrossRef] [PubMed]
43. Dominguez-Salas, P.; Moore, S.E.; Cole, D.; da Costa, K.A.; Cox, S.E.; Dyer, R.A.; Fulford, A.J.C.; Innis, S.M.; Waterland, R.A.; Zeisel, S.H.; et al. DNA methylation potential: dietary intake and blood concentrations of one-carbon metabolites and cofactors in rural African women. *Am. J. Clin. Nutr.* **2013**, *97*, 1217–1227. [CrossRef] [PubMed]
44. Yancey, P.H.; Clark, M.E.; Hand, S.C.; Bowlus, R.D.; Somero, G.N. Living with water stress: Evolution of osmolyte systems. *Science* **1982**, *217*, 1214–1222. [CrossRef] [PubMed]
45. Sheikh-Hamad, D.; García-Pérez, A.; Ferraris, J.D.; Peters, E.M.; Burg, M.B. Induction of gene expression by heat shock versus osmotic stress. *Am. J. Physiol.* **1994**, *267*, F28–F34. [PubMed]
46. Feng, Q.; Kalari, K.; Fridley, B.L.; Jenkins, G.; Ji, Y.; Abo, R.; Hebbring, S.; Zhang, J.; Nye, M.D.; Leeder, J.S.; et al. Betaine-homocysteine methyltransferase: Human liver genotype-phenotype correlation. *Mol. Genet. Metab.* **2011**, *102*, 126–133. [CrossRef] [PubMed]
47. Ganu, R.; Garrow, T.; Koutmos, M.; Rund, L.; Schook, L.B. Splicing variants of the porcine betaine-homocysteine S-methyltransferase gene: Implications for mammalian metabolism. *Gene* **2013**, *529*, 228–237. [CrossRef] [PubMed]
48. Murphy, M.M.; Fernandez-Ballart, J.D. Homocysteine in pregnancy. *Adv. Clin. Chem.* **2011**, *53*, 105–137. [PubMed]
49. Murphy, M.M.; Fernandez-Ballart, J.D.; Molloy, A.M.; Canals, J. Moderately elevated maternal homocysteine at preconception is inversely associated with cognitive performance in children 4 months and 6 years after birth. *Matern. Child. Nutr.* **2016**. [CrossRef] [PubMed]
50. Collinsova, M.; Strakova, J.; Jiracek, J.; Garrow, T.A. Inhibition of betaine-homocysteine S-methyltransferase causes hyperhomocysteinemia in mice. *J. Nutr.* **2006**, *136*, 1493–1497. [PubMed]
51. Murphy, M.M.; Scott, J.M.; McPartlin, J.M.; Fernandez-Ballart, J.D. The pregnancy-related decrease in fasting plasma homocysteine is not explained by folic acid supplementation, hemodilution, or a decrease in albumin in a longitudinal study. *Am. J. Clin. Nutr.* **2002**, *76*, 614–619. [PubMed]
52. Lee, J.E.; Jacques, P.F.; Dougherty, L.; Selhub, J.; Giovannucci, E.; Zeisel, S.H.; Cho, E. Are dietary choline and betaine intakes determinants of total homocysteine concentration? *Am. J. Clin. Nutr.* **2010**, *91*, 1303–1310. [CrossRef] [PubMed]
53. Fiskerstrand, T.; Refsum, H.; Kvalheim, G.; Ueland, P.M. Homocysteine and other thiols in plasma and urine: Automated determination and sample stability. *Clin. Chem.* **1993**, *39*, 263–271. [PubMed]

11

Dietary B Vitamins and a 10-Year Risk of Dementia in Older Persons

Sophie Lefèvre-Arbogast [1,2,*], Catherine Féart [1,2], Jean-François Dartigues [1,2], Catherine Helmer [1,2], Luc Letenneur [1,2] and Cécilia Samieri [1,2]

1 University Bordeaux, Institut de Santé Publique d'Epidémiologie et de Développement (ISPED), Centre INSERM U1219-Bordeaux Population Health, Bordeaux 33076, France; Catherine.Feart@isped.u-bordeaux2.fr (C.F.); Jean-Francois.Dartigues@isped.u-bordeaux2.fr (J.-F.D.); Catherine.Helmer@isped.u-bordeaux2.fr (C.H.); luc.letenneur@inserm.fr (L.L.); Cecilia.Samieri@isped.u-bordeaux2.fr (C.S.)

2 Institut National de la Santé et de la Recherche Médicale (INSERM), Institut de Santé Publique d'Epidémiologie et de Développement (ISPED), Centre INSERM U1219-Bordeaux Population Health, Bordeaux 33076, France

* Correspondence: sophie.lefevre-arbogast@isped.u-bordeaux2.fr

Abstract: B vitamins may lower the risk of dementia, yet epidemiological findings, mostly from countries with folic acid fortification, have remained inconsistent. We evaluated in a large French cohort of older persons the associations between dietary B vitamins and long-term incident dementia. We included 1321 participants from the Three-City Study who completed a 24 h dietary recall, were free of dementia at the time of diet assessment, and were followed for an average of 7.4 years. In Cox proportional hazards models adjusted for multiple potential confounders, including overall diet quality, higher intake of folate was inversely associated with the risk of dementia (p for trend = 0.02), with an approximately 50% lower risk for individuals in the highest compared to the lowest quintile of folate (HR = 0.47; 95% CI 0.28; 0.81). No association was found for vitamins B6 and B12. In conclusion, in a large French cohort with a relatively low baseline folate status (average intake = 278 μg/day), higher folate intakes were associated with a decreased risk of dementia.

Keywords: folate; B vitamins; dementia; aging

1. Introduction

B vitamins have fundamental roles in the function of the central nervous system [1], and have been considered as promising candidates for the prevention of dementia and its major etiology, Alzheimer's disease (AD). B vitamins (B6, folate, and B12) regulate homocysteine (Hcy) levels, and hyperhomocysteinemia is a major vascular risk factor and an established risk factor for dementia [2]. Hyperhomocysteinemia may affect brain function through both vascular mediation and neurotoxicity [3]. B vitamins may also have a direct effect on the brain, independently of homocysteine [4]. Indeed, a lower status in B vitamins decreases *S*-adenosylmethionine, a major intermediate of methylation reactions in the brain which are involved in synaptic transmission and epigenetic regulation [5]. Moreover, tetrahydrofolate, the active form of folate, is involved in DNA repair system [6] and DNA replication, which are both critical for adult hippocampal neurogenesis [7]. Direct mechanistic effects of B vitamins on the brain independent of Hcy may therefore be particularly relevant to folate [8–10].

Prospective epidemiological studies have found associations between higher intakes of B vitamins and a lower risk of dementia and AD; three studies have reported associations with dietary folate (but not with vitamins B6 and B12) [11–13], although inconsistent findings have also been found, with studies reporting null [14,15] or even harmful associations between folate intakes at high levels and cognitive function, when combined with low vitamin B12 status [16]. Findings have also been inconsistent in studies using blood status in B vitamins (see [17] for a review). Moreover, prevention trials have been inconclusive to date [18], with a few exceptions, including the two European FACIT and VITACOG trials, which evidenced the beneficial effect of folic acid on cognitive function and brain atrophy, respectively [19,20]. Although the reasons for such inconsistencies remain unclear, it is possible that the findings of some studies have been influenced by the folic acid fortification of all flour and cereal-grain products that became mandatory starting in 1998 in the US and Canada, leading to a subsequent dramatic increase in folate status in North American populations [21]. The vast majority of observational studies on B vitamins and cognitive aging have been conducted in the US, and limited research has examined European populations. In the present study, we evaluated in a large cohort of older persons from France—a country not subject to folic acid fortification policy—the association between dietary B vitamins and the risk of dementia and AD over 10 years of follow-up.

2. Materials and Methods

2.1. Study Population

Our analysis was based on the Three-City (3C) study, a French population-based cohort on dementia which started in 1999–2000, including 9294 non-institutionalized community dwellers aged 65 years or older in three French cities: Bordeaux (n = 2104), Dijon (n = 4931), and Montpellier (n = 2259). Face-to-face interviews were performed at the cohort baseline with the collection of sociodemographic, lifestyle, and health-related characteristics, neuropsychological testing, and blood sampling. The protocol of the 3C study has been described in detail previously [22]. The Consultative Committee for the Protection of Persons participating in Biomedical Research at Kremlin-Bicêtre University Hospital (Paris, France) approved the 3C study protocol (Project no. 99-28, june 1999) and all participants provided written informed consent. Follow-up examinations were conducted 2 years (2001–2002), 4 years (2003–2004), 7 years (2006–2007), 10 years (2009–2010), and 12 years (2011–2012) after the cohort baseline. The present study is based on data from Bordeaux, the only 3C center with a dietary assessment.

At the 2-year visit in 2001–2002, a comprehensive dietary survey was conducted by trained dieticians, including a food frequency questionnaire (FFQ) and a 24 h dietary recall (which served as baseline in the present analysis). Figure 1 describes the procedure for the study sample selection. Our final study population included 1321 participants followed for 10 years after the dietary assessment.

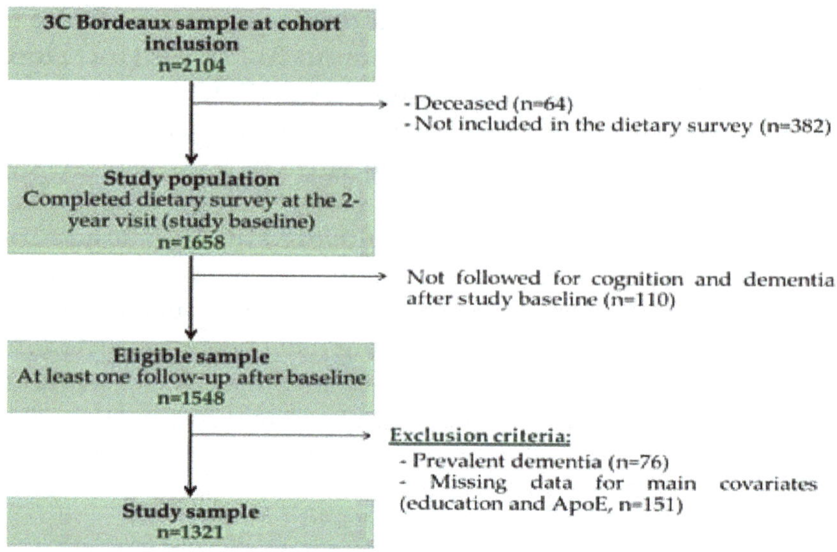

Figure 1. Flow diagram of the study sample selection, the 3C Bordeaux cohort. Abbreviations: 3C: Three-City; ApoE: apolipoprotein genotype.

2.2. Diagnosis of Dementia

Incident dementia was ascertained through a three-stage procedure. First, participants underwent a battery of neuropsychological tests at home conducted by a trained psychologist. Individuals suspected of dementia based on their neuropsychological performances were secondarily examined by a neurologist to establish a clinical diagnosis. Finally, all potential cases of dementia were reviewed by an independent committee of neurologists to set up consensus on dementia diagnosis and etiology, according to the *Diagnostic and Statistical Manual of Mental Disorders* (Fourth Edition) [23] and the *National Institute of Neurological and Communicative Disorders and Stroke and the Alzheimer's Disease and Related Disorders Association* Alzheimer's criteria [24].

2.3. Assessment of Diet and Intake of B-Vitamins

The procedure of the 24 h recall data collection was detailed in a previous publication [25]. Briefly, the 24 h dietary recall consisted in reporting all meals and beverages consumed the day prior to the interview (excluding week-end meals). For each food reported, portion sizes were registered using a book of photographs [26] and were used to estimate the quantity (in grams per day) of intake of each food item. Nutrient and total energy intakes were then estimated using several French food composition tables [27–29]. The contribution of supplemental folic acid (from fortified foods or supplements) to total folate intake is very low and virtually all folic acid is of natural origin in French populations [30]. In our analyses, we focused on intakes of B vitamins involved in one-carbon metabolism, i.e., vitamin B6, folate, and vitamin B12.

2.4. Other Variables

Sociodemographic information included age at study baseline, gender, and level of education. ApoEε4 genotype was defined as carrying at least one ε4 allele vs. no ε4 allele. Lifestyle factors included alcohol consumption, tobacco use, and regular exercise. To control for overall diet quality, we also computed a score of adherence to the Mediterranean diet (MeDi); the methodology for computation of the MeDi score has been described in previous publications [31,32]. Cardiovascular risk factors included body mass index (BMI), hypercholesterolemia (total cholesterol $\geq$6.2 mmol/L or anti-cholesterol medication), diabetes (fasting glucose ≥7.2 mmol/L or antidiabetic medication), history of cardiovascular diseases (including myocardial infarction and stroke), and hypertension (measured blood pressure higher than 140/90 mm Hg or antihypertensive medication). Depressive symptomatology was assessed using the Center for Epidemiological Studies-Depression (CES-D) [33] Scale; we defined high depressive symptoms as having a CES-D score higher than 17 in men and 23 in women (over a maximum of 60 [34]) or when the participant was "too depressed to answer". The number of drugs regularly consumed was recorded and used as a general indicator of comorbidities.

2.5. Statistical Analyses

We used Cox proportional hazards models with delayed entry using age as time-scale [35] to evaluate the multivariate associations between intake of B vitamins and the risk of all-cause dementia over 10 years; we secondarily examined AD specifically. Vitamin B6, folate, and vitamin B12 were modeled simultaneously and considered in quintiles. We first adjusted for the main risk factors of dementia (gender, education, and ApoE genotype), energy intake, and season of the 24 h recall (Model 1). We further controlled for lifestyle factors, cardiovascular risk factors, and other comorbidities (Model 2).

We examined linear trends across quintiles of B vitamins by using a continuous variable taking the median intake value of each quintile. Moreover, we investigated potential interactions of biological relevance between (i) folate and alcohol intakes [36]; (ii) folate and vitamin B12 intakes [37,38]; (iii) B vitamins and long-chain omega-3 fatty acid intakes [39]; and (iv) B vitamin intakes and ApoEε4 genotype. Missing data were treated as follows. For most covariates, data were missing for less than 3% of the sample; we thus assigned to missing data the reference category (for categorical variables) or the median value (for continuous variables). Regular exercise was missing for 11.8% of the sample; we thus created a specific missing category for this variable. The proportional hazard assumption was controlled, as well as the log-linearity assumption for continuous covariates.

In sensitivity analyses, we assessed the robustness of our findings by (i) excluding participants with the highest values for vitamin B intakes, i.e., with intakes >95th percentile of at least one of the 3 B vitamins; (ii) adjusting for regular intake of fruits and vegetables instead of the Mediterranean diet score; and (iii) controlling for other potential confounders with very low prevalence, i.e., consumption of B vitamin supplements. We also controlled for potential reverse causation (which occurs when subtle cognitive impairment modifies dietary intakes) by adjusting our multivariate models for global cognitive performances at baseline, represented by the Mini Mental State Examination score [40].

Statistical analyses were performed using SAS software version 9.3 (SAS Institute Inc., Cary, NC, USA) and R software version 3.2.3 (R Foundation for Statistical Computing, Vienna, Austria).

3. Results

3.1. Characteristics of the Sample

Study participants were 75.8 years old on average (range: 67.7–94.9) at the time of the dietary survey and 62.2% were female (Table 1). Nearly 41% of participants had reached high school level or above, and 18% were ApoEε4 carriers; baseline characteristics including lifestyle and cardiovascular risk factors have been provided in Table 1. A total of 197 individuals (15% of the sample) developed dementia over 7.4 years of follow-up on average (range: 0.9–11.2), including 131 classified with possible or probable AD (351 participants died during follow-up and 192 refused or were lost to follow-up). The incidence rate of dementia was 2.0 cases per 100 person-years, and the incidence of AD was 1.3 per 100 person-years.

Table 1. Baseline characteristics and B vitamin intakes of the participants according to incident all-cause dementia over 10 years, the 3C Bordeaux cohort (n = 1321).

Baseline Characteristics	Overall Sample (n = 1321)	Incident Dementia (n = 197)	No Dementia (n = 1124)	p for Risk of Dementia [a]
Age (years)	75.8 ± 4.8	78.3 ± 4.6	75.4 ± 4.7	<0.001
Gender, female	822 (62.2)	140 (71.1)	682 (60.7)	0.30
Education ≥high school	540 (40.9)	72 (36.5)	468 (41.6)	0.24
ApoEε4, carrier	240 (18.2)	49 (24.9)	191 (17.0)	<0.001
Alcohol intake (g/day)	13.9 ± 15.5	12.9 ± 14.0	14.1 ± 15.8	0.86
Tobacco consumption (pack-year)				
0	861 (65.2)	142 (72.1)	719 (64.0)	
<10	156 (11.8)	20 (10.2)	136 (12.1)	
(10–20)	84 (6.4)	10 (5.1)	74 (6.6)	0.75
(20–30)	71 (5.4)	7 (3.6)	64 (5.7)	
≥30	149 (11.3)	18 (9.1)	131 (11.7)	
Regular exercise [b]	412 (35.3)	46 (28.2)	366 (36.5)	0.14
BMI (kg/m^2)	26.6 ± 4.1	26.1 ± 4.3	26.7 ± 4.1	0.23
Hypercholesterolemia	762 (57.7)	125 (63.5)	637 (56.7)	0.16
Diabetes	125 (9.5)	33 (16.8)	92 (8.2)	<0.001
History of cardiovascular diseases	428 (32.4)	63 (32.0)	365 (32.5)	0.94
Hypertension	998 (75.5)	151 (76.6)	847 (75.4)	0.63
High depressive symptomatology	98 (7.4)	22 (11.2)	76 (6.8)	0.10
Number of drugs consumed	4.8 ± 2.9	5.8 ± 3.2	4.6 ± 2.8	<0.001
B vitamin/multivitamin supplement use	19 (1.4)	2 (1.0)	17 (1.5)	0.59
Energy intake (Kcal/day)	1623.0 ± 514.0	1565.0 ± 500.2	1633.0 ± 515.9	0.44
Vitamin B6 intake (mg/day)	1.5 ± 0.6	1.4 ± 0.6	1.5 ± 0.6	0.52
Folate intake (μg/day)	278.3 ± 134.8	251.9 ± 126.1	283.0 ± 135.8	0.01
Vitamin B12 intake (μg/day)	5.7 ± 11.4	4.9 ± 9.9	5.8 ± 11.7	0.30

Values are mean ± SD or number (percentages). [a] Univariate Cox Proportional Hazards models with delayed entry using age as time scale, except for age which use standard Cox Proportional Hazards models; [b] Percentages are of non-missing values. Abbreviations: ApoEε4: allele ε4 for the apolipoprotein E gene; BMI: body mass index.

Mean daily intakes were 1.5 mg/day for vitamin B6, 278.3 μg/day for folate, and 5.7 μg/day for vitamin B12 (Table 1). Compared with individuals who remained free of dementia during follow-up, those who developed the disease had lower B vitamin intakes at baseline, although the difference was statistically significant for folate only in univariate Cox models (p = 0.01 for risk of dementia for each 1SD-increase of folate intake), without any marked difference in daily energy intake across both groups (p = 0.44).

3.2. Multivariate Associations between Intake of B Vitamins and Risk of Dementia

In multivariate analyses, a higher intake of folate was significantly associated with a lower risk of dementia (p for trend $\leq$ 0.02 across increasing quintiles in multivariate models, Table 2). Adjustments for potential confounders did not markedly alter HRs, suggesting a minimal confounding effect. After controlling for a large set of potential confounders in Model 2, compared with individuals in the lowest quintile of folate, those in the highest quintile had a 47% lower risk of dementia over 10 years (HR (95% CI) = 0.47 (0.28, 0.81)). In contrast, we did not find any significant association between vitamin B6 or vitamin B12 intakes and the risk of dementia (p for trend = 0.38 and 0.73, respectively, in Model 2).

Table 2. Multivariate associations between quintiles of B vitamin intake and risk of all-cause dementia over 10 years, the 3C Bordeaux cohort (n = 1321).

	Number of Dementia Cases	Risk of Dementia (HR [95% CI]) [a]	
		Model 1	Model 2
Vitamin B6 (mg/day)			
Q1 <1.0	50	1.0 (reference)	1.0 (reference)
Q2 (1.0–1.2)	36	0.81 (0.51–1.28)	0.86 (0.54–1.36)
Q3 (1.2–1.5)	36	1.02 (0.63–1.65)	1.08 (0.66–1.77)
Q4 (1.5–1.9)	42	1.26 (0.78–2.04)	1.40 (0.85–2.31)
Q5 ≥1.9	33	1.02 (0.58–1.78)	1.08 (0.60–1.94)
p for trend		0.52	0.38
Folate (µg/day)			
Q1 <168.3	56	1.0 (reference)	1.0 (reference)
Q2 (168.3–225.4)	37	0.66 (0.43–1.02)	0.66 (0.42–1.02)
Q3 (225.4–281.4)	40	0.67 (0.43–1.03)	0.73 (0.47–1.15)
Q4 (281.4–375.6)	35	0.69 (0.43–1.10)	0.76 (0.47–1.24)
Q5 ≥375.6	29	0.47 (0.28–0.79)	0.47 (0.28–0.81)
p for trend		0.01	0.02
Vitamin B12 (µg/day)			
Q1 <1.8	38	1.0 (reference)	1.0 (reference)
Q2 (1.8–2.6)	47	1.42 (0.91–2.21)	1.27 (0.81–1.98)
Q3 (2.6–3.7)	40	1.29 (0.81–2.07)	1.15 (0.71–1.86)
Q4 (3.7–5.7)	40	1.30 (0.81–2.10)	1.26 (0.77–2.05)
Q5 ≥5.7	32	1.17 (0.70–1.94)	1.04 (0.61–1.75)
p for trend		0.95	0.73

[a] Cox proportional hazards models with delayed entry using age as time-scale. The three B vitamins were modeled simultaneously. Model 1: adjusted for gender, level of education, ApoEε4, energy intake, and season of the 24 h recall. Model 2: covariates from Model 1 plus alcohol and tobacco consumptions, regular exercise, the Mediterranean Diet score, BMI, hypercholesterolemia, diabetes, history of cardiovascular diseases, hypertension, depressive symptomatology, and number of drugs consumed.

When we examined the risk of AD, we found similar associations of high folate with a lower risk of AD, although the magnitude of associations was slightly weaker than those found with all-cause dementia (p for trend = 0.08 in the first model, HR for higher versus lower quintile of folate = 0.52, 95% CI = 0.28, 0.97; results are not shown in the tables) and relationships were attenuated and no longer statistically significant after further adjustments (p for trend = 0.17 in Model 2).

We did not detect any significant interaction between B vitamins and alcohol, and omega-3 intakes or with ApoEε4 carrier status. Likewise, there was no significant interaction between folate and vitamin B12 intakes on dementia risk.

3.3. Secondary Analyses

When we conducted sensitivity analysis by further adjusting models for baseline cognition, our results remained unchanged, suggesting that findings may not be due to reverse causation by incipient prodromal dementia. Likewise, a sensitivity analysis excluding the n = 155 participants with higher intake values for at least one of the 3 B vitamins did not modify results, suggesting that findings were not driven by a few particular individuals with extreme intake values. Results were also virtually unchanged when adjusting for regular fruit and vegetable consumption instead of the MeDi score, suggesting minimal confounding by other potentially beneficial nutrients contained in the major food source of dietary folate. Very few people (n = 19) consumed B vitamin/multivitamin supplements in this French population, and the inclusion of B vitamin/multivitamin supplementation in our models did not modify findings.

4. Discussion

In this large French cohort of older persons followed for more than a decade, we found that higher folate intakes were inversely associated with the risk of dementia, independently of intakes of other B vitamins, overall diet quality, and a large set of other potential confounders. Compared with individuals with folate intakes in the lowest quintile, those in the higher quintile had an approximately 50% lower risk of dementia. A similar trend was found with AD risk, although associations were weaker and no longer significant after adjustment for the full set of potential confounders (possibly due to less power to detect a significant relationship with AD cases, which represented only 66% of all-cause dementia cases). In contrast to folate, there was no significant association between dietary vitamins B6 and B12 and the risk of dementia or AD in this large cohort.

Our results are consistent with at least three previous US longitudinal studies, in which higher folate intake was associated with a lower risk of dementia or AD, while associations of dietary vitamins B6 and B12 to dementia risk were not significant [11–13]. In contrast, our results are not consistent with two other previous large US cohorts, the Chicago Health and Aging Project (CHAP) and the Cache County Memory Study (CCMS), which did not evidence any association between quintiles of B vitamin intake and risk of AD [14,15]; harmful associations between higher folate and cognition have also been found among persons with low vitamin B12 status in several cohorts [16,37,38]. The reasons for inconsistencies between studies are unclear. The most evident reason may pertain to differences in baseline intakes between French and US populations, with lower intakes reported in France, a country with limited supplement use and no folic acid fortification (e.g., median total folate intake in the upper quintile was 444 μg/day in our 3C sample, compared to 742 μg/day in the CHAP study [16]). It is thus possible that folate is protective for the brain in lower intake ranges (as those observed in France) and becomes inefficient—and even detrimental for those with low B12 status—at higher ranges. Otherwise, findings of US cohorts have remained difficult to interpret due to the fortification policy introduced in the late 1990s. Indeed, part of the dietary data in the CHAP study was collected after folic acid fortification; furthermore, although diet was ascertained in 1995 (i.e., pre-folic acid fortification) in the CCMS, follow-up for cognition and dementia was conducted through 2004, with >70% of the follow-up period for cognition covering post-folic acid fortification. It is thus possible that the increase in folate status in the US population which occurred after folic acid fortification have biased these studies towards the null.

Additionally, although most trials failed to evidence any benefit of B vitamin supplementation on cognitive function, our results are nonetheless consistent with three European trials which found a protective effect of B vitamins on brain aging outcomes among persons with raised Hcy or with low folate status [19,20,41–43]. In Italy, a small pilot trial found a benefit of folic acid supplementation on memory and attention among older persons selected with low initial status in folate [43]. In The Netherlands, the large FACIT trial included participants aged ≥50 years old with high levels of Hcy and found a significant benefit of folic acid supplementation over three years on memory and processing speed [19]; in the UK, the VITACOG study included older persons aged ≥70 years old with mild cognitive impairment (without a priori selection based on Hcy levels) and found an efficacy of B vitamins on brain atrophy [20,41], and on cognition limited to those with raised Hcy at baseline [42]. Finally, in the single largest French study to date based on secondary analyses on cognition from the large SU.FOL.OM3 trial on B vitamins and omega-3 fatty acids for secondary prevention of cardiovascular diseases, a protective effect of B vitamins was evidenced on global cognition and memory in the older age group (65–80 years) [44]. Together with our own study, these results suggest a beneficial effect of B vitamins on cognition in older persons (especially among those with raised Hcy or low folate status).

In contrast to folate, dietary vitamins B6 and B12 were not significantly associated with the risk of dementia or AD in the present study. Although several longitudinal studies found inverse associations between blood markers of vitamin B12 and brain health [45–49] (associations potentially fully mediated by Hcy [47,48]), studies generally found, as in our study, null results when examining dietary B6 and

B12 and cognitive health [11–16]. Indeed, studies based on intake data (including our own study) may not capture food-bound vitamin B12 malabsorption, which is common in older persons and adversely affects vitamin B12 status in healthy older people irrespective of dietary intakes [50]. Thus, circulating vitamin B12 may be a better marker of vitamin B12 deficiency than vitamin B12 intakes in older populations.

A limitation of the present study is that a single 24 h recall was used to assess B vitamin intake. A reported single day of intake does not fully capture intra-individual variation in dietary intakes, and might lead to misclassification, especially for foods consumed occasionally (such as offal, a top source for vitamin B12). However, in large samples, a single 24 h provides acceptable estimations of average intakes in subgroups of a population [51]; accordingly, we observed in our study average intake values similar to other studies in older populations for macronutrients [25] and for micronutrients including B vitamins (e.g., average intake values for B vitamins in our sample were close to those observed among older persons from the French Individual and National Study on Food Consumption (INCA 2) [52]—a national representative survey). In addition, the use of dietary supplements may not have been accurately recorded by our questionnaire [53]. Moreover, as in any observational study, there might be residual confounding. In particular, B vitamin intake may reflect an overall healthy diet, and we did not adjust for other healthy nutrients which may exert protective effects to the brain. However, we were able to control for a well-established index of overall diet quality, the MeDi score, and further adjustment for the MeDi revealed minimal confounding by global diet quality.

Our study also has important strengths. Obvious strengths include a longitudinal design with a decade of follow-up, and a multi-step procedure of diagnosis of dementia including a validation of cases by an independent committee of neurologists. The long lag period between the ascertainment of B vitamin intakes and the diagnosis of dementia minimizes the possibility of reverse causation. Finally, we considered a large range of potential confounders, including cardiovascular and lifestyle factors, such as the overall diet quality, and adjusting for these factors did not markedly decrease our risk estimate, suggesting minimal confounding effect.

5. Conclusions

In conclusion, we found in a large cohort of older persons from France—a country with no folic acid fortification and relatively low average intake levels—a strong association between a higher intake of folate and a lower long-term risk of dementia, while there was no evidence of association of vitamin B6 and B12 intake to dementia risk; however, vitamin B12 malabsorption has not been explored through circulating level data in this cohort of older persons and deserves further research. The protective role of folate in populations with relatively low basal folate status such as France may be worth exploring in future dementia prevention trials.

Acknowledgments: The Three-City Study is conducted under a partnership agreement between the Institut National de la Santé et de la Recherche Médicale (INSERM), the Institut de Santé Publique et Développement of the Victor Segalen Bordeaux 2 University and Sanofi-Aventis. The Fondation pour la Recherche Médicale funded the preparation and initiation of the study. The 3C Study is also supported by the Caisse Nationale Maladie des Travailleurs Salariés, Direction Générale de la Santé, Mutuelle Générale de l'Education Nationale, Institut de la Longévité, Regional Governments of Aquitaine and Bourgogne, Fondation de France, Ministry of Research-INSERM Programme "Cohortes et collections de données biologiques", the French National Research Agency COGINUT ANR-06-PNRA-005, the Fondation Plan Alzheimer (FCS 2009–2012), and the Caisse Nationale pour la Solidarité et l'Autonomie (CNSA).

Author Contributions: S.L.-A. performed statistical analyses and drafted the manuscript; C.S. contributed to the drafting of the manuscript and supervised the research project; C.F., J.-F.D., C.H., and L.L. critically reviewed the manuscript; J.F.D., C.H., and L.L. participated in the design and the protocol of the 3C study.

References

1. Reynolds, E. Vitamin B12, folic acid, and the nervous system. *Lancet Neurol.* **2006**, *5*, 949–960. [CrossRef]
2. Seshadri, S.; Beiser, A.; Selhub, J.; Jacques, P.F.; Rosenberg, I.H.; D'Agostino, R.B.; Wilson, P.W.F.; Wolf, P.A. Plasma Homocysteine as a Risk Factor for Dementia and Alzheimer's Disease. *N. Engl. J. Med.* **2002**, *346*, 476–483. [CrossRef] [PubMed]

3. Morris, M.S. Homocysteine and Alzheimer's disease. *Lancet Neurol.* **2003**, *2*, 425–428. [CrossRef]
4. Smith, A.D.; Refsum, H. Homocysteine, B Vitamins, and Cognitive Impairment. *Annu. Rev. Nutr.* **2016**, *36*, 211–239. [CrossRef] [PubMed]
5. Selhub, J.; Troen, A.; Rosenberg, I.H. B vitamins and the aging brain. *Nutr. Rev.* **2010**, *68* (Suppl. 2), S112–S118. [CrossRef] [PubMed]
6. Araújo, J.R.; Martel, F.; Borges, N.; Araújo, J.M.; Keating, E. Folates and aging: Role in mild cognitive impairment, dementia and depression. *Ageing Res. Rev.* **2015**, *22*, 9–19. [CrossRef] [PubMed]
7. Morris, M.S. The Role of B Vitamins in Preventing and Treating Cognitive Impairment and Decline. *Adv. Nutr. Int. Rev. J.* **2012**, *3*, 801–812. [CrossRef] [PubMed]
8. Ravaglia, G.; Forti, P.; Maioli, F.; Martelli, M.; Servadei, L.; Brunetti, N.; Porcellini, E.; Licastro, F. Homocysteine and folate as risk factors for dementia and Alzheimer disease. *Am. J. Clin. Nutr.* **2005**, *82*, 636–643. [PubMed]
9. Ramos, M.I.; Allen, L.H.; Mungas, D.M.; Jagust, W.J.; Haan, M.N.; Green, R.; Miller, J.W. Low folate status is associated with impaired cognitive function and dementia in the Sacramento Area Latino Study on Aging. *Am. J. Clin. Nutr.* **2005**, *82*, 1346–1352. [PubMed]
10. De Lau, L.M.L.; Refsum, H.; Smith, A.D.; Johnston, C.; Breteler, M.M.B. Plasma folate concentration and cognitive performance: Rotterdam Scan Study. *Am. J. Clin. Nutr.* **2007**, *86*, 728–734. [PubMed]
11. Agnew-Blais, J.C.; Wassertheil-Smoller, S.; Kang, J.H.; Hogan, P.E.; Coker, L.H.; Snetselaar, L.G.; Smoller, J.W. Folate, vitamin B-6, and vitamin B-12 intake and mild cognitive impairment and probable dementia in the Women's Health Initiative Memory Study. *J. Acad. Nutr. Diet.* **2015**, *115*, 231–241. [CrossRef] [PubMed]
12. Corrada, M.M.; Kawas, C.H.; Hallfrisch, J.; Muller, D.; Brookmeyer, R. Reduced risk of Alzheimer's disease with high folate intake: The Baltimore Longitudinal Study of Aging. *Alzheimers Dement. J. Alzheimers Assoc.* **2005**, *1*, 11–18. [CrossRef] [PubMed]
13. Luchsinger, J.A.; Tang, M.-X.; Miller, J.; Green, R.; Mayeux, R. Relation of higher folate intake to lower risk of Alzheimer disease in the elderly. *Arch. Neurol.* **2007**, *64*, 86–92. [CrossRef] [PubMed]
14. Nelson, C.; Wengreen, H.J.; Munger, R.G.; Corcoran, C.D. Dietary folate, vitamin B-12, vitamin B-6 and incident Alzheimer's disease: The cache county memory, health and aging study. *J. Nutr. Health Aging* **2009**, *13*, 899–905. [CrossRef] [PubMed]
15. Morris, M.C.; Evans, D.A.; Schneider, J.A.; Tangney, C.C.; Bienia, J.L.; Aggarwal, N.T. Dietary folate and vitamins B-12 and B-6 not associated with incident Alzheimer's disease. *J. Alzheimers Dis.* **2006**, *9*, 435–443. [PubMed]
16. Morris, M.C.; Evans, D.A.; Bienias, J.L.; Tangney, C.C.; Hebert, L.E.; Scherr, P.A.; Schneider, J.A. Dietary folate and vitamin B12 intake and cognitive decline among community-dwelling older persons. *Arch. Neurol.* **2005**, *62*, 641–645. [CrossRef] [PubMed]
17. Hinterberger, M.; Fischer, P. Folate and Alzheimer: When time matters. *J. Neural Transm.* **2013**, *120*, 211–224. [CrossRef] [PubMed]
18. Clarke, R.; Bennett, D.; Parish, S.; Lewington, S.; Skeaff, M.; Eussen, S.J.P.M.; Lewerin, C.; Stott, D.J.; Armitage, J.; Hankey, G.J.; et al. B-Vitamin Treatment Trialists' Collaboration Effects of homocysteine lowering with B vitamins on cognitive aging: Meta-analysis of 11 trials with cognitive data on 22,000 individuals. *Am. J. Clin. Nutr.* **2014**, *100*, 657–666. [CrossRef] [PubMed]
19. Durga, J.; van Boxtel, M.P.; Schouten, E.G.; Kok, F.J.; Jolles, J.; Katan, M.B.; Verhoef, P. Effect of 3-year folic acid supplementation on cognitive function in older adults in the FACIT trial: A randomised, double blind, controlled trial. *Lancet* **2007**, *369*, 208–216. [CrossRef]
20. Douaud, G.; Refsum, H.; de Jager, C.A.; Jacoby, R.E.; Nichols, T.; Smith, S.M.; Smith, A.D. Preventing Alzheimer's disease-related gray matter atrophy by B-vitamin treatment. *Proc. Natl. Acad. Sci. USA* **2013**, *110*, 9523–9528. [CrossRef] [PubMed]
21. Jacques, P.F.; Selhub, J.; Bostom, A.G.; Wilson, P.W.F.; Rosenberg, I.H. The Effect of Folic Acid Fortification on Plasma Folate and Total Homocysteine Concentrations. *N. Engl. J. Med.* **1999**, *340*, 1449–1454. [CrossRef] [PubMed]
22. 3C Study Group. Vascular factors and risk of dementia: Design of the Three-City Study and baseline characteristics of the study population. *Neuroepidemiology* **2003**, *22*, 316–325.
23. American Psychiatric Association. *DSM-IV: Diagnostic and Statistical Manual of Mental Disorders*, 4th ed.; American Psychiatric Association: Washington, DC, USA, 1994.

24. McKhann, G.; Drachman, D.; Folstein, M.; Katzman, R.; Price, D.; Stadlan, E.M. Clinical diagnosis of Alzheimer's disease: Report of the NINCDS-ADRDA Work Group under the auspices of Department of Health and Human Services Task Force on Alzheimer's Disease. *Neurology* **1984**, *34*, 939–944. [CrossRef] [PubMed]
25. Féart, C.; Jutand, M.A.; Larrieu, S.; Letenneur, L.; Delcourt, C.; Combe, N.; Barberger-Gateau, P. Energy, macronutrient and fatty acid intake of French elderly community dwellers and association with socio-demographic characteristics: Data from the Bordeaux sample of the Three-City Study. *Br. J. Nutr.* **2007**, *98*, 1046–1057. [CrossRef] [PubMed]
26. Hercberg, S.; Deheeger, M.; Preziosi, P. *Portions Alimentaires: Manuel Photos Pour L'estimation des Quantités*; Economica: Paris, France, 2000.
27. Favier, J.-C.; Ireland-Ripert, J.; Toque, C.; Feinberg, M. *Répertoire Général des Aliments: Table de Composition*, 2nd ed.; Technique & Documentation; Institut National de la Recherche Agronomique: Paris, France, 1995.
28. Souci, S.W.; Fachmann, W.; Kraut, H. *Food Composition and Nutrition Tables*; Medpharm Scientific Publishers: Stuttgart, Germany, 2000.
29. Renaud, S.; Godsey, F.; Ortchanian, E.; Baudier, F. *Table de Composition des Aliments*; ASTRA-CALVE: Courbevoie, France, 1979.
30. Agence Nationale de Sécurité Sanitaire, de l'alimentation, de l'environnement et du travail (ANSES). *AVIS Relatif à L'évaluation des Apports en Vitamines et Minéraux Issus de L'alimentation non Enrichie, de L'alimentation Enrichie et des Compléments Alimentaires dans la Population Française: Estimation des Apports Usuels, des Prévalences D'inadéquation et des Risques de Dépassement des Limites de Sécurité; Avis de l'ANSES. Saisine n°2012-SA-0142*; ANSES: Maisons-Alfort, France, 2015.
31. Trichopoulou, A.; Costacou, T.; Bamia, C.; Trichopoulos, D. Adherence to a Mediterranean Diet and Survival in a Greek Population. *N. Engl. J. Med.* **2003**, *348*, 2599–2608. [CrossRef] [PubMed]
32. Féart, C.; Samieri, C.; Rondeau, V.; Amieva, H.; Portet, F.; Dartigues, J.F.; Scarmeas, N.; Barberger-Gateau, P. Adherence to a mediterranean diet, cognitive decline, and risk of dementia. *JAMA* **2009**, *302*, 638–648. [CrossRef] [PubMed]
33. Radloff, L.S. The CES-D Scale A Self-Report Depression Scale for Research in the General Population. *Appl. Psychol. Meas.* **1977**, *1*, 385–401. [CrossRef]
34. Fuhrer, R.; Rouillon, F. The French version of the CES-D (Center for Epidemiologic Studies-Depression Scale). *Psychiatr. Psychobiol.* **1989**, *4*, 163–166.
35. Lamarca, R.; Alonso, J.; Gómez, G.; Muñoz, Á. Left-truncated Data with Age as Time Scale: An Alternative for Survival Analysis in the Elderly Population. *J. Gerontol. A Biol. Sci. Med. Sci.* **1998**, *53*, M337–M343. [CrossRef] [PubMed]
36. Halsted, C.H.; Villanueva, J.A.; Devlin, A.M.; Chandler, C.J. Metabolic Interactions of Alcohol and Folate. *J. Nutr.* **2002**, *132*, 2367S–2372S. [PubMed]
37. Morris, M.S.; Jacques, P.F.; Rosenberg, I.H.; Selhub, J. Folate and vitamin B-12 status in relation to anemia, macrocytosis, and cognitive impairment in older Americans in the age of folic acid fortification. *Am. J. Clin. Nutr.* **2007**, *85*, 193–200. [PubMed]
38. Moore, E.M.; Ames, D.; Mander, A.G.; Carne, R.P.; Brodaty, H.; Woodward, M.C.; Boundy, K.; Ellis, K.A.; Bush, A.I.; Faux, N.G.; et al. Among vitamin B12 deficient older people, high folate levels are associated with worse cognitive function: Combined data from three cohorts. *J. Alzheimers Dis.* **2014**, *39*, 661–668. [PubMed]
39. Jernerén, F.; Elshorbagy, A.K.; Oulhaj, A.; Smith, S.M.; Refsum, H.; Smith, A.D. Brain atrophy in cognitively impaired elderly: The importance of long-chain ω-3 fatty acids and B vitamin status in a randomized controlled trial. *Am. J. Clin. Nutr.* **2015**, *102*, 215–221. [CrossRef] [PubMed]
40. Folstein, M.F.; Folstein, S.E.; McHugh, P.R. "Mini-mental state": A practical method for grading the cognitive state of patients for the clinician. *J. Psychiatr. Res.* **1975**, *12*, 189–198. [CrossRef]
41. Smith, A.D.; Smith, S.M.; de Jager, C.A.; Whitbread, P.; Johnston, C.; Agacinski, G.; Oulhaj, A.; Bradley, K.M.; Jacoby, R.; Refsum, H. Homocysteine-lowering by B vitamins slows the rate of accelerated brain atrophy in mild cognitive impairment: A randomized controlled trial. *PLoS ONE* **2010**, *5*, e12244. [CrossRef] [PubMed]
42. De Jager, C.A.; Oulhaj, A.; Jacoby, R.; Refsum, H.; Smith, A.D. Cognitive and clinical outcomes of homocysteine-lowering B-vitamin treatment in mild cognitive impairment: A randomized controlled trial. *Int. J. Geriatr. Psychiatry* **2012**, *27*, 592–600. [CrossRef] [PubMed]
43. Fioravanti, M.; Ferrario, E.; Massaia, M.; Cappa, G.; Rivolta, G.; Grossi, E.; Buckley, A.E. Low folate levels

in the cognitive decline of elderly patients and the efficacy of folate as a treatment for improving memory deficits. *Arch. Gerontol. Geriatr.* **1997**, *26*, 1–13. [CrossRef]
44. Andreeva, V.A.; Kesse-Guyot, E.; Barberger-Gateau, P.; Fezeu, L.; Hercberg, S.; Galan, P. Cognitive function after supplementation with B vitamins and long-chain omega-3 fatty acids: Ancillary findings from the SU.FOL.OM3 randomized trial. *Am. J. Clin. Nutr.* **2011**, *94*, 278–286. [CrossRef] [PubMed]
45. Vogiatzoglou, A.; Refsum, H.; Johnston, C.; Smith, S.M.; Bradley, K.M.; de Jager, C.; Budge, M.M.; Smith, A.D. Vitamin B12 status and rate of brain volume loss in community-dwelling elderly. *Neurology* **2008**, *71*, 826–832. [CrossRef] [PubMed]
46. Hooshmand, B.; Mangialasche, F.; Kalpouzos, G.; Solomon, A.; Kåreholt, I.; Smith, A.D.; Refsum, H.; Wang, R.; Mühlmann, M.; Ertl-Wagner, B.; et al. Association of vitamin B12, folate, and sulfur amino acids with brain magnetic resonance imaging measures in older adults: A longitudinal population-based study. *JAMA Psychiatry* **2016**, *73*, 606–613. [CrossRef] [PubMed]
47. Morris, M.S.; Selhub, J.; Jacques, P.F. Vitamin B-12 and Folate Status in Relation to Decline in Scores on the Mini-Mental State Examination in the Framingham Heart Study. *J. Am. Geriatr. Soc.* **2012**, *60*, 1457–1464. [CrossRef] [PubMed]
48. Clarke, R.; Birks, J.; Nexo, E.; Ueland, P.M.; Schneede, J.; Scott, J.; Molloy, A.; Evans, J.G. Low vitamin B-12 status and risk of cognitive decline in older adults. *Am. J. Clin. Nutr.* **2007**, *86*, 1384–1391. [PubMed]
49. Moorthy, D.; Peter, I.; Scott, T.M.; Parnell, L.D.; Lai, C.-Q.; Crott, J.W.; Ordovás, J.M.; Selhub, J.; Griffith, J.; Rosenberg, I.H.; et al. Status of Vitamins B-12 and B-6 but Not of Folate, Homocysteine, and the Methylenetetrahydrofolate Reductase C677T Polymorphism Are Associated with Impaired Cognition and Depression in Adults123. *J. Nutr.* **2012**, *142*, 1554–1560. [CrossRef] [PubMed]
50. McNulty, H.; Scott, J.M. Intake and status of folate and related B-vitamins: Considerations and challenges in achieving optimal status. *Br. J. Nutr.* **2008**, *99*, S48–S54. [CrossRef] [PubMed]
51. Willett, W. *Nutritional Epidemiology*; Oxford University Press: New York, NY, USA, 1998.
52. ANSES. Food Consumption Data from the Individual and National Study on Food Consumption 2 (INCA2). Available online: Data.gouv.fr/fr/datasets/donnees-de-consommations-et-habitudes-alimentaires-de-letude-inca-2-3/ (accessed on 2 June 2016).
53. Bates, C.J.; Prentice, A.; van der Pols, J.C.; Walmsley, C.; Pentieva, K.D.; Finch, S.; Smithers, G.; Clarke, P.C. Estimation of the use of dietary supplements in the National Diet and Nutrition Survey: People aged 65 years and Over. An observed paradox and a recommendation. *Eur. J. Clin. Nutr.* **1998**, *52*, 917–923. [CrossRef] [PubMed]

12

Association of Vitamin B12 with Pro-Inflammatory Cytokines and Biochemical Markers Related to Cardiometabolic Risk in Saudi Subjects

Nasser M. Al-Daghri [1,2,*], Shakilur Rahman [1,2], Shaun Sabico [1,2], Sobhy Yakout [1,2], Kaiser Wani [1,2], Omar S. Al-Attas [1,2], Ponnusamy Saravanan [3], Gyanendra Tripathi [1,2,4,5], Philip G. McTernan [4] and Majed S. Alokail [1,2]

1 Biomarkers Research Program, Biochemistry Department, College of Science, King Saud University, Riyadh 11451, Saudi Arabia; shakilhamdard@gmail.com (S.R.); eaglescout01@yahoo.com (S.S.); sobhy.yakout@gmail.com (S.Y.); wani.kaiser@gmail.com (K.W.); omrattas@ksu.edu.sa (O.S.A.-A.); g.tripathi@warwick.ac.uk (G.T.); msa85@yahoo.co.uk (M.S.A.)

2 Prince Mutaib Chair for Biomarkers of Osteoporosis, Biochemistry Department, College of Science, King Saud University, Riyadh 11451, Saudi Arabia

3 Division of Health Sciences, Warwick Medical School, University of Warwick, Coventry CV4 7AL, UK; p.saravanan@warwick.ac.uk

4 Division of Biomedical Sciences, Warwick Medical School, University of Warwick, UHCW Trust, Clifford Bridge Road, Walsgrave, Coventry CV2 2DX, UK; p.g.mcternan@warwick.ac.uk

5 Department of Biomedical Sciences, University of Westminster, London W1W 6UW, UK

* Correspondence: aldaghri2011@gmail.com

Abstract: Background: This study aimed to examine the relationship between changes in systemic vitamin B12 concentrations with pro-inflammatory cytokines, anthropometric factors and biochemical markers of cardiometabolic risk in a Saudi population. Methods: A total of 364 subjects (224 children, age: 12.99 ± 2.73 (mean ± SD) years; BMI: 20.07 ± 4.92 kg/m^2 and 140 adults, age: 41.87 ± 8.82 years; BMI: 31.65 ± 5.77 kg/m^2) were studied. Fasting blood, anthropometric and biochemical data were collected. Serum cytokines were quantified using multiplex assay kits and B12 concentrations were measured using immunoassay analyzer. Results: Vitamin B12 was negatively associated with TNF-α ($r = -0.14$, $p < 0.05$), insulin ($r = -0.230$, $p < 0.01$) and HOMA-IR ($r = -0.252$, $p < 0.01$) in all subjects. In children, vitamin B12 was negatively associated with serum resistin ($r = -0.160$, $p < 0.01$), insulin ($r = -0.248$, $p < 0.01$), HOMA-IR ($r = -0.261$, $p < 0.01$). In adults, vitamin B12 was negatively associated with TNF-α ($r = -0.242$, $p < 0.01$) while positively associated with resistin ($r = 0.248$, $p < 0.01$). Serum resistin was the most significant predictor for circulating vitamin B12 in all subjects ($r^2 = -0.17$, $p < 0.05$) and in children ($r^2 = -0.167$, $p < 0.01$) while HDL-cholesterol was the predictor of B12 in adults ($r^2 = -0.78$, $p < 0.05$). Conclusions: Serum vitamin B12 concentrations were associated with pro-inflammatory cytokines and biochemical markers of cardiometabolic risks in adults. Maintaining adequate vitamin B12 concentrations may lower inflammation-induced cardiometabolic risk in the Saudi adult population.

Keywords: vitamin B12; resistin; TNF-α; cardiometabolic diseases

---

1. Introduction

Vitamin B12 is an essential micronutrient required for optimal hemopoetic, neurologic and cardiometabolic function [1,2]. Human beings are dependent upon bacterial and protozoal sources to maintain adequate serum concentrations [3]. Vitamin B12 absorption is a complex process and any dysfunction can result in its deficiency, despite adequate dietary intake [4]. Vitamin B12 deficiency affects two principal enzymatic pathways, i.e., methylation process of homocysteine to methionine and the conversion of methylmalonyl coenzyme A (CoA) to succinyl-CoA [2,5], which lead to accumulation of methylmalonic acid (MMA) and/or homocysteine (Hcy) [2,5]. Excessive accumulation of homocysteine in blood (hyperhomocysteinemia) is associated with an increased risk of cardiovascular disease due to its cellular and vasculo-toxic effects [1,5]; whilst, increase in circualting methylmalonic acid (MMA) level is associated with defective fatty acid synthesis of neuronal membranes [3,5].

Current evidence demonstrated that vitamin B12 deficiency is linked to various atherogenic processes, mainly, but not exclusively, through B12 deficiency-induced hyperhomosyteinemia [6]. Hyperhomocysteinemia is a possible independent risk factor for cardiovascular disease, mechanisms of which include reduction of nitric oxide thereby promoting endothelial dysfunction [7,8]. On the other hand, cytokines, such as tumor necrosis factor (TNF-α) and resistin, play an important role in cardiovascular risk and insulin resistance [9,10].

Unfortunately, there is limited information available as to whether circulating vitamin B12 concentrations affect the cardiometabolic status of the Arab population. In fact, while it has been previously observed that vitamin B12 is inversely associated with homocysteine in the general Saudi population [11], homocysteine itself is not a risk factor for endothelial function, at least amongst Saudi Arabs [12]. Therefore, in this study we aimed to examine the associations between serum vitamin B12 concentrations, pro-inflammatory cytokines and biochemical markers of cardiovascular and metabolic risk in the general population of Saudi Arabia.

2. Materials and Methods

2.1. *Subjects and Experimental Design*

In this cross-sectional study, a total of 364 Saudi subjects (224 children aged 8–17 years and 140 adults aged 30–59 years) were recruited from four Primary Health Care Centers (PHCCs) within Riyadh, Saudi Arabia. Written informed consent was obtained prior to inclusion in the study. Inclusion criteria were apparently healthy children (N = 224) and adults (N = 140), nonsmokers, non-diabetic, non-hypertensive and without morbid obesity. Ethical approval was obtained from the Ethics Committee of the College of Science Research Center (Ethics Approval Code: 8/25/36681), King Saud University, Riyadh, Saudi Arabia.

2.2. *Anthropometric Measurements*

A generalized questionnaire was given to all participating subjects aimed at seeking demographic information, general health status and past medical history. Physical examination was carried out by a physician who ensured exclusion of subjects with chronic conditions (cardiac, kidney or liver disease, hypertension, psychiatric conditions) or use of medications known to affect body weight (e.g., steroids). Weight and height were recorded to the nearest 0.2 kg and 0.5 cm, respectively, using an appropriate international standard scale (Digital Pearson Scale, ADAM Equipment Inc., Oxford, CT, USA). Both measurements were done while subjects were standing upright and wearing light clothing. Body mass index (BMI) was calculated as weight in kg divided by height in squared meters (kg/m^2). Additionally, waist and hip circumferences were measured using a standardized measuring tape in centimeters (cm) and the waist-to-hip ratio (WHR) was estimated. Blood pressure was measured using an appropriate mercury sphygmomanometer, measured twice with 5-min intervals and the mean of the two readings was recorded.

2.3. *Blood Collection and Biochemical Measurements*

Fasting blood samples were collected and stored at -20 °C. Serum insulin, leptin, adiponectin, TNF-α and resistin were quantified using multiplex assay kits that utilize fluorescent microbead technology, allowing simultaneous quantification of several target proteins within a single serum sample of 50–100 μL. These included pre-mixed and fully customized panels that utilized the Luminex's xMAP Technology platform (Luminexcorp, TX, USA). For parameters measured using the multiplex assay, the intra-assay variation was 1.4%–7.9% and inter-assay variation of <21%. Minimum detectable concentrations (MDC) were as follows: insulin, 50.9 pg/mL; leptin, 85.4 pg/mL; adiponectin, 145.4 pg/mL; resistin, 6.7 pg/mL, and TNF-α, 0.14 pg/mL.

Vitamin B12 was measured using Roche Elecsys immunoassay analyzer, Cobas e 411 (Roche Diagnsotics GmbH, Mannheim, Germany) that employs the test principle of competitive electrochemiluminiscence immunoassay. The assay has a linearity range of 30–2000 pg/mL. The assay involves binding of vitamin B12 in the sample to the ruthenium labeled antibody. Streptavidin coated microparticles (solid phase), binds the biotin labeled vitamin B12 and ruthenium labeled antibody. A further wash period leaves the solid phase magnetic microparticles bound with vitamin B12-biotin and ruthenium labeled antibody, which generates chemiluminiscent emission signal that is inversely proportional to the concentration of vitamin B12 present in the patient sample. The inter- and intra-assay coefficients of variation (CV) for Vitamin B12 were 3.0% and 3.7%, respectively.

Fasting serum glucose concentrations and complete lipid profile (triglycerides, total cholesterol, high density lipoprotein (HDL)-cholesterol were determined using a biochemical analyzer) (Konelab, Espoo, Finland). This biochemical analyzer was calibrated routinely prior to the analysis of all serum samples using quality control samples provided by the manufacturer (Thermo-Fisher Scientific, Espoo, Finland). Low density lipoprotein (LDL)-cholesterol was calculated using the Friedman formula.

2.4. Statistical Analyses

Statistical analyses were carried out using the SPSS software version 16.0 (SPSS Inc., Chicago, IL, USA). Data were expressed as mean ± standard deviation. Kolmogorov-Smirnov statistics was performed to test continuous variables for normality. All non-Gaussian parameters were logarithmically or square-root transformed to normalize data. Independent Student T-test was used to compare means between groups of normally distributed data. Pearson correlations between serum vitamin B12 and the rest of the variables were determined. Stepwise linear regression models were performed using vitamin B12 as dependent variable and age, gender, BMI, systolic and diastolic blood pressure, waist and hip circumference, glucose, insulin, HDL, LDL, triglycerides, total cholesterol, leptin, adiponectin, TNF-α, resistin, HOMA-IR as independent variables to determine significant predictors. In all statistical tests, p-values < 0.05 were considered significant.

3. Results

A total of 364 Saudi subjects (224 children and 140 adults) satisfied the inclusion criteria and were included in the analysis. All the anthropometric and laboratory characteristics of the study participants are presented in Table 1.

Table 1. Clinical characteristics, glycemic, lipid and metabolic profiles of subjects.

Parameters	Children	Adults
	Clinical Characteristics	
N	224	140
M/F (%)	122/102 (54.5/45.5)	37/103 (26.4/73.6)
Age (years)	12.99 ± 2.73	41.87 ± 8.82
Body Mass Index (kg/m^2)	20.07 ± 4.92	31.65 ± 5.77
Waist circumference (cm)	66.37 ± 15.50	88.51 ± 15.65
Hip circumference (cm)	82.06 ± 15.59	99.01 ± 15.77
Systolic Blood Pressure	105.54 ± 10.21	114.25 ± 13.53
Diastolic Blood Pressure	68.85 ± 7.12	75.73 ± 8.81
	Glycemic Profile	
Glucose (mmol/L)	5.11 ± 0.61	5.37 ± 0.81
Insulin (IU/mL) #	6.5 (4.1–10.8)	9.3 (7.1–13.2)
HOMA-IR #	1.46 (0.88–2.41)	2.37 (1.50–3.22)

Table 1. *Cont.*

Parameters	Children	Adults
	Lipid Profile	
Triglycerides (mmol/L) #	1.06 ± 0.55	1.54 ± 0.71
Total Cholesterol (mmol/L)	4.23 ± 0.77	4.65 ± 0.98
HDL-Cholesterol (mmol/L)	1.02 ± 0.34	0.87 ± 0.33
LDL-Cholesterol (mmol/L)	2.72 ± 0.69	3.07 ± 0.77
	Metabolic Profile	
Leptin (ng/mL) #	9.10 (1.94–27.62)	15.73 (7.52–25.67)
Adiponectin (mg/mL) #	20.22 (12.66–28.42)	17.37 (5.19–431)
Resistin (ng/mL) #	15.10 (9.97–20.88)	5.01 (2.89–14.47)
TNF-α (pg/mL) #	7.51 (4.91–9.79)	15.34 (5.08–74.02)
Vitamin B12 (Pg/mL) #	421 (290.6–530.6)	371.25 (288.6–496.3)

Note: Data presented as N (%) for frequencies; mean ± standard deviation for normal continuous variables; # denotes continuous variables with non-Gaussian distribution and presented as median (25th–75th Percentile).

Correlations between vitamin B12 and clinical parameters measured are presented in Table 2. In children, vitamin B12 level was negatively associated with age ($r = -0.19$, $p < 0.01$), hip circumference ($r = -0.20$, $p < 0.01$), systolic BP ($r = -0.21$, $p < 0.01$), insulin ($r = -0.24$, $p < 0.01$), HOMA-IR ($r = -0.26$, $p < 0.01$) and resistin ($r = -0.16$, $p < 0.01$). In adults, vitamin B12 was positively associated with serum resistin ($r = 0.24$, $p < 0.01$), whereas it was negatively associated with TNF-α ($r = -0.24$, $p < 0.01$). Mean serum concentrations of vitamin B12 were plotted against quartiles of HOMA-IR (supplementary materials Figure S1) and resistin (supplementary materials Figure S2) in children and adults.

Table 2. Associations between vitamin B12 and clinical, glycemic, lipid and metabolic profiles.

Parameters	Coefficients of Correlation (r)	
	Children (N = 224)	Adults (N = 140)
Age (years)	−0.192 **	0.022
Body Mass Index (kg/m^2)	−0.132	0.006
Waist circumference (cm)	−0.105	0.089
Hip circumference (cm)	−0.207 **	0.050
Systolic Blood Pressure (mmHg)	−0.211 **	0.116
Diastolic Blood Pressure (mmHg)	−0.119	−0.029
Glucose (mmol/L)	−0.102	−0.071
Insulin (IU/mL) #	−0.248 **	−0.118
HOMA-IR	−0.261 **	−0.156
Triglyceride (mmol/L) #	−0.104	0.041
Cholesterol (mmol/L)	0.010	0.177
HDL-Cholesterol (mmol/L)	0.139 *	0.030
LDL-Cholesterol (mmol/L)	−0.046	0.117
Leptin (ng/mL) #	−0.130	0.060
Adiponectin (mg/mL) #	0.054	0.036
Resistin (ng/mL) #	−0.160 **	0.248 **
TNF-α (pg/mL) #	−0.062	−0.242 **

Note: Data presented as coefficient (r); * denotes significance at 0.05 level; ** denotes significance at 0.01 level; # log transformed values.

Stepwise linear regression analysis, using vitamin B12 as the dependent variable and all the parameters as independent variables, is presented in Table 3. In adults, HDL-cholesterol was the significant predictor of vitamin B12 ($r^2 = 0.78$, $p = 0.044$) whilst, serum resistin ($r^2 = -0.16$, $p = 0.004$), gender ($r^2 = -0.15$, $p = 0.001$) and age ($r^2 = -0.22$, $p = 0.02$) were independent predictors of vitamin B12 level in children.

Table 3. Stepwise linear regression analysis using vitamin B12 as a dependent variable.

	Predictor	Unstandardized β	SE	*p*-Value
Adults	HDL-cholesterol	0.781	0.169	0.044
Children	Gender	−0.155	0.036	0.001
	Age	−0.022	0.007	0.02
	Resistin	−0.167	0.069	0.004

Note: Independent variables entered: age, gender, BMI, systolic and diastolic blood pressure, waist and hip circumference, glucose, insulin, HDL-cholesterol, LDL-cholesterol, triglycerides, total cholesterol, leptin, adiponectin, TNF-α, resistin, HOMA-IR. Significant at $p < 0.05$.

4. Discussion

The present study represents the first in a Saudi population and highlights a relationship between circulating vitamin B12 concentrations, cytokines and biomarkers associated with cardiometabolic risk. For this study we recruited a total of 364 subjects (224 children, and 140 adults). Fasting blood, anthropometric and biochemical data were collected. Serum cytokines were quantified using multiplex assay kits and B12 concentrations were measured using immunoassay analyzer. Our observations are of considerable clinical importance, as any irregularity in the metabolism of vitamin B12 is known to be associated with a wide spectrum of hematologic, metabolic and cardiovascular disorders and early intervention appears key [1,4,5,9].

TNF-α is a hallmark of inflammation [13] and several lines of evidence suggest the association of vitamin B12 deficiency with an increased incidence of inflammation and associated metabolic complications [3,13]. In the current study we observed a significant inverse correlation between serum vitamin B12 and TNF-α level in adults. However, in children, there was no such correlation. Elevated systemic TNF-α level is observed to be associated with depletion of primary antioxidants that cells use to protect themselves against free radicals' damaging effects [14]. Depletion of antioxidants further induces pro-inflammatory cytokines and other inflammatory by-products like prostaglandins and leukotrienes, known risk factors for metabolic and cardiovascular diseases [14,15]. Earlier studies suggest that consistent chronic inflammation may lead to insulin resistance, type 2 diabetes mellitus (T2DM) and cardiovascular disease (CVD) [10]. Deficiency of vitamin B12 causes hyperhomocysteinemia (HHcy) [5,16], and elevated homocysteine is known to lead to an inflammatory state, a risk factor for coronary heart disease [16] and insulin resistance [17,18]. In mice, HHcy promotes insulin resistance by directly inducing the expression and secretion of TNF-α and resistin [19]. TNF-α then activates c-Jun N-terminal kinase (JNK), which, in turn, inhibits Akt activity and leads to insulin resistance [20,21].

The study also observed an inverse association between vitamin B12, HOMA-IR and insulin levels in children, indicating that deficiency of vitamin B12 at an early age may cause insulin resistance. Consistent with our observation, a similar association between vitamin B12 and HOMA-IR was observed by Mahalle et al. [1] and Kaya et al. [22], in Indian subjects with coronary artery disease and in women with polycystic ovary syndrome, respectively. Furthermore, Stewart et al. found in Nepalese subjects that low maternal vitamin B12 status was associated with insulin resistance in offspring [23]. Contrary to these, a cross-sectional study conducted in 135 Asian-Indian women found no correlation between serum vitamin B12 and HOMA-IR [24].

Resistin, originally described as an adipocyte-specific hormone, has been suggested to be an important link between obesity, insulin resistance and diabetes [25,26]. It was observed that serum concentrations of resistin are significantly increased in obese and diabetic patients [27,28]. Resistin has also been linked to the development of atherosclerosis and CVD [23,29]. In our study, a significant inverse association between vitamin B12 concentrations and resistin was observed in children, whereas, in adults, it was positively associated. Stepwise linear regression analysis revealed that resistin was the most significant predictor of vitamin B12 in children. In another study, 220 patients with acute coronary syndrome (ACS) had significantly higher serum resistin concentrations than patients classified as normal [30]. However, research on resistin has also been controversial in understanding their pathological relevance and its association with T2DM and cardiovascular diseases [31,32]. Hence, conclusive data await new strong evidence to elucidate the role of resistin in various disease processes. Nevertheless, resistin has primarily been shown to be relevant to inflammation-related diseases like atherosclerosis and arthritis [33] and may have a role in the regulation of pro-inflammatory cytokines' (IL-6 and TNF-α) expression in human peripheral blood mononuclear cells (PBMC) via NF-κB pathway [33,34]. In yet another study conducted by Stejskal et al., it was observed that persons with clinical signs of severe inflammation showed significantly higher concentrations of resistin than healthy individuals [35]. Since resistin and TNF-α are pro-inflammatory in action, and inflammation has a central role in cardiovascular diseases and insulin resistance, deficiency of vitamin B12 may, therefore, have importance in the development of cardiometabolic diseases in Saudi population.

The limitations of this study include its cross-sectional nature and, thus, we cannot determine causality. Furthermore, information on diet is lacking and would have provided added value as to whether adequate B12 concentrations lead to better cardiometabolic parameters independent of a healthy diet. Lastly, the findings may not be a true representation of the general healthy population, since women were over represented in the current study, and whether the associations are true for those with chronic diseases also cannot be answered in the study's present scope. Despite these limitations, this is the first study particularly from the Arab region, which reflects direct link between vitamin B12 with adipocytokines and biochemical markers of cardiometabolic risks. The present findings warrant further investigation addressing how interventional therapies with vitamin B12 affect cardiovascular and metabolic diseases.

5. Conclusions

In conclusion, our study suggests weak but significant associations between circulating vitamin B12 concentrations with serum insulin and HOMA-IR in children, and inflammatory cytokines such as TNF-α and resistin in adults. Our findings have significant clinical importance, since these biochemical markers and cytokines are independent risk factors for cardiovascular and metabolic diseases in adults. Thus, determination of vitamin B12 status and treatment in cases of deficiency could be a clinically useful strategy in the prevention of cardiometabolic diseases.

Acknowledgments: The study was supported by King Saud University, Deanship of Scientific Research, Prince Mutaib Bin Abdullah Chair for Biomarkers of Osteoporosis (PMCO). The authors are also thankful for Malak Nawaz Khan Khattak for the statistical analyses of data.

Author Contributions: N.M.A., M.S.A., O.S.A., and S.P. conceptualized the study, K.W. and S.Y. performance of experiments, S.R. and S.S. researched the data, wrote the manuscript and contributed to the final version of the manuscript, G.T., P.G.M., S.P., and S.S. provided intellectual input and contributed to the final version of the manuscript.

References

1. Mahalle, N.; Kulkarni, M.V.; Garg, M.K.; Naik, S.S. Vitamin B12 deficiency and hyperhomocysteinemia as correlates of cardiovascular risk factors in Indian subjects with coronary artery disease. *J. Cardiol.* **2013**, *61*, 289–294. [CrossRef] [PubMed]
2. Oh, R.; Brown, D.L. Vitamin B12 deficiency. *Am. Fam. Physician* **2003**, *67*, 979–986. [PubMed]
3. Guéant, J.-L.; Alpers, D.H. Vitamin B12, a fascinating micronutrient, which influences human health in the very early and later stages of life. *Biochimie* **2013**, *95*, 967–969. [CrossRef] [PubMed]
4. Sadeghian, S.; Fallahi, F.; Salarifar, M.; Davoodi, G.; Mahmoodian, M.; Fallah, N.; Darvish, N.; Karimi, S.; Tehran Heart Center. Homocysteine, vitamin B12 and folate levels in premature coronary artery disease. *BMC Cardiovas. Disord.* **2006**, *6*, 38. [CrossRef] [PubMed]

5. Battaglia-Hsu, S.F.; Akchiche, N.; Noel, N.; Alberto, J.M.; Jeannesson, E.; Orozco-Barrios, C.E.; Martinez-Fong, D.; Daval, J.L.; Gueant, J.L. Vitamin B12 deficiency reduces proliferation and promotes differentiation of neuroblastoma cells and up-regulates PP2A, proNGF, and TACE. *Proc. Natl. Acad. Sci. USA* **2009**, *106*, 21930–21935. [CrossRef] [PubMed]
6. Pawlak, R. Is vitamin B12 deficiency a risk factor for cardiovascular disease in vegatarians? *Am. J. Prev. Med.* **2015**, *48*, e11–e26. [CrossRef] [PubMed]
7. Lai, W.K.; Kan, M.Y. Homocysteine-induced endothelial dysfunction. *Ann. Nutr. Metab.* **2015**, *67*, 1–12. [CrossRef] [PubMed]
8. Fratoni, V.; Brandi, M.L. B vitamins, homocysteine and bone health. *Nutrients* **2015**, *7*, 2176–2192. [CrossRef] [PubMed]
9. Smits, M.M.; Woudstra, P.; Utzschneider, K.M.; Tong, J.; Gerchman, F.; Faulenbach, M.; Carr, D.B.; Aston-Mourney, K.; Chait, A.; Knopp, R.H.; et al. Adipocytokines as features of the metabolic syndrome determined using confirmatory factor analysis. *Ann. Epidemiol.* **2013**, *23*, 415–421. [CrossRef] [PubMed]
10. Piya, M.K.; McTernan, P.G.; Kumar, S. Adipokine inflammation and insulin resistance: The role of glucose, lipids and endotoxin. *J. Endocrinol.* **2013**, *216*, T1–T15. [CrossRef] [PubMed]
11. Ardawi, M.S.; Rouzi, A.A.; Qari, M.H.; Dahlawi, F.M.; Al-Raddadi, R.M. Influence of age, sex, folate and vitamin B12 status on plasma homocysteine in Saudis. *Saudi Med. J.* **2002**, *23*, 959–968. [PubMed]
12. Abdulle, A.M.; Pathan, J.Y.; Moussa, N.; Gariballa, S. Association between homocysteine and endothelial dysfunction markers in stroke disease. *Nutr. Neursci.* **2010**, *13*, 2–6. [CrossRef] [PubMed]
13. Popa, C.; Netea, M.G.; van Riel, P.L.; van der Meer, J.W.; Stalenhoef, A.F. The role of TNF-alpha in chronic inflammatory conditions, intermediary metabolism, and cardiovascular risk. *J. Lipid Res.* **2007**, *48*, 751–762. [CrossRef] [PubMed]
14. Chen, X.; Andresen, B.T.; Hill, M.; Zhang, J.; Booth, F.; Zhang, C. Role of Reactive Oxygen Species in Tumor Necrosis Factor-alpha Induced Endothelial Dysfunction. *Curr. Hypertens Rev.* **2008**, *4*, 245–255. [CrossRef] [PubMed]
15. Weiss, N. Mechanisms of increased vascular oxidant stress in hyperhomocys-teinemia and its impact on endothelial function. *Curr. Drug Metab.* **2005**, *6*, 27–36. [CrossRef] [PubMed]
16. Lawrence de Koning, A.B.; Werstuck, G.H.; Zhou, J.; Austin, R.C. Hyperhomocysteinemia and its role in the development of atherosclerosis. *Clin. Biochem.* **2003**, *36*, 431–441. [CrossRef]
17. Buysschaer, M.; Dramais, A.S.; Wallemacq, P.E.; Hermans, M.P. Hyperhomocysteinemia in type 2 diabetes: Relationship to macroangiopathy, nephropathy, and insulin resistance. *Diabetes Care* **2000**, *23*, 1816–1822. [CrossRef]
18. Al-Daghri, N.M. Hyperhomocysteinemia, coronary heart disease, and diabetes mellitus as predicted by various definitions for metabolic syndrome in a hypertensive Saudi population. *Saudi Med. J.* **2007**, *28*, 339–346. [PubMed]
19. Li, Y.; Jiang, C.; Xu, G.; Wang, N.; Zhu, Y.; Tang, C.; Wang, X. Homocysteine upregulates resistin production from adipocytes in vivo and in vitro. *Diabetes* **2008**, *57*, 817–827. [CrossRef] [PubMed]
20. Hotamisligil, G.S. Mechanisms of TNF-alpha-induced insulin resistance. *Exp. Clin. Endocrinol. Diabetes* **1999**, *107*, 119–125. [CrossRef] [PubMed]
21. Moller, D.E. Potential role of TNF-alpha in the pathogenesis of insulin resistance and type 2 diabetes. *Trends Endocrinol. Metab.* **2000**, *11*, 212–217. [CrossRef]
22. Kaya, C.; Cengiz, S.D.; Satiroglu, H. Obesity and insulin resistance associated with lower plasma vitamin B12 in PCOS. *Reprod. Biomed. Online* **2009**, *19*, 721–726. [CrossRef] [PubMed]
23. Stewart, C.P.; Christian, P.; Schulze, K.J.; Arguello, M.; LeClerq, S.C.; Khatry, S.K.; West, K.P., Jr. Low maternal vitamin B-12 status is associated with offspring insulin resistance regardless of antenatal micronutrient supplementation in rural Nepal. *J. Nutr.* **2011**, *141*, 1912–1917. [CrossRef] [PubMed]
24. Gammon, C.S.; von Hurst, P.R.; Coad, J.; Kruger, R.; Stonehouse, W. Vegetarianism, vitamin B12 status, and insulin resistance in a group of predominantly overweight/obese South Asian women. *Nutrition* **2012**, *28*, 20–24. [CrossRef] [PubMed]
25. Jamaluddin, M.S.; Weakley, S.M.; Yao, Q.; Chen, C. Resistin: Functional roles and therapeutic considerations for cardiovascular disease. *Brit. J. Pharmacol.* **2012**, *165*, 622–632. [CrossRef] [PubMed]
26. Sheng, C.H.; Di, J.; Jin, Y.; Zhang, Y.C.; Wu, M.; Sun, Y.; Zhang, G.Z. Resistin is expressed in human hepatocytes and induces insulin resistance. *Endocrine* **2008**, *33*, 135–143. [CrossRef] [PubMed]

27. Steppan, C.M.; Bailey, S.T.; Bhat, S.; Brown, E.J.; Banerjee, R.R.; Wright, C.M.; Patel, H.R.; Ahima, R.S.; Lazar, M.A. The hormone resistin links obesity to diabetes. *Nature* **2001**, *409*, 307–312. [CrossRef] [PubMed]
28. Gerber, M.; Boettner, A.; Seidel, B.; Lammert, A.; Bar, J.; Schuster, E.; Thiery, J.; Kiewss, W.; Kratzsch, J. Serum resistin levels of obese and lean children and adolescents: Biochemical analysis and clinical relevance. *J. Clin. Endocrinol. Metab.* **2005**, *90*, 4503–4509. [CrossRef] [PubMed]
29. Filková, M.; Haluzík, M.; Gay, S.; Šenolt, L. The role of resistin as a regulator of inflammation: Implications for various human pathologies. *Clin. Immunol.* **2009**, *133*, 157–170. [CrossRef] [PubMed]
30. Wang, H.; Chen, D.Y.; Cao, J.; He, Z.Y.; Zhu, B.P.; Long, M. High serum resistin level may be an indicator of the severity of coronary disease in acute coronary syndrome. *Chin. Med. Sci. J.* **2009**, *24*, 161–166. [CrossRef]
31. Hotamisligil, G.S. The irresistible biology of resistin. *J. Clin. Investig.* **2003**, *111*, 173–174. [CrossRef] [PubMed]
32. McTernan, C.L.; McTernan, P.G.; Harte, A.L.; Levick, P.L.; Barnett, A.H.; Kumar, S. Resistin, central obesity, and type 2 diabetes. *Lancet* **2002**, *359*, 46–47. [CrossRef]
33. Pang, S.S.; Le, Y.Y. Role of resistin in inflammation and inflammation-related diseases. *Cell. Mol. Immunol.* **2006**, *3*, 29–34. [PubMed]
34. Bokarewa, M.; Nagaev, I.; Dahlberg, L.; Smith, U.; Tarkowski, A. Resistin, an adipokine with potent proinflammatory properties. *J. Immunol.* **2005**, *174*, 5789–5795. [CrossRef] [PubMed]
35. Stejskal, D.; Adamovska, S.; Bartek, J.; Jurakova, R.; Proskova, J. Resistin - concentrations in persons with type 2 diabetes mellitus and in individuals with acute inflammatory disease. *Biomed. Pap.* **2003**, *147*, 63–69. [CrossRef]

13

Causes, Consequences and Public Health Implications of Low B-Vitamin Status in Ageing

Kirsty Porter, Leane Hoey, Catherine F. Hughes, Mary Ward and Helene McNulty *

Northern Ireland Centre for Food and Health, Ulster University, Cromore Road, Coleraine BT52 1SA, UK; porter-k7@email.ulster.ac.uk (K.P.); l.hoey@ulster.ac.uk (L.H.); c.hughes@ulster.ac.uk (C.F.H.); mw.ward@ulster.ac.uk (M.W.)

* Correspondence: h.mcnulty@ulster.ac.uk

Abstract: The potential protective roles of folate and the metabolically related B-vitamins (vitamins B12, B6 and riboflavin) in diseases of ageing are of increasing research interest. The most common cause of folate and riboflavin deficiencies in older people is low dietary intake, whereas low B12 status is primarily associated with food-bound malabsorption, while sub-optimal vitamin B6 status is attributed to increased requirements in ageing. Observational evidence links low status of folate and the related B-vitamins (and/or elevated concentrations of homocysteine) with a higher risk of degenerative diseases including cardiovascular disease (CVD), cognitive dysfunction and osteoporosis. Deficient or low status of these B-vitamins alone or in combination with genetic polymorphisms, including the common *MTHFR* 677 C $\rightarrow$ T polymorphism, could contribute to greater disease risk in ageing by causing perturbations in one carbon metabolism. Moreover, interventions with the relevant B-vitamins to optimise status may have beneficial effects in preventing degenerative diseases. The precise mechanisms are unknown but many have been proposed involving the role of folate and the related B-vitamins as co-factors for one-carbon transfer reactions, which are fundamental for DNA and RNA biosynthesis and the maintenance of methylation reactions. This review will examine the evidence linking folate and related B-vitamins with health and disease in ageing, associated mechanisms and public health implications.

Keywords: B-vitamins; ageing; degenerative diseases; cardiovascular disease; cognitive dysfunction; dementia; osteoporosis; methylenetetrahydrofolate reductase (MTHFR)

---

1. Introduction

An estimated 900 million people are aged $\geq$65 years globally, equating with 8% of the world's population, and by 2050, this is predicted to exceed two billion (16%) [1]. Approximately one quarter of the total global burden of disease is in older people, with a higher prevalence in high income countries [2]. Hypertension, the leading risk factor of cardiovascular disease (CVD) affects an estimated one billion people worldwide and CVD is the most common cause of death in older people [3]. Globally, osteoporotic fractures affect over nine million older people annually [4], while 46.8 million older people are reported to have dementia worldwide [5]. The prevalence of these diseases of ageing is expected to substantially increase as a result of the ever-increasing ageing population. In addition, these degenerative diseases cause multiple co-morbidities in older people which in turn has important societal and economic consequences. Maintaining good health in older age has therefore become a major public health priority. Poor nutrition is recognised as a modifiable risk factor in the development of degenerative diseases in ageing, and improved nutrition may prevent or delay the onset of adverse health outcomes as people age. In this context, the potential adverse effect of elevated homocysteine and/or the protective roles of folate and the metabolically related B-vitamins (B12 and B6), have received much attention.

This review will examine the emerging evidence linking folate and the metabolically related B-vitamins with ageing, the potential roles of these nutrients in preventing or delaying diseases of ageing and the associated mechanisms. The challenges and opportunities in achieving optimal B-vitamin status in older people will also be considered with particular emphasis on the role of food fortification.

2. Metabolic Role of B-Vitamins in One-Carbon Metabolism

Folate along with vitamins B12, B6 and riboflavin in their co-enzymatic forms are all essential in one-carbon metabolism (Figure 1), a network of reactions involving the transfer of one-carbon units. In the folate cycle, tetrahydrofolate obtains a carbon unit from serine in a vitamin B6 (plasma pyridoxal phosphate; PLP) dependent reaction forming 5,10-methylenetetrahydrofolate which is used for the synthesis of thymidine and purines or converted to 5-methyltetrahydrofolate. 5-methyltetrahydrofolate is the principal circulating form of folate, and this reaction is catalysed by methylenetetrahydrofolate reductase (MTHFR) using riboflavin (flavin adenine dinucleotide, FAD) as a co-factor. At this point, the folate cycle links with the methionine cycle, 5-methyltetrahydrofolate donates its methyl group to homocysteine for the formation of methionine in a reaction catalysed by methionine synthase which uses vitamin B12 (methylcobalamin) as a cofactor. Methionine is the precursor for *S*-adenosyl-methionine (SAM), the universal methyl donor for DNA and RNA, proteins and numerous central nervous system methylation reactions involving neurotransmitters, membrane phospholipid synthesis and myelin methylation [6,7]. SAM is converted to *S*-adenosylhomocysteine and then homocysteine which is either remethylated back to methionine or conversely metabolised in the transsulphuration pathway to form cysteine through another vitamin B6-dependent process [8]. The metabolism of the B-vitamins is closely related; folate and vitamin B12 are both intrinsically linked via the enzyme methionine synthase [9]. In vitamin B12 depletion, methionine synthase activity is reduced and the formation of tetrahydrofolate is blocked, with folate essentially becoming trapped as 5-methyltetrahydrofolate because the conversion by MTHFR is physiologically irreversible [10]. There is also an important metabolic inter-relationship between vitamin B6 and riboflavin. The conversion of dietary vitamin B6 in tissues to its functional enzyme, pyridoxal 5′ phosphate (PLP), requires the enzyme pyridoxine phosphate oxidase (PPO), which is dependent on the riboflavin in its co-factor form, flavin mononucleotide (FMN).

Deficiencies in any of these B-vitamins can perturb the complex regulatory network maintaining one-carbon metabolism resulting in reduced methylation status within the relevant tissue, hyperhomocysteinemia, and/or increased misincorporation of uracil into DNA as a result of thymidylate synthesis being impaired owing to low 5,10-methylene-THF concentrations and thus uracil is inserted instead during DNA synthesis which in turn may contribute to adverse health outcomes in ageing [11,12]. In addition, genetic polymorphisms, including the common 677 C $\rightarrow$ T polymorphism in the gene encoding the folate-metabolising enzyme MTHFR, can interact adversely with sub-optimal status of one or more of the B-vitamins in one-carbon metabolism and thus contribute to a greater disease risk [13]. The *MTHFR* 677TT genotype affects an estimated 10% of individuals worldwide (ranging from 3% to 32% depending on ethnicity) [14] and 12% in Ireland [15].

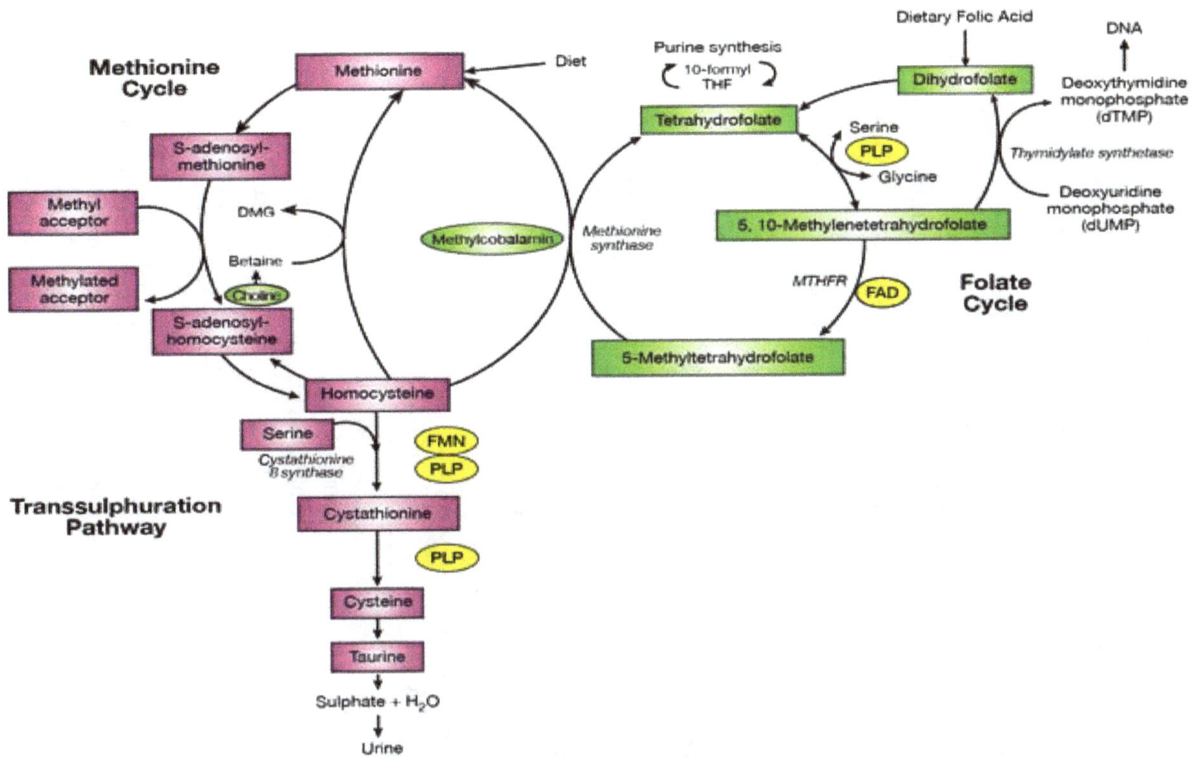

Figure 1. One-carbon metabolism. Abbreviations: PLP, plasma pyridoxal phosphate; MTHFR, methylenetetrahydrofolate reductase; FAD, flavin adenine dinucleotide; FMN, flavin mononucleotide. Adapted from [16].

3. Causes of B-Vitamin Deficiency

Depending on the particular vitamin, there are a number of potential causes of B-vitamin deficiency including inadequate intake, increased requirements, malabsorption, drug–nutrient interactions and others including genetic disorders or medical conditions (Table 1). In addition, the ageing process itself can negatively affect the absorption, transport and metabolism of B-vitamins and thus older people have increased requirements. A recent systematic review in community dwelling older adults in developed Western countries (n = 28,000) reported a high prevalence of low dietary intakes for B-vitamins (i.e., below the estimated average requirement, EAR), including folate (29%–35%), vitamin B6 (24%–31%) and identified riboflavin (31%–41%) among six nutrients of potential public health concern [17]. An estimated 9%–12% of older people in the UK are considered to suffer from folate deficiency [18], with the most common cause being low dietary intake.

Table 1. Causes of B vitamin deficiency.

B Vitamin	Inadequate Intake	Increased Requirement	Malabsorption	Drug–Nutrient Interactions	Other
Folate [19–24]	Common Poor cooking techniques	Elderly Pathological conditions	Intestinal diseases Coeliac disease Crohn's disease Ulcerative Colitis	Phenytoin Phenobarbital/Primidone Trimethoprim Methotrexate Sulfasalazine Metformin	Alcohol abuse Genetic disorders Haemolytic anaemia
B12 [19,21,22,25,26]	Common Vegan diets	Elderly	Intestinal diseases Coeliac disease Crohn's disease Gastric/intestinal resection Atrophic gastritis Bacterial overgrowth Helicobacter pylori Pancreatic insufficiency Pernicious anaemia Zollinger–Ellison Syndrome	Proton pump inhibitors H2-receptor antagonists Metformin Nitrous oxide Colchicine	Alcohol abuse Genetic disorders Tropical or non-tropical sprue
B6 [21,22,25,26]	Rare Chronic dieters	Elderly	HIV	Isoniazid Anti-Convulsants Steroids	Alcohol abuse Genetic disorders Liver disease Renal dialysis Rheumatoid arthritis
B2 [21,25–27]	Common Chronic dieters	Elderly	Diabetes Liver disease Thyroid and renal insufficiency GI and biliary obstruction	Phenothiazines, e.g., chlorpromazine Theophylline	Alcohol abuse Genetic disorders Hypochromic anaemia Metals such as zinc, copper and iron

There is a high prevalence of vitamin B12 deficiency in older people globally [28], with two early studies finding 75% of Asian Indians demonstrating metabolic evidence of vitamin B12 deficiency [29,30]. Numerous population surveys have also identified varying levels of vitamin B12 deficiency and sub-optimal status in older people from the UK (5%–20% deficient) [31–33], US (6% deficient, >20% marginal status) [34,35] Canada (5% deficient) [36], New Zealand (12% deficient, 28% marginal deficiency) [37] and Finland (6% low B12 and 32% borderline) [38]. The variation in prevalence may in part be explained by the diagnostic criteria used and different studies have used different biomarkers and cut off points. Pernicious anaemia, the classic form of B12 deficiency, caused by a lack of intrinsic factor is thought to account for just 1%–2% of cases of insufficiency in older people [39]. The maintenance of vitamin B12 status in older people is not only dependent on adequate dietary intake but more critically on the normal absorption of the vitamin which is dependent on the normal functioning of the gastrointestinal tract, gastric acid secretion and a number of transport proteins including intrinsic factor [40]. Food-bound malabsorption, primarily as a result of atrophic gastritis, an age-related disorder affects up to 30% of older people [41], leads to a reduction in gastric acid secretion which prevents the release of B12 from food and thus absorption. Deficiency is less pronounced and the limitations of the conventional vitamin B12 assays may also mean that a significant proportion of the older population may have low vitamin B12 status which is not detected [40,42].

Medications including proton pump inhibitors (PPI) and H2-receptor antagonists (H_2RA) are commonly prescribed (for conditions such as reflux and peptic ulcers) in older people, resulting in gastric acid suppression, this mimics atrophic gastritis and leads to food-bound malabsorption. There is evidence to suggest that these medications have been associated with up to 4.5 times higher risk of vitamin B12 deficiency in case control studies [43,44]. Recently in the USA, a large community survey (25,956 cases and 184,199 controls) found that the long term use (>2 years) of H_2RAs and PPIs was associated with a 25%–65% greater risk of a subsequent diagnosis of vitamin B12 deficiency [45]. In addition, metformin usage in Type 2 Diabetes can also result in vitamin B12 deficiency, possibly interfering with calcium-dependent membrane action in the terminal ileum required for the absorption of the vitamin B12-intrinsic factor complex [46,47].

Vitamin B6 and riboflavin in older people have not been as widely investigated. There is a high prevalence of vitamin B6 deficiency in older people as evident in three large population based surveys in Europe (Survey in Europe Nutrition and the Elderly, a Concerted Action, SENECA; 23%) [48], the UK (National Diet and Nutrition survey; NDNS; 11%–27% free living, 30%–65% institutionalised) [49], and the US (National Health and Nutrition Examination Survey, NHANES; 15%–23% males, 14%–49% females) [50] This deficiency in older age has been attributed to increased requirements as a result of reduced absorption, increased catabolism and impaired phosphorylation as opposed to inadequate dietary intake [51,52].

Riboflavin deficiency is thought to mainly arise from inadequate dietary intake, particularly in those who do not consume dairy products or fortified foods [17,27,53]. A high prevalence of riboflavin deficiency is acknowledged in the developing world; less well recognised is the emerging evidence to suggest that sub-optimal status is also evident in developed countries. To date, most population based surveys only report dietary intake data, and relatively few include biomarker data. Despite dietary intakes being reported to be sufficient in the NDNS (5% below reference nutrient intake, RNI) [54] and in the Irish National Adult Nutrition Survey (NANS, 13% below EAR) [55], 39%–43% of older people had biochemical deficiency in the NDNS and 19%–22% in NANS. Thus, further population based surveys are still required to investigate the intake and requirements of older people based on robust biomarker data of both vitamin B6 and riboflavin.

4. Assessment of B-Vitamin Biomarker Status

There are a number of direct and functional biomarkers available to determine B-vitamin status each with various strengths and limitations (Table 2). Plasma homocysteine accumulates with folate deficiency, it has been used as a biomarker of status but it lacks specificity as it can also be elevated by other B-vitamin deficiencies, including vitamins B12 [56], B6 [57] and riboflavin [58]. Serum folate is the earliest indicator of altered folate exposure and reflects recent dietary intake [59]. Red blood cell (RBC) folate is a sensitive indicator of long term folate status (during the preceding 120 days) [60,61]. It parallels liver concentrations this is considered to reflect tissue folate stores [20,62]. One recent meta-analysis demonstrated that both serum folate (27 RCTs) and RBC folate (12 RCTs) respond to interventions with folic acid in a dose-dependent manner and concluded that both indicators were robust measures of folate status [63]. To date, there is no gold standard biomarker for the assessment of vitamin B12 status despite there being a number of direct and functional measures available. Serum B12, although still widely used both clinically and in research, measures the total amount of the vitamin, however only 20% of this is metabolically active [64]. Serum total vitamin B12 can under-report the true prevalence of vitamin B12 deficiency [65,66] and up to 40% of older people can have low serum vitamin B12 but normal metabolic status [41,67]. Holo-transcobalamin (holoTC) measures the biologically active fraction of vitamin B12 and is considered to have superior diagnostic value to total B12 [68,69] although it can be affected by inborn errors altering intracellular vitamin B12 metabolism [68]. Plasma homocysteine can be used as a functional measure of vitamin B12 status but as previously discussed it is not specific to vitamin B12 (Table 2). Methylmalonic acid (MMA) is a more specific and sensitive functional biomarker of vitamin B12 status [31], the conversion of methylmalonyl-CoA to succinyl-CoA is a B12 dependant process, impaired B12 status leads to an accumulation of methymalonyl-CoA which then is metabolised to MMA and excreted in the urine. However, MMA is also elevated in renal dysfunction, which is common in older people [69] and so limits its use. Two reviews have recommended that at least 2 biomarkers are required in the diagnosis of vitamin B12 deficiency [42,70].

Plasma PLP concentration is the most widely used measure of vitamin B6 [71] with good specificity [72]. It is considered to reflect PLP concentrations in the liver [73]. Other markers of B6 are available including 4-pyridoxic acid and erythrocyte pyridoxal-5-phosphate. Erythrocyte glutathione reductase activation (EGRac) assay is the most widely used functional assay for riboflavin status and is generally regarded as the gold standard. EGRac measures glutathione reductase activity in erythrocytes before and after reactivation with its prosthetic group flavin adenine dinucleotide (FAD). A systematic review (14 RCTs) concluded that EGRac was a sensitive biomarker of change in riboflavin intake in populations with status ranging from deficient to normal [74].

In general, the use of different biomarkers or different cut off points for defining deficiency/suboptimal status when assessing individual B-vitamins can influence the interpretation and conclusion of relevant studies. This can make direct comparisons among studies difficult and may explain some inconsistencies in the literature as regards the role of B-vitamins in diseases in ageing.

Table 2. Assessment of B-vitamin biomarker status.

		Biomarker	Strengths	Limitations
Homocysteine [20]	**Functional**	Plasma homocysteine	Sensitive functional biomarker Highly responsive to intervention with B-vitamins Responds within 3–4 weeks of B-vitamin depletion and subsequent repletion Very stable analyte Can be stored frozen for extended periods of time	Lacks specificity as affected by other B-vitamins Requires separation from RBCs within one hour of blood collection, or <8 h if whole blood is kept on ice Influenced by other factors such as lifestyle, genetics, renal insufficiency, age and medications
Folate [20,21,60,63,75]	**Direct**	Serum/Plasma folate	Earliest indicator of altered folate exposure Reflects recent dietary folate intake Requires less time processing at time of blood collection vs. RBC folate Can be measured in the field	Inconsistent use of cut off values makes comparisons across different methods and labs difficult Fasting blood samples are recommended
		Red cell folate	Sensitive indicator of long-term folate status Reflects folate status over half-life of RBCs Reflects tissue folate stores as parallels liver concentrations Highly correlated with habitual intake when expressed as DFEs	Affected by vitamin B12 deficiency Inconsistent use of cut off values makes comparisons across different methods and labs difficult Cannot be measured in the field
B12 [21,34,60,70,75,76]	**Direct**	Serum/Plasma total B12	Serum standard clinical test Variety of assays available Measures all forms of vitamin B12	Does not reflect intracellular vitamin B12 Falsely elevated B12 caused by factors including liver disorders, bacterial overgrowth, renal failure Falsely low B12 caused by factors such as iron deficiency, HIV infection and pregnancy Inconsistent use of cut off values makes comparisons across different methods and labs difficult
		Serum/Plasma Holo-transcobalamin (HoloTC)	Represents metabolically active fraction of B12 Decrease in holoTC can indicate earliest sign of B12 depletion Considered better indicator of B12 status in elderly	Highly sensitive to altered renal function and influenced by factors including genetics
	Functional	Serum/plasma/urine Methylmalonic acid (MMA)	Reflects availability of intracellular B12 Early detection of functional B12 deficiency Not affected by folate deficiency	Lacks sensitivity as can be elevated in those with renal impairment High running costs

Table 2. *Cont.*

		Biomarker	Strengths	Limitations
B6 [21,60,72,77,78]	**Direct**	Plasma Pyridoxal-Phosphate (PLP)	Most widely used Good specificity and reflects PLP content in liver Responds quickly within 1–2 weeks of B6 depletion and subsequent repletion Reference ranges available for younger and older adults Fairly stable at low temperatures	Does not represent PLP content in the muscle which is resistant to B6 depletion Influenced by other factors such as age, sex, pregnancy, protein and alcohol intake PLP declines in samples stored at room temperature and exposure to light Fasting blood samples are recommended Plasma PLP concentrations affected by use of certain drugs
		Erythrocyte PLP	Positively correlated with B6 dietary intake Responds within weeks of B6 depletion and subsequent repletion Appears more responsive than plasma PLP to supplementation May be more reliable marker than plasma PLP under conditions and disease associated with inflammation	Affected by haemoglobin variants Assay is cumbersome, with variable recovery and low precision
B2 [21,60,74,78]	**Direct**	Serum/Plasma/Erythrocyte Riboflavin/Flavine Adenine Dinucleotide (FAD)/Flavin Mononucleotide (FMN)	Riboflavin vitamers are stable for several years when plasma samples are stored at −80 ° CSerum/plasma can be used retrospectively in a hospital setting	Influenced by other factors such as age, sex, pregnancy, protein and alcohol intake Serum/plasma riboflavin concentrations affected by use of certain drugs High variability within and between-subjects compared to the cofactor forms of riboflavin (plasma/erythrocyte)
	Functional	Erythrocyte glutathione reductase activation (EGRac) assay	Most widely used marker of status Measures tissue saturation and long term status Enzyme is stable for several years when erythrocyte lysates are stored at −80 °C	Poor index of optimum riboflavin status Assay is not linear against status Difficult make comparisons across different methods and labs

5. Consequences of B-Vitamin Deficiency

There are established clinical signs of B-vitamin deficiency (Table 3). The haematological manifestation of folate and vitamin B12 deficiency is indistinguishable, as both vitamins are linked through the enzyme methionine synthase [9] which catalyses the remethylation of homocysteine to methionine and thus are metabolically interrelated [79]. Deficiency of either vitamin results in a reduction of the active form of folate which subsequently results in megaloblastic anaemia [80], characterised by megaloblasts in the bone marrow, macrocytes in the peripheral blood and gigantism in the morphology of proliferating cells [25]. Vitamin B12 deficiency can also result in diverse neurological symptoms including irreversible nerve damage and sub-acute combined degeneration of the spinal cord if left untreated, as patients are often asymptomatic [81]. Neuropathy is quite specific to vitamin B12 and does not occur in folate deficiency [79]. Although severe vitamin B6 deficiency is relatively uncommon, it can present with notable symptoms such as anaemia, depression and sores or ulcers of the mouth [22]. The classical signs of riboflavin deficiency are angular stomatitis, cheilosis and glossitis, but these are rarely encountered in isolation and may be as a result of other B-vitamin deficiencies [27].

Apart from clinical deficiency signs, deficient or low status of B-vitamins can be associated with various adverse health outcomes throughout the lifecycle [82]. It should be noted that these can arise in the absence of more classical deficiency signs, and can occur within the range of what may be classed as "normal" within the clinical setting.

Table 3. Consequences of deficient or low status of B-vitamins.

	Clinical Deficiency Signs [19–22]
Folate	Megaloblastic anaemia, clinical features characterised by megaloblasts in the bone marrow macrocytes in the peripheral blood gigantism in the morphology of proliferating cells
B12	Megaloblastic anaemia indistinguishable from folate-related megaloblastic anaemia Irreversible nerve damage/neuropathy Sub-acute combined degeneration of the spinal cord (SCD)
B6	Notable symptoms include: Microcytic anaemia Inflammation of the tongue Sores or ulcers of the mouth Dermatitis Nervous/muscular signs Irritability, fatigue, numbness Headache, muscle twitching Difficulty walking, convulsions Depression and confusion
B2	Classic signs arbioflavinosis, rarely encountered in isolation Anaemia Cheliosis, Angular stomatitis Glossitis Redness and swelling of the lining of the mouth and throat Seborrheic dermatitis particularly affecting the nose, cheeks and forehead Eyes burning and itching Sensitivity to light Loss of visual acuity Gritty sensation under the eyelids
	Health Consequences of Low Status of Folate and/or Other B-Vitamins [83–89]
	Elevated homocysteine CVD and stroke Cognitive decline/dementia/Alzheimer's Osteoporosis and risk of fractures

6. Emerging Roles of B-Vitamin Status in Preventing Diseases of Ageing

6.1. Cardiovascular Health in Ageing

Clinical evidence has linked elevated plasma homocysteine concentrations and/or low folate with an increased risk of CVD. Early meta-analyses of observational studies concluded that lowering homocysteine would reduce the risk of heart disease by 11%–16% [83,84]. Homocysteine may however be a marker of suboptimal B-vitamin status and thus simply reflect a perturbation in one-carbon metabolism, rather than playing a causative role in CVD, but this is not universally accepted [90]. In any case, several secondary prevention randomised controlled trials (RCTs) published between 2004 and 2012 have failed to demonstrate a benefit of homocysteine-lowering by B-vitamin supplementation on CVD events generally [91–97]. These studies, however, typically involved patients with existing optimal B-vitamin status and/or advanced CVD, and thus a significant effect of B-vitamin supplementation on CVD risk may have been unlikely.

The evidence however is generally much stronger for stroke than heart disease, with meta-analyses of earlier observational studies concluding that lowering homocysteine would reduce the risk of stroke by 19%–24% [83,84]. Furthermore, population data from the USA and Canada, reported an improvement in stroke mortality corresponding to the time that mandatory food fortification was introduced; in contrast, no similar improvement was found over the same time period in England and Wales where no mandatory fortification policy exists [98]. Of greatest relevance however are the findings of RCTs in relation to stroke risk, with meta-analyses of folic acid interventions showing a reduced risk of stroke by 18% overall [99], but with much greater reductions in risk noted in studies with longer folic acid treatment duration, with greater homocysteine reduction and in particular in those with no history of stroke [99,100]. More recent evidence including the China Stroke Primary Prevention Trial (CSPPT) [101] and a meta-analysis of 30 RCTs [102] also support a significant beneficial effect of folic acid supplementation on CVD risk (especially stroke), particularly in those with lower baseline folate status and without pre-existing CVD. Thus, optimisation of folate and the related B-vitamins might be beneficial in lowering CVD risk, particularly stroke, and most convincingly in primary prevention.

In addition, genetic studies are now providing stronger evidence for the potential role of folate and the related B-vitamins in CVD, primarily through the investigation of the common 677 C $\rightarrow$ T polymorphism in the gene encoding the folate-metabolising enzyme MTHFR. Epidemiological evidence suggests that this common polymorphism increases the risk of CVD, especially stroke by up to 40% overall [84,103–105]. Furthermore, evidence is emerging to suggest that the excess genetic risk of CVD may be driven by higher blood pressure (rather than higher homocysteine), with meta-analyses of observational studies showing that the *MTHFR* 677 C $\rightarrow$ T polymorphism increases the risk of hypertension by 36%–87% [106,107]. This is also supported by recent evidence from a large study of Irish adults (n = 6069), which estimated that the *MTHFR* 677TT genotype was associated with an almost two-fold increased hypertension risk, a risk which was further increased when the genotype occurred in combination with low riboflavin status [15]. In addition, intervention studies from this centre, conducted in participants with premature CVD or hypertension showed that those with the *MTHFR* 677TT genotype were highly responsive to blood-pressure lowering through riboflavin supplementation, whilst no response was observed in participants with CC or CT genotypes [108–110]. Therefore, sub-populations worldwide with the *MTHFR* 677TT genotype (ranging from 3% to 32%) [14], may particularly be at greater risk of CVD via a blood pressure effect, and could benefit from a more optimal riboflavin status ideally before hypertension has developed.

6.2. Bone Health in Ageing

The role of B-vitamins in bone health has been extensively reviewed [16]. Briefly, observational evidence in older people has found independent associations of elevated homocysteine with bone mineral density (BMD) [111,112] and fracture risk [89,113]. Meta-analyses of observational studies have confirmed these relationships, with one (n = 14,863) concluding that homocysteine was an independent risk factor [114]. Another dose response meta-analysis (n = 11,511) estimated a 4% increased fracture risk for every 1 μmol/L increase of homocysteine concentration [115]. Low BMD has also been associated with sub-optimal status or dietary intakes of folate [111,116] or vitamin B12 [112,117]. Likewise, studies have also found an increased fracture risk in older people with sub-optimal status/intake of folate [118], vitamin B12 [119,120], or vitamin B6 [121,122]. Only one study to date in coeliac patients (n = 110) has examined riboflavin biomarker status with bone health (BMD), and found no relationship [16]. Although, low riboflavin intake in women (aged ≥55 years, n = 5035) was associated with a 1.8 times increased risk of osteoporotic facture and 2.6 times increased risk of fragility fractures [119]. The evidence is not entirely consistent, however, as some observational studies have shown no relationships with B-vitamin biomarkers on BMD [123] or fracture risk [124]. To date, there is limited RCT evidence linking B-vitamins with bone health and disease. One notable two-year RCT of combined folic acid and vitamin B12 supplementation (n = 628) resulted in a 75% reduction in the risk of hip fractures in older post-stroke Japanese patients, with low baseline folate status [125]. Certain RCTs with B-vitamins, which are not designed to examine bone outcomes (but rather other health outcomes), have reported no significant associations with fracture risk [126,127]. Additionally, interventions involving participants with generally higher baseline folate status have also reported no significant associations with BMD [128] or fracture risk [129]. This suggests that the benefit of interventions with B-vitamins may be confined to at-risk groups such as those with sub-optimal status.

Genetic studies also support the potential role of folate and the related B-vitamins in bone health. The potential influence of *MTHFR* 677TT polymorphism on bone health may be mediated through impaired DNA methylation as a result of impaired DNA structure and stability [130,131], expression and the silencing of genes [132–134]. Epidemiological studies have reported that the *MTHFR* 677TT genotype is associated with significantly lower BMD [135,136] and a 2- to 2.5-fold increased risk of fractures [135,137]. This is also strengthened by one meta-analysis (3525 cases and 17,909 controls) which concluded that the *MTHFR* 677 C → T polymorphism was associated with BMD at multiple sites and individuals with the TT genotype had a 23% increased risk of all fractures [138]. Furthermore, the association appears to be influenced by prevailing B-vitamin intake, an interaction between the *MTHFR* 677TT genotype and low intakes of folate or riboflavin has been linked with lower BMD [139–141], higher bone loss and up to a three-fold increased fracture risk [118,142], although the majority of these studies do not consider B-vitamin biomarker status. This suggests that individuals with the *MTHFR* 677TT genotype and low B-vitamin status may be most vulnerable to poor bone health in later life.

6.3. Brain Health in Ageing

Cognitive Dysfunction

Cognitive dysfunction ranges from mild cognitive impairment (MCI) to dementia and can result in a progressive loss of a number of specific cognitive functions [143,144]. The rate of cognitive decline varies between individuals [145], and it is estimated that 50% of older people with MCI will go on to develop dementia within five years of diagnosis [146]. Dementia has a number of distinct pathologies, although mixed pathologies in individuals have been shown at brain autopsies [147,148]. These include reduced/blocked flow to the brain [149], neuronal loss and damage to the connection between neurones [150] and the presence of Lewy bodies which has also been associated with neurotransmitter depletion [151]. Extra-neuronal β amyloid plaques and intra-neuronal neurofibrillary tangles [152] can also be present. Brain atrophy is a normal part of the ageing process, but with dementia, the rate is significantly higher overall and particularly in the hippocampus region [153,154]. Grey and white matter loss, thinning of cortical gyri and enlarged ventricles can also be evident in those with dementia [155].

Prospective studies make a strong case for elevated homocysteine and/or low B-vitamin status as potential causative factors in cognitive decline [156,157] and dementia [85]. This is further supported by three recent reviews and meta-analyses [87,158,159]. Epidemiological studies have also investigated the role of the relevant B-vitamins, with the focus mainly on folate and vitamin B12. Studies involving populations with lower baseline folate status in general support the role of folate in cognitive dysfunction [160–162] and cognitive decline [163,164], whereas those in countries with food fortification policies and thus overall higher mean concentrations of folate, are generally less supportive for a role in cognitive dysfunction [165,166], cognitive decline [167–169] or dementia [170]. Similarly, a number of large cohort studies have associated low vitamin B12 status (using more sensitive biomarkers of status including MMA and HoloTC) with cognitive dysfunction [160,166,171] and cognitive decline [162,172,173] in older people. However, the evidence for B12 is less convincing, and one meta-analysis has shown no association of vitamin B12 with cognitive decline or dementia (n = 14,325) [174]. This lack of significant association for B12 may be explained the fact that some of the included studies had methodological shortcomings (including limitations in the biomarkers used to determine B12 status). Thus, when sub-analysis of the data was carried out based on studies using more sensitive biomarkers of vitamin B12 status the results indicated that low vitamin B12 was in fact significantly associated with an increased risk of cognitive decline and dementia [174]. Relatively few studies have examined the role of vitamin B6 in cognition and even fewer have examined riboflavin. Low status of vitamin B6 has been shown to contribute to cognitive dysfunction [175,176] and cognitive decline [177]. Low vitamin B6 intake has been associated with a reduced risk of Alzheimer's disease [178] in older Americans. Only one study from Taiwan has investigated the role of riboflavin status and found a significant association with cognitive dysfunction, which was assessed using only a short portable mental status questionnaire and cognition was not the primary outcome [179].

Several RCTs have investigated the potential role of folate alone or in combination, with vitamins B12 and/or B6 in maintaining cognitive health in ageing, although to date most include high pharmacological doses and none include riboflavin (Table 4). One meta-analysis of nine RCTs in healthy people (n = 2835) concluded that folic acid had no effect on cognitive function [180]. However, in this meta-analysis, only two studies had more than 275 participants and were longer than 12 months in duration (five were $\leq$ 6 months). Additionally, one recent controversial meta-analysis in almost 22,000 healthy older people concluded that neither folic acid nor vitamin B12 had a beneficial effect on "cognitive ageing" [181]. The results have been widely criticised, mainly due to the inclusion criteria used to select the trials [182–184]. Only three of the RCTs had final cognitive test scores and two thirds of the baseline results were not available. MMSE, a screening tool that is considered as a crude measure of global cognition, was the main cognitive assessment tool used. Furthermore, this meta-analysis did not identify subgroups or at risk groups in each trial that may have benefited from B-vitamins. The recent B-Vitamins for the Prevention of Osteoporotic Fractures (B-PROOF) study did show a slower rate of global cognitive decline, this was attributed to chance by the authors [185]. In general, greatest cognitive benefits have been demonstrated in RCTs involving participants with lower baseline folate status [186,187], higher homocysteine concentrations [188,189] and lower B-vitamin intake [190]. In contrast, RCTs in individuals with higher baseline folate status [191] or higher cognitive status [185] have shown no significant benefit on cognitive performance. This supports the view that baseline B-vitamin status is a critical consideration in the outcome of trials examining cognition, and further is supported by a systematic review involving 14 RCTs, which found no overall benefit of B-vitamin interventions, but reported a benefit in cognitive function in those with lower baseline folate status [192]. Thus, well designed RCTs are still required, particularly in those with sub-optimal B-vitamin status as they might benefit most in optimising B-vitamin status to maintain cognitive health in ageing.

Table 4. Summary of Randomised Controlled Trials of 2 years or more assessing the effect of B vitamins on cognitive function in ageing.

Author/Year/Trial	Country	Sample Size (*n*)	Age (Years)	Population Studied Plasma tHcy (μmol/L)	Treatment (mg/day)	Duration	Cognitive Outcomes
Questionnaire based assessment							
McMahon 2006 [191]	New Zealand	276	≥65	Healthy tHcy > 13	1.0 FA, 0.5 B12, 10 B6	2 years	No significant effect on cognition
FACIT Durga 2007 [186]	The Netherlands	818	50–70	Healthy tHcy 13–26	0.8 FA or placebo	3 years	Improvement in domains including memory, information-processing and sensorimotor speed No improvement in global cognition or domains of complex speed or word fluency
WAFACS Kang 2008 [190]	USA	2009	≥65	CVD/high risk women tHcy not provided	2.5 FA, 1.0 B12, 50 B6 or placebo	6.6 years	Reduced risk of cognitive decline among women with low baseline dietary intake of B-vitamins Overall no significant effect on rate of cognitive decline
Brady 2009 [193]	USA	659	Mean 67.3	Advanced renal disease tHcy ≥ 15	40 FA, 2.0 B12, 100 B6 or placebo	5 years	No significant effect on cognition
Health in Men Study: sub set Ford 2010 [194]	Australia	299	≥75	Hypertensive men Mean tHcy 13.1–14	2.0 FA, 0.4 B12, 25 B6 or placebo	2 years	No significant effect on cognition
Kwok 2011 [189]	Hong Kong	140	≥60	Dementia diagnosis Mean tHcy 14.1	5.0 FA, 1.0 B12 or placebo	2 years	Improvement in domain of construction No change in global cognitive decline, attention, memory or conceptualisation
Beyond ageing project Walker 2012 [187]	Australia	900	60–74	Elevated psychological distress Mean tHcy 9.7	0.4 FA, 0.1 B12 or placebo	2 years	Improvement in overall global cognition and in domains of immediate and delayed recall scores No significant change in other cognitive domains
VITACOG De Jager 2012 [195]	UK	168	≥70	MCI Mean tHcy 11.3	0.8 FA, 0.5 B12, 20 B6 or placebo	2 years	Slower decline in global cognition and in domains of semantic and episodic memory Clinical benefit in global clinical dementia rating score
BPROOF Van Der Zwaluw 2014 [185]	The Netherlands	2919	≥65	Healthy tHcy 12–50	0.4 FA, 0.5 B12, 0.15 D3 or placebo + D3	2 years	Slower rate of decline in global cognition No change in domains of memory
Brain-imaging assessment							
VITACOG Smith 2010 Douaud 2013 [188,196]	UK	168	≥70	MCI Mean tHcy 11.3	0.8 FA, 0.5 B12, 20 B6 or placebo	2 years	Slowed shrinkage of brain Marked reduction in cerebral atrophy in grey matter regions
BPROOF Van Der Zwaluw 2014 [185]	The Netherlands	2919	≥65	Healthy tHcy 12–50	0.4 FA, 0.5 B12, 0.15 D3 or placebo + D3	2 years	*Awaiting MRI scan results*

Abbreviations: tHcy, homocysteine; FA, folic acid; MMA, methylmalonic acid; holoTC, holo-transcobalamin; EPA, eicosapentaenoic; DHA, docosahexaenoic acid; MCI, mild cognitive impairment; MRI, magnetic resonance imaging; CVD, cardiovascular disease.

Apart from evidence from observational studies and RCTs, genetic studies also provide support for the role of B-vitamins in maintaining cognitive health in ageing. The *MTHFR* 677TT genotype has been associated with poorer cognitive performance in Chinese males [197] and a 42% increased risk of cognitive impairment in older Australian males [198], but not in older Americans [166]. Meta-analyses have also associated the *MTHFR* C677T polymorphism with an increased risk of Alzheimer's disease [199], and dementia albeit in Asian populations only [200,201]. These results may be attributed to the varying prevalence of the *MTHFR* 677TT genotype worldwide and the modulating effect of B-vitamin status. To date, no studies have investigated interactions between this gene and B-vitamin status in relation to cognitive health.

6.4. Future Directions

While questionnaire based tools tests are typically used to assess cognitive performance in observational studies and RCTs, they do have inherent limitations. The use of brain imaging technology is considered a more robust measure of cognitive and brain health as it can overcome the inherent weaknesses of cognitive questionnaire based tools. MRI scans have shown that vitamin B12 status is inversely related to the rate of overall brain atrophy [202], and lower B12 status has been associated with a reduced microstructure integrity of the hippocampus [203], increased rate of brain volume losses [204,205], and a greater severity of white matter lesions [206]. Likewise, lower folate status has also been associated with severe cortical and hippocampal brain atrophy [207] and white matter lesions [161]. Furthermore, the VITACOG trial demonstrated that combined folate, B12 and B6 supplementation over two years markedly reduced (by up to 53%) the rate of brain atrophy. This effect was modulated by baseline homocysteine concentration, with the greatest impact observed in those with concentrations $\geq$ 13 μmol/L [196]. A reduction in cerebral atrophy by as much as seven fold was also observed in grey matter regions, which are the most relevant regions for Alzheimer's disease pathology [188]. More recently, the use of a new functional neuroimaging technique, magnetoencephalography (MEG), has emerged which can map brain activity and assess cognitive processes and specific functions of the brain [208]. MEG is currently being used in some clinical studies, including cognitive studies in ageing, but to date none have examined B-vitamins. Brain imaging could therefore help further elucidate the role and underlying mechanism linking B-vitamins with brain health and disease.

Future studies are therefore warranted to investigate the effects (and interactions) of folate, the related B-vitamins, and relevant genetic variants, particularly in cohorts with lower B-vitamin status. Longitudinal studies are also required to explore differential effects on cognition over time. Targeted RCTs of sufficient duration, with lower doses of B-vitamins at levels achievable through dietary means, are also indicated.

7. Potential Mechanisms Linking B-Vitamins with Diseases of Ageing

Although no clear mechanisms have been established, a variety of biologically plausible mechanisms have been suggested to explain the role of B-vitamins in the diseases of ageing [85,156]. In the brain and other tissues, folate and the metabolically related B-vitamins are required as co-factors for one-carbon transfer reactions, which in turn are fundamental for the synthesis of DNA and RNA nucleotides, the metabolism of amino acids and the maintenance of methylation reactions [6,7]. Thus, the proposed mechanisms by which sub-optimal B-vitamins status or deficiency could contribute to greater risk of cognitive impairment and other diseases of ageing, involve perturbations in the complex regulatory network maintaining one-carbon metabolism [11,12]. This can result in hyperhomocysteinemia [209] and/or reduced methylation status within the relevant tissue [210,211], increased misincorporation of uracil into DNA, and altered RNA [212–214] and neurotransmitter products [215]. Vitamin B6 is important in brain health as pyridoxine is a co-factor in transamination and decarboxylation reactions required for the metabolism of several neurotransmitters, including serotonin, dopamine, and histamine [216]. Elevated homocysteine and/or lower B-vitamins can also impact on the immune system and cause increased inflammation and antioxidant damage, alone or in synergy, which can have adverse effects on the disease of ageing through the vascular system and atherosclerosis [217–219]. B-vitamins have also been shown to have an indirect role on bone remodelling and protective effects on bone formation which help to maintain bone health in ageing [220–222]. Cognitive deficits and Alzheimer's disease has also been observed in B-vitamin deficient rats and been attributed to abnormal methylation [223,224].

Specific genetic polymorphisms, including the common *MTHFR* 677 C $\rightarrow$ T polymorphism can disrupt normal one-carbon metabolism and thus have an impact on diseases of ageing, independent of homocysteine, as a result of impairments in methylation activity; improved B-vitamin status could help to modulate this risk [13,225,226]. Furthermore, this polymorphism has more recently been associated with blood pressure while riboflavin has emerged as having a novel role in lowering blood pressure in hypertensive patients with the variant *MTHFR* 677TT genotype [110]. The effect of the *MTHFR* 677 C $\rightarrow$ T polymorphism on blood pressure might be mediated by nitric oxide, a potent vasodilator, and riboflavin has been demonstrated as a means to restoring MTHFR activity in vivo [58]. The interaction between the *MTHFR* genotype, B-vitamin status and risk of hypertension requires further exploration.

8. Public Health Implications

Folic acid food fortification was instigated primarily to reduce the prevalence of neural tube defects (NTDs) but it may also have additional benefits for the ageing population. Currently, 80 countries have mandatory folic acid food fortification policies in place, including America and Canada [227]. As a result of fortification, there has been a dramatic fall in NTDs [228] and folate deficiency in the USA and Canada is practically non-existent [34,36,229]. Mandatory folic acid food fortification has also lead to an improvement in stroke mortality in the US and Canada [98] and could have additional beneficial effects in maintaining better cognitive function [230] and bone health [231] in older people. No European country has a mandatory folic acid food fortification policy but most do allow voluntary food fortification. The UK and Ireland have quite liberal voluntary fortification polices and are currently considering mandatory fortification. Voluntary food fortification has resulted in significantly higher dietary intakes and biomarker status of folate and related B-vitamins in Irish adults of all ages [232,233]. The NANS dietary survey however highlighted that the overall 21% of Irish adults who were non-consumers of fortified foods were at higher risk of sub-optimal status of folate and related B-vitamins [233]. Regular fortified food consumption therefore has the potential to improve dietary and biomarker status of B-vitamins but a mandatory food fortification would ensure that the whole population were protected.

Low vitamin B12 status in older people is also a concern. Current dietary recommendations for vitamin B12 range between 2.4 μg/day in the USA [234] and 4 μg/day in Europe [235]. However, the European recommendations do not account for the high prevalence of food-bound malabsorption in older people, whereas people aged $\geq$50 years in the USA are recommended to consume most of their vitamin B12 from crystalline sources (i.e., fortified food and supplements) in order to overcome food-bound B12 malabsorption [234]. The synthetic form of vitamin B12, found in fortified foods and supplements, is freely available and thus has no gastric acid requirement [40]. Furthermore, there was a previous safety concern that the high folic acid intake may potentially mask the anaemia of vitamin B12 deficiency and thus delay diagnosis resulting in irreversible nerve damage [79,236]. Mandatory food fortification in the USA however has not led to these adverse events [237–239]. Therefore, from a public health perspective, there are significant challenges in relation to maintaining vitamin B12 in older people and vitamin B12 food fortification could help address some of these challenges.

Concerns have been raised as regards a possible adverse interaction of high folate with low vitamin B12 leading to an increased risk of cognitive impairment in the USA and Australia [230,240,241], but this is rather controversial. Two studies in the UK and USA failed to detect such an adverse interaction [238,242] and one study in the Netherlands in fact found that this combination (i.e., high folate and low B12) was associated with a reduced risk of cognitive impairment [243]. Discrepancies among studies in this regard may in part be attributed to the relatively low numbers in most studies with this folate/vitamin B12 combination and the type of biomarker used or the cut off value used to define low status in each study. Additionally, a recent US review concluded that the current observational data was limited and that no RCTs had investigated this folate–B12 interaction in cognitive health [244]. Concerns have also been raised that excessively high folate intakes could have cancer promoting effects in segments of the ageing population [245–247]. A Scientific Advisory Committee on Nutrition (SACN) review in the UK however found insufficient evidence to support the view that mandatory folic acid fortification would promote cancer [248]. Excessive folic acid intakes have also been reported to increase un-metabolized folic acid in the circulation with potential adverse effects on health [34,249], although a recent international review did not find any health concerns even at very high folic acid levels [20]. Suggestions have been made to include both folic acid and vitamin B12 in mandatory food fortification policies, to prevent adverse health outcomes and address food-bound malabsorption but the costs of such an approach may be prohibitive. Furthermore, vitamin B6 and riboflavin status in older people is also of concern and may be much more important than previously appreciated for public health in ageing. Therefore, those contemplating public health issues worldwide need to consider a balanced approach and should endeavour to achieve optimal status of all relevant B-vitamins throughout all stages of life.

9. Conclusions

In summary, folate and the metabolically related B-vitamins, B12, B6 and riboflavin, have a vital role in maintaining one-carbon metabolism and any perturbation in this pathway as a result of low/deficient B-vitamin status can impact on health through a number of related mechanisms. Evidence is accumulating to support the beneficial role of B-vitamins in maintaining cardiovascular, bone and brain health in ageing, with the most at risk sub-populations benefiting from optimising one/more B-vitamins involved in one-carbon metabolism. To date, studies investigating the role of B-vitamins in health and disease have tended to focus predominantly on folate and vitamin B12. Future well designed research is warranted to further investigate the metabolically linked B-vitamins B6 and riboflavin, and should include robust and sensitive measures of B-vitamins as well as novel measures of the health outcome of interest (e.g., imaging techniques to assess brain function). In an era where personalised nutrition has gained much attention, further work is also needed to explore the role of the interaction of the *MTHFR* 677 C $\rightarrow$ T polymorphism with both folate and riboflavin, given that this gene–nutrient interaction has the potential to modulate the risk of disease.

Acknowledgments: K.P.'s Ph.D. studentship was funded by the Northern Ireland Department for Employment and Learning who had no role in the design, analysis or writing of this paper.

Author Contributions: K.P. drafted the manuscript. H.M., L.H., C.F.H. and M.W. critically revised the manuscript for important intellectual content. All the authors have read and approved the final manuscript.

References

1. Beard, J.R.; Bloom, D.E. Towards a comprehensive public health response to population ageing. *Lancet* **2015**, *385*, 658–661. [CrossRef]
2. Prince, M.; Wu, F.; Guo, Y.; Gutierrez Robledo, L.; O'Donnell, M.; Sullivan, R.; Yusuf, S. The burden of disease in older people and implications for health policy and practice. *Lancet* **2015**, *385*, 549–562. [CrossRef]
3. A Global Brief on Hypertension. Available online: http://ish-world.com/news/a/World-Health-Organization-A-Global-Brief-on-Hypertension/ (accessed on 1 August 2016).
4. Johnell, O.; Kanis, J.A. An estimate of the worldwide prevalence and disability associated with osteoporotic fractures. *Osteoporos. Int.* **2006**, *17*, 1726–1733. [CrossRef] [PubMed]
5. Prince, M.; Wimo, A.; Guerchet, M.; Ali, G.C.; Wu, Y.-T.; Prina, M.; International, A.D. *World Alzheimer's Report—The Global Impact of Dementia*; Alzheimer's Disease International: London, UK, 2015.

6. Selhub, J. Folate, vitamin B12 and vitamin B6 and one carbon metabolism. *J. Nutr. Health Aging* **2002**, *6*, 39–42. [PubMed]
7. Kennedy, D.O. B Vitamins and the Brain: Mechanisms, Dose and Efficacy—A Review. *Nutrients* **2016**, *8*, 68. [CrossRef] [PubMed]
8. McGarel, C.; Pentieva, K.; Strain, J.J.; McNulty, H. Emerging roles for folate and related B-vitamins in brain health across the lifecycle. *Proc. Nutr. Soc.* **2015**, *74*, 46–55. [CrossRef] [PubMed]
9. Molloy, A. Folate-vitamin B12 interrelationships; links to disease risk. In *Folate in Health and Disease*, 2nd ed.; Bailey, L., Ed.; CRC Press: Boca Raton, FL, USA, 2010; pp. 381–408.
10. Scott, J.; Weir, D. The methyl folate trap: A physiological response in man to prevent methyl group deficiency in kwashiorkor (methionine deficiency) and an explanation for folic-acid-induced exacerbation of subacute combined degeneration in pernicious anaemia. *Lancet* **1981**, *318*, 337–340. [CrossRef]
11. Brachet, P.; Chanson, A.; Demigne, C.; Batifoulier, F.; Alexandre-Gouabau, M.C.; Tyssandier, V.; Rock, E. Age-associated B vitamin deficiency as a determinant of chronic diseases. *Nutr. Res. Rev.* **2004**, *17*, 55–68. [CrossRef] [PubMed]
12. Araujo, J.R.; Martel, F.; Borges, N.; Araujo, J.M.; Keating, E. Folates and aging: Role in mild cognitive impairment, dementia and depression. *Ageing Res. Rev.* **2015**, *22*, 9–19. [CrossRef] [PubMed]
13. Lai, C.; Parnell, L.D.; Troen, A.M.; Shen, J.; Caouette, H.; Warodomwichit, D.; Lee, Y.; Crott, J.W.; Qiu, W.Q.; Rosenberg, I.H.; et al. MAT1A variants are associated with hypertension, stroke, and markers of DNA damage and are modulated by plasma vitamin B-6 and folate. *Am. J. Clin. Nutr.* **2010**, *91*, 1377–1386. [CrossRef] [PubMed]
14. Wilcken, B.; Bamforth, F.; Li, Z.; Zhu, H.; Ritvanen, A.; Redlund, M.; Stoll, C.; Alembik, Y.; Dott, B.; Czeizel, A.E.; et al. Geographical and ethnic variation of the 677C > T allele of 5,10-methylenetetrahydrofolate reductase (*MTHFR*): Findings from over 7000 newborns from 16 areas Worldwide. *J. Med. Genet.* **2003**, *40*, 619–625. [CrossRef] [PubMed]
15. Reilly, R.; Hopkins, S.; Ward, M.; McNulty, H.; McCann, A.; McNulty, B.; Walton, J.; Molloy, A.; Strain, J.J.; Flynn, A.; et al. *MTHFR 677TT* genotype and related B-vitamins: Novel determinants of hypertension in healthy Irish adults. *J. Inherit. Metab. Dis.* **2013**, *36*, 35.
16. Clarke, M.; Ward, M.; Dickey, W.; Hoey, L.; Molloy, A.M.; Waldron, L.; Varghese, A.; McCann, A.; Blayney, J.K.; McNulty, H. B-vitamin status in relation to bone mineral density in treated celiac disease patients. *Scand. J. Gastroenterol.* **2015**, *50*, 975–984. [CrossRef] [PubMed]
17. Ter Borg, S.; Verlaan, S.; Hemsworth, J.; Mijnarends, D.M.; Schols, J.M.G.A.; Luiking, Y.C.; De Groot, L.C.P.G.M. Micronutrient intakes and potential inadequacies of community-dwelling older adults: A systematic review. *Br. J. Nutr.* **2015**, *113*, 1195–1206. [CrossRef] [PubMed]
18. Bates, B.; Lennox, A.; Bates, C. *National Diet and Nutrition Survey: Results from Years 1–4 (Combined) of the Rolling Programme (2008/2009–2011/12)*; Public Health England: London, UK, 2014.
19. Lindenbaum, J.; Allen, R. Clinical spectrum and diagnosis of folate deficiency. In *Folate in Health and Disease*, 2nd ed.; Bailey, L., Ed.; CRC Press: London, UK, 2009; pp. 43–67.
20. Bailey, L.B.; Stover, P.J.; McNulty, H.; Fenech, M.F.; Gregory, J.F., III; Mills, J.L.; Pfeiffer, C.M.; Fazili, Z.; Zhang, M.; Ueland, P.M.; et al. Biomarkers of Nutrition for Development-Folate Review. *J. Nutr.* **2015**, *145*, 1636–1680. [CrossRef] [PubMed]
21. Gibson, R. Assessment status of riboflavin, B6, folate and B12 status. In *Principles of Nutritional Assessment*, 2nd ed.; Oxford University: New York, NY, USA, 2005; pp. 554–562, 575–640.
22. Carmel, R.; Jacobsen, D. (Eds.) *Homocysteine in Health and Disease*; Cambridge University Press: Cambridge, UK, 2001.
23. Selhub, J.; Jacques, P.F.; Bostom, A.G.; Wilson, P.W.; Rosenberg, I.H. Relationship between plasma homocysteine and vitamin status in the Framingham study population. Impact of folic acid fortification. *Public Health Rev.* **2000**, *28*, 117–145. [PubMed]
24. McKillop, D.; Pentieva, K.; Daly, D.; McPartlin, J.; Hughes, J.; Strain, J.; Scott, J.; McNulty, H. The effect of different cooking methods on folate retention in various foods that are amongst the major contributors to folate intake in the UK diet. *Br. J. Nutr.* **2002**, *88*, 681–688. [CrossRef] [PubMed]
25. McNulty, H.; Scott, J.M. Intake and status of folate and related B-vitamins: Considerations and challenges in achieving optimal status. *Br. J. Nutr.* **2008**, *99*, S48–S54. [CrossRef] [PubMed]
26. Selhub, J.; Bagley, L.C.; Miller, J.; Rosenberg, I.H. B vitamins, homocysteine, and neurocognitive function in the elderly. *Am. J. Clin. Nutr.* **2000**, *71*, 614S–620S. [PubMed]

27. Powers, H.J. Riboflavin (vitamin B-2) and health. *Am. J. Clin. Nutr.* **2003**, *77*, 1352–1360. [PubMed]
28. Allen, L.H. How common is vitamin B-12 deficiency? *Am. J. Clin. Nutr.* **2009**, *89*, 693S–696S. [CrossRef] [PubMed]
29. Refsum, H.; Yajnik, C.S.; Gadkari, M.; Schneede, J.; Vollset, S.E.; Orning, L.; Guttormsen, A.B.; Joglekar, A.; Sayyad, M.G.; Ulvik, A.; et al. Hyperhomocysteinemia and elevated methylmalonic acid indicate a high prevalence of cobalamin deficiency in Asian Indians. *Am. J. Clin. Nutr.* **2001**, *74*, 233–241. [PubMed]
30. Antony, A.C. Prevalence of cobalamin (vitamin B-12) and folate deficiency in India—Audi alteram partem. *Am. J. Clin. Nutr.* **2001**, *74*, 233–241.
31. Clarke, R.; Refsum, H.; Birks, J.; Evans, J.G.; Johnston, C.; Sherliker, P.; Ueland, P.M.; Schneede, J.; McPartlin, J.; Nexo, E.; et al. Screening for vitamin B-12 and folate deficiency in older persons. *Am. J. Clin. Nutr.* **2003**, *77*, 1241–1247. [PubMed]
32. Clarke, R.; Sherliker, P.; Hin, H.; Nexo, E.; Hvas, A.M.; Schneede, J.; Birks, J.; Ueland, P.M.; Emmens, K.; Scott, J.M.; et al. Detection of vitamin B-12 deficiency in older people by measuring vitamin B-12 or the active fraction of vitamin B-12, holotranscobalamin. *Clin. Chem.* **2007**, *53*, 963–970. [CrossRef] [PubMed]
33. Clarke, R.; Grimley Evans, J.; Schneede, J.; Nexo, E.; Bates, C.; Fletcher, A.; Prentice, A.; Johnston, C.; Ueland, P.M.; Refsum, H.; et al. Vitamin B12 and folate deficiency in later life. *Age Ageing* **2004**, *33*, 34–41. [CrossRef] [PubMed]
34. Pfeiffer, C.M.; Caudill, S.P.; Gunter, E.W.; Osterloh, J.; Sampson, E.J. Biochemical indicators of B vitamin status in the US population after folic acid fortification: Results from the National Health and Nutrition Examination Survey 1999–2000. *Am. J. Clin. Nutr.* **2005**, *82*, 442–450. [PubMed]
35. Pfeiffer, C.M.; Johnson, C.L.; Jain, R.B.; Yetley, E.A.; Picciano, M.F.; Rader, J.I.; Fisher, K.D.; Mulinare, J.; Osterloh, J.D. Trends in blood folate and vitamin B-12 concentrations in the United States, 1988–2004. *Am. J. Clin. Nutr.* **2007**, *86*, 718–727. [PubMed]
36. MacFarlane, A.J.; Greene-Finestone, L.S.; Shi, Y. Vitamin B-12 and homocysteine status in a folate-replete population: Results from the Canadian Health Measures Survey. *Am. J. Clin. Nutr.* **2011**, *94*, 1079–1087. [CrossRef] [PubMed]
37. Green, T.J.; Venn, B.J.; Skeaff, C.M.; Williams, S.M. Serum vitamin B-12 concentrations and atrophic gastritis in older New Zealanders. *Eur. J. Clin. Nutr.* **2005**, *59*, 205–210. [CrossRef] [PubMed]
38. Loikas, S.; Koskinen, P.; Irjala, K.; Lopponen, M.; Isoaho, R.; Kivela, S.; Pelliniemi, T. Vitamin B12 deficiency in the aged: A population-based study. *Age Ageing* **2007**, *36*, 177–183. [CrossRef] [PubMed]
39. Carmel, R. Cobalamin, the stomach, and aging. *Am. J. Clin. Nutr.* **1997**, *66*, 750–759. [PubMed]
40. Hughes, C.F.; Ward, M.; Hoey, L.; McNulty, H. Vitamin B-12 and ageing: Current issues and interaction with folate. *Ann. Clin. Biochem.* **2013**, *50*, 315–329. [CrossRef] [PubMed]
41. Van Asselt, D.Z.B.; De Groot, L.C.P.G.M.; Van Staveren, W.A.; Blom, H.J.; Wevers, R.A.; Biemond, I.; Hoefnagels, W.H.L. Role of cobalamin intake and atrophic gastritis in mild cobalamin deficiency in older Dutch subjects. *Am. J. Clin. Nutr.* **1998**, *68*, 328–334. [PubMed]
42. Hannibal, L.; Lysne, V.; Bjørke-Monsen, A.L.; Behringer, S.; Grünert, S.C.; Spiekerkoetter, U.; Jacobsen, D.W.; Blom, H.J. Biomarkers and algorithms for the diagnosis of vitamin B12 deficiency. *Front. Mol. Biosci.* **2016**, *3*, 27. [CrossRef] [PubMed]
43. Valuck, R.J.; Ruscin, J.M. A case-control study on adverse effects: H2 blocker or proton pump inhibitor use and risk of vitamin B-12 deficiency in older adults. *J. Clin. Epidemiol.* **2004**, *57*, 422–428. [CrossRef] [PubMed]
44. Masclee, G.M.C.; Sturkenboom, M.C.J.M.; Kuipers, E.J. A Benefit-Risk Assessment of the Use of Proton Pump Inhibitors in the Elderly. *Drugs Aging* **2014**, *31*, 263–282. [CrossRef] [PubMed]
45. Lam, J.R.; Schneider, J.L.; Zhao, W.; Corley, D.A. Proton pump inhibitor and histamine 2 receptor antagonist use and vitamin B-12 deficiency. *JAMA* **2013**, *310*, 2435–2442. [CrossRef] [PubMed]
46. Chapman, L.E.; Darling, A.L.; Brown, J.E. Association between metformin and vitamin B12 deficiency in patients with type 2 diabetes: A systematic review and meta-analysis. *Diabetes Metab.* **2016**. [CrossRef] [PubMed]
47. Aroda, V.R.; Edelstein, S.L.; Goldberg, R.B.; Knowler, W.C.; Marcovina, S.M.; Orchard, T.J.; Bray, G.A.; Schade, D.S.; Temprosa, M.G.; White, N.H.; et al. Long-term metformin use and vitamin B12 deficiency in the diabetes prevention program outcomes study. *J. Clin. Endocrinol. Metab.* **2016**, *101*, 1754–1761. [CrossRef] [PubMed]
48. Haller, J. The vitamin status and its adequacy in the elderly: An international overview. *Int. J. Vitam. Nutr. Res.* **1999**, *69*, 160–168. [CrossRef] [PubMed]

49. Bates, C.; Pentieva, K.; Prentice, A.; Mansoor, M.; Finch, S. Plasma pyridoxal phosphate and pyridoxic acid and their relationship to plasma homocysteine in a representative sample of British men and women aged 65 years and over. *Br. J. Nutr.* **1999**, *81*, 191–201. [PubMed]
50. Morris, M.S.; Picciano, M.F.; Jacques, P.F.; Selhub, J. Plasma pyridoxal 5′-phosphate in the US population: The National Health and Nutrition Examination Survey, 2003–2004. *Am. J. Clin. Nutr.* **2008**, *87*, 1446–1454. [PubMed]
51. Ribayamercado, J.; Russell, R.; Sahyoun, N.; Morrow, F.; Gershoff, S. Vitamin-B6 requirements of elderly men and women. *J. Nutr.* **1991**, *121*, 1062–1074.
52. Van Den Berg, H. Vitamin B6 status and requirements in older adults. *Br. J. Nutr.* **1999**, *81*, 175–176. [PubMed]
53. Troesch, B.; Hoeft, B.; McBurney, M.; Eggersdorfer, M.; Weber, P. Dietary surveys indicate vitamin intakes below recommendations are common in representative Western countries. *Br. J. Nutr.* **2012**, *108*, 692–698. [CrossRef] [PubMed]
54. Bates, B.; Cox, L.; Page, S.; Prentice, A.; Steer, T.; Swan, G. *National Diet and Nutrition Survey: Results from Years 5 and 6 (Combined) of the Rolling Programme (2012/2013–2013/2014)*; Public Health England: London, UK, 2016.
55. Walton, J.; Flynn, A. *NANS: Food and Nutrient Intakes, Physical Measurements, Physical Activity Patterns and Food Choice Motives*; Irish Universities Nutrition Alliance: Dublin, Ireland, 2011; pp. 1–40.
56. Eussen, S.J.P.M.; De Groot, C.P.G.M.; Clarke, R.; Schneede, J.; Ueland, P.M.; Hoefnagels, W.H.L.; Van Staveren, W.A. Oral cyanocobalamin supplementation in older people with vitamin B-12 deficiency—A dose-finding trial. *Arch. Intern. Med.* **2005**, *165*, 1167–1172. [CrossRef] [PubMed]
57. McKinley, M.C.; McNulty, H.; McPartlin, J.; Strain, J.J.; Pentieva, K.; Ward, M.; Weir, D.G.; Scott, J.M. Low-dose vitamin B-6 effectively lowers fasting plasma homocysteine in healthy elderly persons who are folate and riboflavin replete. *Am. J. Clin. Nutr.* **2001**, *73*, 759–764. [PubMed]
58. McNulty, H.; Dowey, L.R.C.; Strain, J.J.; Dunne, A.; Ward, M.; Molloy, A.M.; McAnena, L.B.; Hughes, J.P.; Hannon-Fletcher, M.; Scott, J.M. Riboflavin lowers homocysteine in individuals homozygous for the *MTHFR 677C* → T polymorphism. *Circulation* **2006**, *113*, 74–80. [CrossRef] [PubMed]
59. Pfeiffer, C.; Fazili, Z.; Zhang, M. Folate analytical methodology. In *Folate in Health and Disease*, 2nd ed.; Bailey, L.B., Ed.; CRC Press: Boca Raton, FL, USA, 2010; pp. 517–574.
60. Mason, J.B. Biomarkers of nutrient exposure and status in one-carbon (methyl) metabolism. *J. Nutr.* **2003**, *133*, 941S–947S. [PubMed]
61. Clifford, A.J.; Noceti, E.M.; Block-Joy, A.; Block, T.; Block, G. Erythrocyte folate and its response to folic acid supplementation is assay dependent in women. *J. Nutr.* **2005**, *135*, 137–143. [PubMed]
62. Wu, A.; Chanarin, I.; Slavin, G.; Levi, A.J. Folate-Deficiency in alcoholic—Relationship to clinical and hematological abnormalities, liver-disease and folate stores. *Br. J. Haematol.* **1975**, *29*, 469–478. [CrossRef] [PubMed]
63. Duffy, M.E.; Hoey, L.; Hughes, C.F.; Strain, J.J.; Rankin, A.; Souverein, O.W.; Dullemeijer, C.; Collings, R.; Hooper, L.; McNulty, H. Biomarker responses to folic acid intervention in healthy adults: A meta-analysis of randomized controlled trials. *Am. J. Clin. Nutr.* **2014**, *99*, 96–106. [CrossRef] [PubMed]
64. Carmel, R. Current concepts in cobalamin deficiency. *Annu. Rev. Med.* **2000**, *51*, 357–375. [CrossRef] [PubMed]
65. Lindenbaum, J.; Rosenberg, I.H.; Wilson, P.W.F.; Stabler, S.P.; Allen, R.H. Prevalence of cobalamin deficiency in the Framingham elderly population. *Am. J. Clin. Nutr.* **1994**, *60*, 2–11. [PubMed]
66. Naurath, H.J.; Joosten, E.; Riezler, R.; Stabler, S.P.; Allen, R.H.; Lindenbaum, J. Effects of vitamin-B12, folate, and vitamin-B6 supplements in elderly people with normal serum vitamin concentrations. *Lancet* **1995**, *346*, 85–89. [CrossRef]
67. Carmel, R.; Green, R.; Jacobsen, D.W.; Rasmussen, K.; Florea, M.; Azen, C. Serum cobalamin, homocysteine, and methylmalonic acid concentrations in a multiethnic elderly population: Ethnic and sex differences in cobalamin and metabolite abnormalities. *Am. J. Clin. Nutr.* **1999**, *70*, 904–910. [PubMed]
68. Riedel, B.M.; Molloy, A.M.; Meyer, K.; Fredriksen, A.; Ulvik, A.; Schneede, J.; Nexo, E.; Hoff, G.; Ueland, P.M. Transcobalamin Polymorphism 67A → G, but Not 776C → G, Affects serum holotranscobalamin in a cohort of healthy middle-aged men and women. *J. Nutr.* **2011**, *141*, 1784–1790. [CrossRef] [PubMed]
69. Iqbal, N.; Azar, D.; Yun, Y.; Ghausi, O.; Ix, J.; Fitzgerald, R.L. Serum methylmalonic Acid and holotranscobalamin-II as markers for vitamin b12 deficiency in end-stage renal disease patients. *Ann. Clin. Lab. Sci.* **2013**, *43*, 243–249. [PubMed]

70. Carmel, R. Biomarkers of cobalamin (vitamin B-12) status in the epidemiologic setting: A critical overview of context, applications, and performance characteristics of cobalamin, methylmalonic acid, and holotranscobalamin II. *Am. J. Clin. Nutr.* **2011**, *94*, 348S–358S. [CrossRef] [PubMed]
71. Leklem, J.E. Vitamin-B6—A status-report. *J. Nutr.* **1990**, *120*, 1503–1507. [PubMed]
72. Ueland, P.M.; Ulvik, A.; Rios-Avila, L.; Midttun, O.; Gregory, J.F. Direct and functional biomarkers of vitamin b6 status. *Annu. Rev. Nutr.* **2015**, *35*, 33–70. [CrossRef] [PubMed]
73. Chiang, E.P.; Smith, D.E.; Selhub, J.; Dallal, G.; Wang, Y.C.; Roubenoff, R. Inflammation causes tissue-specific depletion of vitamin B-6. *Arthritis Res. Ther.* **2005**, *7*, R1254–R1262. [CrossRef] [PubMed]
74. Hoey, L.; McNulty, H.; Strain, J.J. Studies of biomarker responses to intervention with riboflavin: A systematic review. *Am. J. Clin. Nutr.* **2009**, *89*, 1960S–1980S. [CrossRef] [PubMed]
75. Yetley, E.A.; Johnson, C.L. Folate and vitamin B-12 biomarkers in NHANES: History of their measurement and use. *Am. J. Clin. Nutr.* **2011**, *94*, 322S–331S. [CrossRef] [PubMed]
76. Hoey, L.; Strain, J.J.; McNulty, H. Studies of biomarker responses to intervention with vitamin B-12: A systematic review of randomized controlled trials. *Am. J. Clin. Nutr.* **2009**, *89*, 1981S–1996S. [CrossRef] [PubMed]
77. Bisp, M.R.; Bor, M.V.; Heinsvig, E.M.; Kall, M.A.; Nexo, E. Determination of vitamin B6 vitamers and pyridoxic acid in plasma: Development and evaluation of a high-performance liquid chromatographic assay. *Anal. Biochem.* **2002**, *305*, 82–89. [CrossRef] [PubMed]
78. Apeland, T.; Mansoor, M.A.; Pentieva, K.; McNulty, H.; Strandjord, R.E. Fasting and post-methionine loading concentrations of homocysteine, vitamin B2, and vitamin B6 in patients on antiepileptic drugs. *Clin. Chem.* **2003**, *49*, 1005–1008. [CrossRef] [PubMed]
79. Reynolds, E. Vitamin B12, folic acid, and the nervous system. *Lancet Neurol.* **2006**, *5*, 949–960. [CrossRef]
80. Scott, J.; Weir, D. Folate/vitamin B12 inter-relationships. *Essays Biochem.* **1994**, *28*, 63–72. [PubMed]
81. Healton, E.; Brust, J.; Garrett, T.; Lindenbaum, J. Neurologic aspects of coabalmin deficiency. *Medicine* **1991**, *70*, 229–245. [CrossRef] [PubMed]
82. Rampersaud, G.C.; Kauwell, G.P.A.; Bailey, L.B. Folate: A key to optimizing health and reducing disease risk in the elderly. *J. Am. Coll. Nutr.* **2003**, *22*, 1–8. [CrossRef] [PubMed]
83. Homocysteine Studies Collaboration. Homocysteine and risk of ischemic heart disease and stroke: A meta-analysis. *JAMA* **2002**, *288*, 2015–2022.
84. Wald, D.S.; Law, M.; Morris, J.K. Homocysteine and cardiovascular disease: Evidence on causality from a meta-analysis. *Br. Med. J.* **2002**, *325*, 1202K–1206K. [CrossRef]
85. Smith, D.A.; Refsum, H. Homocysteine, B Vitamins, and Cognitive Impairment. *Annu. Rev. Nutr.* **2016**, *36*, 211–239. [CrossRef] [PubMed]
86. Wald, D.S.; Morris, J.K.; Wald, N.J. Reconciling the Evidence on Serum Homocysteine and Ischaemic Heart Disease: A Meta-Analysis. *PLoS ONE* **2011**, *6*, e16473. [CrossRef] [PubMed]
87. Wald, D.S.; Kasturiratne, A.; Simmonds, M. Serum homocysteine and dementia: Meta-analysis of eight cohort studies including 8669 participants. *Alzheimer's Dement.* **2011**, *7*, 412–417. [CrossRef] [PubMed]
88. Yang, H.; Lee, M.; Hong, K.; Ovbiagele, B.; Saver, J.L. Efficacy of folic acid supplementation in cardiovascular disease prevention: An updated meta-analysis of randomized controlled trials. *Eur. J. Intern. Med.* **2012**, *23*, 745–754. [CrossRef] [PubMed]
89. Enneman, A.W.; Swart, K.M.; Van Wijngaarden, J.P.; Zillikens, M.C.; Dhonukshe-Rutten, R.A.; De Groot, L.C.; Van Schoor, N.M.; Lips, P.; Van Meurs, J.B.; Uitterlinden, A.G.; et al. Association between plasma homocysteine and bone density and quality parameters in the elderly. *Bone* **2012**, *50*, S134. [CrossRef]
90. McNulty, H.; Strain, J.J.; Pentieva, K.; Ward, M. C-1 metabolism and CVD outcomes in older adults. *Proc. Nutr. Soc.* **2012**, *71*, 213–221. [CrossRef] [PubMed]
91. Toole, J.F.; Malinow, M.R.; Chambless, L.E.; Spence, J.D.; Pettigrew, L.C.; Howard, V.J.; Sides, E.G.; Wang, C.; Stampfer, M. Lowering homocysteine in patients with ischemic stroke to prevent recurrent stroke, myocardial infarction, and death: The Vitamin Intervention for Stroke Prevention (VISP) randomized controlled trial. *JAMA* **2004**, *291*, 565–575. [CrossRef] [PubMed]
92. Bonaa, K.H.; Njolstad, I.; Ueland, P.M.; Schirmer, H.; Tverdal, A.; Steigen, T.; Wang, H.; Nordrehaug, J.E.; Arnesen, E.; Rasmussen, K. Homocysteine lowering and cardiovascular events after acute myocardial infarction. *N. Engl. J. Med.* **2006**, *354*, 1578–1588. [CrossRef] [PubMed]
93. Lonn, E.; Yusuf, S.; Arnold, M.J.; Sheridan, P.; Pogue, J.; Micks, M.; McQueen, M.J.; Probstfield, J.; Fodor, G.;

Held, C.; et al. Homocysteine lowering with folic acid and B vitamins in vascular disease. *N. Engl. J. Med.* **2006**, *354*, 1567–1577. [PubMed]

94. Albert, C.M.; Cook, N.R.; Gaziano, J.M.; Zaharris, E.; MacFadyen, J.; Danielson, E.; Buring, J.E.; Manson, J.E. Effect of folic acid and B vitamins on risk of cardiovascular events and total mortality among women at high risk for cardiovascular disease: A randomized trial. *JAMA* **2008**, *299*, 2027–2036. [CrossRef] [PubMed]
95. Ebbing, M.; Bleie, O.; Ueland, P.M.; Nordrehaug, J.E.; Nilsen, D.W.; Vollset, S.E.; Refsum, H.; Pedersen, E.K.R.; Nygard, O. Mortality and cardiovascular events in patients treated with homocysteine-lowering B vitamins after coronary angiography—A Randomized controlled trial. *JAMA* **2008**, *300*, 795–804. [CrossRef] [PubMed]
96. Hankey, G.J.; Eikelboom, J.W.; Baker, R.I.; Gelavis, A.; Hickling, S.C.; Jamrozik, K.; Van Bockxmeer, F.M.; Vasikaran, S.; Hankey, G.J.; Chen, C.; et al. B vitamins in patients with recent transient ischaemic attack or stroke in the VITAmins TO Prevent Stroke (VITATOPS) trial: A randomised, double-blind, parallel, placebo-controlled trial. *Lancet Neurol.* **2010**, *9*, 855–865.
97. Clarke, R.; Bennett, D.A.; Parish, S.; Verhoef, P.; Dotsch-Klerk, M.; Lathrop, M.; Xu, P.; Nordestgaard, B.G.; Holm, H.; Hopewell, J.C.; et al. Homocysteine and Coronary Heart Disease: Meta-analysis of MTHFR Case-Control Studies, Avoiding Publication Bias. *PLoS Med.* **2012**, *9*, e1001177. [CrossRef] [PubMed]
98. Yang, Q.H.; Botto, L.D.; Erickson, J.D.; Berry, R.J.; Sambell, C.; Johansen, H.; Friedman, J.M. Improvement in stroke mortality in Canada and the United States, 1990 to 2002. *Circulation* **2006**, *113*, 1335–1343. [CrossRef] [PubMed]
99. Wang, X.; Qin, X.; Demirtas, H.; Li, J.; Mao, G.; Huo, Y.; Sun, N.; Liu, L.; Xu, X. Efficacy of folic acid supplementation in stroke prevention: A meta-analysis. *Lancet* **2007**, *369*, 1876–1882. [CrossRef]
100. Lee, M.; Hong, K.; Chang, S.; Saver, J.L. Efficacy of homocysteine-lowering therapy with folic acid in stroke prevention: A meta-analysis. *Stroke* **2010**, *41*, 1205–1212. [CrossRef] [PubMed]
101. Huo, Y.; Li, J.; Qin, X.; Huang, Y.; Wang, X.; Gottesman, R.F.; Tang, G.; Wang, B.; Chen, D.; He, M.; et al. Efficacy of folic acid therapy in primary prevention of stroke among adults with hypertension in China the CSPPT Randomized Clinical Trial. *JAMA* **2015**, *313*, 1325–1335. [CrossRef] [PubMed]
102. Li, Y.; Huang, T.; Zheng, Y.; Muka, T.; Troup, J.; Hu, F.B. Folic acid supplementation and the risk of cardiovascular diseases: A meta-Analysis of randomized controlled trials. *J. Am. Heart Assoc.* **2016**, *5*, e003768. [CrossRef] [PubMed]
103. Klerk, M.; Verhoef, P.; Clarke, R.; Blom, H.J.; Kok, F.J.; Schouten, E.G.; MTHFR Studies Collaboration Group. MTHFR 677C $\rightarrow$ T polymorphism and risk of coronary heart disease—A meta-analysis. *JAMA* **2002**, *288*, 2023–2031. [CrossRef] [PubMed]
104. Lewis, S.J.; Ebrahim, S.; Smith, G.D. Meta-analysis of MTHFR 677C $\rightarrow$ T polymorphism and coronary heart disease: Does totality of evidence support causal role for homocysteine and preventive potential of folate? *Br. Med. J.* **2005**, *331*, 1053A–1056A. [CrossRef] [PubMed]
105. Holmes, M.V.; Newcombe, P.; Hubacek, J.A.; Sofat, R.; Ricketts, S.L.; Cooper, J.; Breteler, M.M.B.; Bautista, L.E.; Sharma, P.; Whittaker, J.C.; et al. Effect modification by population dietary folate on the association between *MTHFR* genotype, homocysteine, and stroke risk: A meta-analysis of genetic studies and randomised trials. *Lancet* **2011**, *378*, 584–594. [CrossRef]
106. Niu, W.-Q.; You, Y.-G.; Qi, Y. Strong association of methylenetetrahydrofolate reductase gene *C677T* polymorphism with hypertension and hypertension-in-pregnancy in Chinese: A meta-analysis. *J. Hum. Hypertens.* **2012**, *26*, 259–267. [CrossRef] [PubMed]
107. Yang, K.; Jia, J.; Mao, L.; Men, C.; Tang, K.; Li, Y.; Ding, H.; Zhang, Y. Methylenetetrahydrofolate reductase *C677T* gene polymorphism and essential hypertension: A meta-analysis of 10,415 subjects. *Biomed. Rep.* **2014**, *2*, 699–708. [CrossRef] [PubMed]
108. Horigan, G.; McNulty, H.; Ward, M.; Strain, J.J.; Purvis, J.; Scott, J.M. Riboflavin lowers blood pressure in cardiovascular disease patients homozygous for the 677C $\rightarrow$ T polymorphism in MTHFR. *J. Hypertens.* **2010**, *28*, 478–486. [CrossRef] [PubMed]
109. Wilson, C.P.; Ward, M.; McNulty, H.; Strain, J.J.; Trouton, T.G.; Horigan, G.; Purvis, J.; Scott, J.M. Riboflavin offers a targeted strategy for managing hypertension in patients with the *MTHFR 677TT* genotype: A 4-y follow-up. *Am. J. Clin. Nutr.* **2012**, *95*, 766–772. [CrossRef] [PubMed]
110. Wilson, C.P.; McNulty, H.; Ward, M.; Strain, J.J.; Trouton, T.G.; Hoeft, B.A.; Weber, P.; Roos, F.F.; Horigan, G.; McAnena, L.; et al. Blood pressure in treated hypertensive individuals with the MTHFR 677TT genotype is

responsive to intervention with riboflavin: Findings of a targeted randomized trial. *Hypertension* **2013**, *61*, 1302–1308. [CrossRef] [PubMed]

111. Gjesdal, C.G.; Vollset, S.E.; Ueland, P.M.; Refsum, H.; Drevon, C.A.; Gjessing, H.K.; Tell, G.S. Plasma total homocysteine level and bone mineral density: The hordaland homocysteine study. *Arch. Intern. Med.* **2006**, *166*, 88–94. [CrossRef] [PubMed]
112. Morris, M.S.; Jacques, P.F.; Selhub, J. Relation between homocysteine and B-vitamin status indicators and bone mineral density in older Americans. *Bone* **2005**, *37*, 234–242. [CrossRef] [PubMed]
113. McLean, R.R.; Jacques, P.F.; Selhub, J.; Tucker, K.L.; Samelson, E.J.; Broe, K.E.; Hannan, M.T.; Cupples, L.A.; Kiel, D.P. Homocysteine as a predictive factor for hip fracture in older persons. *N. Engl. J. Med.* **2004**, *350*, 2042–2049. [CrossRef] [PubMed]
114. Yang, J.; Hu, X.; Zhang, Q.; Cao, H.; Wang, J.; Liu, B. Homocysteine level and risk of fracture: A meta-analysis and systematic review. *Bone* **2012**, *51*, 376–382. [CrossRef] [PubMed]
115. Van Wijngaarden, J.P.; Doets, E.L.; Szczecinska, A.; Souverein, O.W.; Duffy, M.E.; Dullemeijer, C.; Cavelaars, A.E.J.M.; Pietruszka, B.; Van't Veer, P.; Brzozowska, A.; et al. Vitamin B12, folate, homocysteine, and bone health in adults and elderly people: A systematic review with meta-analyses. *J. Nutr. Metab.* **2013**, *2013*, 486186. [CrossRef] [PubMed]
116. Cagnacci, A.; Baldassari, F.; Rivolta, G.; Arangino, S.; Volpe, A. Relation of homocysteine, folate, and vitamin B-12 to bone mineral density of postmenopausal women. *Bone* **2003**, *33*, 956–959. [CrossRef] [PubMed]
117. Tucker, K.L.; Hannan, M.T.; Qiao, N.; Jacques, P.F.; Selhub, J.; Cupples, L.A.; Kiel, D.P. Low plasma vitamin B12 is associated with lower BMD: The Framingham Osteoporosis Study. *J. Bone Miner. Res.* **2005**, *20*, 152–158. [CrossRef] [PubMed]
118. Gjesdal, C.G.; Vollset, S.E.; Ueland, P.M.; Refsum, H.; Meyer, H.E.; Tell, G.S. Plasma homocysteine, folate, and vitamin B 12 and the risk of hip fracture: The hordaland homocysteine study. *J. Bone Miner. Res.* **2007**, *22*, 747–756. [CrossRef] [PubMed]
119. Yazdanpanah, N.; Zillikens, M.C.; Rivadeneira, F.; De Jong, R.; Lindemans, J.; Uitterlinden, A.G.; Pols, H.A.P.; Van Meurs, J.B.J. Effect of dietary B vitamins on BMD and risk of fracture in elderly men and women: The Rotterdam Study. *Bone* **2007**, *41*, 987–994. [CrossRef] [PubMed]
120. Dhonukshe-Rutten, R.A.M.; De Vries, J.H.M.; De Bree, A.; Van Der Put, N.; Van Staveren, W.A.; De Groot, L.C.P.G.M. Dietary intake and status of folate and vitamin B12 and their association with homocysteine and cardiovascular disease in European populations. *Eur. J. Clin. Nutr.* **2009**, *63*, 18–30. [CrossRef] [PubMed]
121. Dai, Z.; Wang, R.; Ang, L.W.; Yuan, J.-M.; Koh, W.-P. Dietary B vitamin intake and risk of hip fracture: The Singapore Chinese Health Study. *Osteoporos. Int.* **2013**, *24*, 2049–2059. [CrossRef] [PubMed]
122. McLean, R.R.; Jacques, P.F.; Selhub, J.; Fredman, L.; Tucker, K.L.; Samelson, E.J.; Kiel, D.P.; Cupples, L.A.; Hannan, M.T. Plasma B vitamins, homocysteine, and their relation with bone loss and hip fracture in elderly men and women. *J. Clin. Endocrinol. Metab.* **2008**, *93*, 2206–2212. [CrossRef] [PubMed]
123. Rumbak, I.; Zizic, V.; Sokolic, L.; Cvijetic, S.; Kajfez, R.; Baric, I.C. Bone mineral density is not associated with homocysteine level, folate and vitamin B-12 status. *Arch. Gynecol. Obstet.* **2012**, *285*, 991–1000. [CrossRef] [PubMed]
124. Zhu, K.; Beilby, J.; Dick, I.M.; Devine, A.; Soos, M.; Prince, R.L. The effects of homocysteine and *MTHFR* genotype on hip bone loss and fracture risk in elderly women. *Osteoporos. Int.* **2009**, *20*, 1183–1191. [CrossRef] [PubMed]
125. Sato, Y.; Honda, Y.; Iwamoto, J.; Kanoko, T.; Satoh, K. Effect of folate and mecobalamin on hip fractures in patients with stroke: A randomized controlled trial. *JAMA* **2005**, *293*, 1082–1088. [CrossRef] [PubMed]
126. Sawka, A.M.; Ray, J.G.; Yi, Q.; Josse, R.G.; Lonn, E. Randomized clinical trial of homocysteine level-lowering therapy and fractures. *Arch. Intern. Med.* **2007**, *167*, 2136–2139. [CrossRef] [PubMed]
127. Gommans, J.; Yi, Q.; Eikelboom, J.W.; Hankey, G.J.; Chen, C.; Rodgers, H.; VITATOPS Trial Study Group. The effect of homocysteine-lowering with B-vitamins on osteoporotic fractures in patients with cerebrovascular disease: Substudy of VITATOPS, a randomised placebo-controlled trial. *BMC Geriatr.* **2013**, *13*, 88. [CrossRef] [PubMed]
128. Enneman, A.W.; Swart, K.M.A.; Van Wijngaarden, J.P.; Van Dijk, S.C.; Ham, A.C.; Brouwer-Brolsma, E.M.; Van Der Zwaluw, N.L.; Dhonukshe-Rutten, R.A.M.; van der Cammen, T.J.M.; De Groot, L.C.P.G.M.; et al. Effect of vitamin b12 and folic acid supplementation on bone mineral density and quantitative ultrasound

parameters in older people with an elevated plasma homocysteine level: B-PROOF, a randomized controlled trial. *Calcif. Tissue Int.* **2015**, *96*, 401–409. [CrossRef] [PubMed]

129. Van Wijngaarden, J.P.; Swart, K.M.A.; Enneman, A.W.; Dhonukshe-Rutten, R.A.M.; Van Dijk, S.C.; Ham, A.C.; Brouwer-Brolsma, E.M.; Van der Zwaluw, N.L.; Sohl, E.; Van Meurs, J.B.J.; et al. Effect of daily vitamin B-12 and folic acid supplementation on fracture incidence in elderly individuals with an elevated plasma homocysteine concentration: B-PROOF, a randomized controlled trial. *Am. J. Clin. Nutr.* **2014**, *100*, 1578–1586. [CrossRef] [PubMed]
130. Wolffe, A.P.; Matzke, M.A. Epigenetics: Regulation through repression. *Science* **1999**, *286*, 481–486. [CrossRef] [PubMed]
131. Robertson, K.D.; Wolffe, A.P. DNA methylation in health and disease. *Nat. Rev. Genet.* **2000**, *1*, 11–19. [CrossRef] [PubMed]
132. Kass, S.U.; Pruss, D.; Wolffe, A.P. How does DNA methylation repress transcription? *Trends Genet.* **1997**, *13*, 444–449. [CrossRef]
133. Bird, A.P.; Wolffe, A.P. Methylation-induced repression—Belts, braces, and chromatin. *Cell* **1999**, *99*, 451–454. [CrossRef]
134. Jones, P.A.; Takai, D. The role of DNA methylation in mammalian epigenetics. *Science* **2001**, *293*, 1068–1070. [CrossRef] [PubMed]
135. Abrahamsen, B.; Madsen, J.S.; Tofteng, C.L.; Stilgren, L.; Bladbjerg, E.M.; Kristensen, S.R.; Brixen, K.; Mosekilde, L. A common methylenetetrahydrofolate reductase (*C677T*) polymorphism is associated with low bone mineral density and increased fracture incidence after menopause: Longitudinal data from the Danish osteoporosis prevention study. *J. Bone Miner. Res.* **2003**, *18*, 723–729. [CrossRef] [PubMed]
136. Miyao, M.; Morita, H.; Hosoi, T.; Kurihara, H.; Inoue, S.; Hoshino, S.; Shiraki, M.; Yazaki, Y.; Ouchi, Y. Association of methylenetetrahydrofolate reductase (*MTHFR*) polymorphism with bone mineral density in postmenopausal Japanese women. *Calcif. Tissue Int.* **2000**, *66*, 190–194. [CrossRef] [PubMed]
137. Hong, X.; Hsu, Y.; Terwedow, H.; Tang, G.; Liu, X.; Jiang, S.; Xu, X.; Xu, X. Association of the methylenetetrahydrofolate reductase *C677T* polymorphism and fracture risk in Chinese postmenopausal women. *Bone* **2007**, *40*, 737–742. [CrossRef] [PubMed]
138. Wang, H.; Liu, C. Association of *MTHFR C667T* polymorphism with bone mineral density and fracture risk: An updated meta-analysis. *Osteoporos. Int.* **2012**, *23*, 2625–2634. [CrossRef] [PubMed]
139. Macdonald, H.M.; McGuigan, F.E.; Fraser, W.D.; New, S.A.; Ralston, S.H.; Reid, D.M. Methylenetetrahydrofolate reductase polymorphism interacts with riboflavin intake to influence bone mineral density. *Bone* **2004**, *35*, 957–964. [CrossRef] [PubMed]
140. McLean, R.R.; Karasik, D.; Selhub, J.; Tucker, K.L.; Ordovas, J.M.; Russo, G.T.; Cupples, L.A.; Jacques, P.F.; Kiel, D.P. Association of a common polymorphism in the methylenetetrahydrofolate reductase (*MTHFR*) gene with bone phenotypes depends on plasma folate status. *J. Bone Miner. Res.* **2004**, *19*, 410–418. [CrossRef] [PubMed]
141. Abrahamsen, B.; Madsen, J.S.; Tofteng, C.L.; Stilgren, L.; Bladbjerg, E.M.; Kristensen, S.R.; Brixen, K.; Mosekilde, L. Are effects of MTHFR (C677T) genotype on BMD confined to women with low folate and riboflavin intake? Analysis of food records from the Danish osteoporosis prevention study. *Bone* **2005**, *36*, 577–583. [CrossRef] [PubMed]
142. Yazdanpanah, N.; Uitterlinden, A.G.; Zillikens, M.C.; Jhamai, M.; Rivadeneira, F.; Hofman, A.; De Jonge, R.; Lindemans, J.; Pols, H.A.; Van Meurs, J.B. Low dietary riboflavin but not folate predicts increased fracture risk in postmenopausal women homozygous for the *MTHFR 677 T* allele. *J. Bone Miner. Res.* **2008**, *23*, 86–94. [CrossRef] [PubMed]
143. Hedden, T.; Gabrieli, J. Insights into the ageing mind: A view from cognitive neuroscience. *Nat. Rev. Neurosci.* **2004**, *5*, 87–96. [CrossRef] [PubMed]
144. Park, D.C.; Reuter-Lorenz, P. The Adaptive Brain: Aging and Neurocognitive Scaffolding. *Annu. Rev. Psychol.* **2009**, *60*, 173–196. [CrossRef] [PubMed]
145. Busse, A.; Bischkopf, J.; Riedel-Heller, S.G.; Angermeyer, M.C. Mild cognitive impairment: Prevalence and incidence according to different diagnostic criteria. Results of the Leipzig Longitudinal Study of the Aged (LEILA75+). *Br. J. Psychiatry* **2003**, *182*, 449–454. [CrossRef] [PubMed]
146. Gauthier, S.; Reisberg, B.; Zaudig, M.; Petersen, R.C.; Ritchie, K.; Broich, K.; Belleville, S.; Brodaty, H.; Bennett, D.; Chertkow, H.; et al. Mild cognitive impairment. *Lancet* **2006**, *367*, 1262–1270. [CrossRef]

147. Esiri, M.; Matthews, F.; Brayne, C.; Ince, P.; Matthews, F.; Xuereb, J.; Broome, J.; McKenzie, J.; Rossi, M.; McKeith, I.; et al. Pathological correlates of late-onset dementia in a multicentre, community-based population in England and Wales. *Lancet* **2001**, *357*, 169–175.

148. Stevens, T.; Livingston, G.; Kitchen, G.; Manela, M.; Walker, Z.; Katona, C. Islington study of dementia subtypes in the community. *Br. J. Psychiatry* **2002**, *180*, 270–276. [CrossRef] [PubMed]

149. Gorelick, P.B.; Scuteri, A.; Black, S.E.; DeCarli, C.; Greenberg, S.M.; Iadecola, C.; Launer, L.J.; Laurent, S.; Lopez, O.L.; Nyenhuis, D.; et al. Vascular contributions to cognitive impairment and dementia: A statement for healthcare professionals from the American Heart Association/American Stroke Association. *Stroke* **2011**, *42*, 2672–2713. [CrossRef] [PubMed]

150. Van der Flier, W.; Scheltens, P. Epidemiology and risk factors of dementia. *J. Neurol. Neurosurg. Psychiatry* **2005**, *76*, V2–V7. [CrossRef] [PubMed]

151. Barber, R.; Panikkar, A.; McKeith, I. Dementia with Lewy bodies: Diagnosis and management. *Int. J. Geriatr. Psychiatry* **2001**, *16*, S12–S18. [CrossRef]

152. Querfurth, H.W.; LaFerla, F.M. Alzheimer's Disease. *N. Engl. J. Med.* **2010**, *362*, 329–344. [CrossRef] [PubMed]

153. O'Brien, J.; Paling, S.; Barber, R.; Williams, E.; Ballard, C.; McKeith, I.; Gholkar, A.; Crum, W.; Rossor, M.; Fox, N. Progressive brain atrophy on serial MRI in dementia with Lewy bodies, AD, and vascular dementia. *Neurology* **2001**, *56*, 1386–1388. [CrossRef] [PubMed]

154. De Wilde, M.C.; Kamphuis, P.J.G.H.; Sijben, J.W.C.; Scheltens, P. Utility of imaging for nutritional intervention studies in Alzheimer's disease. *Eur. J. Pharmacol.* **2011**, *668*, S59–S69. [CrossRef] [PubMed]

155. Miller, J.W.; Green, R.; Mungas, D.M.; Reed, B.R.; Jagust, W.J. Homocysteine, vitamin B6, and vascular disease in AD patients. *Neurology* **2002**, *58*, 1471–1475. [CrossRef] [PubMed]

156. Smith, A.D. The worldwide challenge of the dementias: A role for B vitamins and homocysteine? *Food Nutr. Bull.* **2008**, *29*, S143–S172. [CrossRef] [PubMed]

157. Oulhaj, A.; Refsum, H.; Beaumont, H.; Williams, J.; King, E.; Jacoby, R.; Smith, A.D. Homocysteine as a predictor of cognitive decline in Alzheimer's disease. *Int. J. Geriatr. Psychiatry* **2010**, *25*, 82–90. [CrossRef] [PubMed]

158. Nie, T.; Lu, T.; Xie, L.; Huang, P.; Lu, Y.; Jiang, M. Hyperhomocysteinemia and risk of cognitive decline: A meta-analysis of prospective cohort studies. *Eur. Neurol.* **2014**, *72*, 241–248. [PubMed]

159. Beydoun, M.A.; Beydoun, H.A.; Gamaldo, A.A.; Teel, A.; Zonderman, A.B.; Wang, Y. Epidemiologic studies of modifiable factors associated with cognition and dementia: Systematic review and meta-analysis. *BMC Public Health* **2014**, *14*, 643. [CrossRef] [PubMed]

160. Horvat, P.; Gardiner, J.; Kubinova, R.; Pajak, A.; Tamosiunas, A.; Schoettker, B.; Pikhart, H.; Peasey, A.; Jansen, E.; Bobak, M. Serum folate, vitamin B-12 and cognitive function in middle and older age: The HAPIEE study. *Exp. Gerontol.* **2016**, *76*, 33–38. [CrossRef] [PubMed]

161. De Lau, L.M.L.; Refsum, H.; Smith, A.D.; Johnston, C.; Breteler, M.M.B. Plasma folate concentration and cognitive performance: Rotterdam scan study. *Am. J. Clin. Nutr.* **2007**, *86*, 728–734. [PubMed]

162. Hooshmand, B.; Solomon, A.; Kareholt, I.; Rusanen, M.; Hanninen, T.; Leiviska, J.; Winblad, B.; Laatikainen, T.; Soininen, H.; Kivipelto, M. Associations between serum homocysteine, holotranscobalamin, folate and cognition in the elderly: A longitudinal study. *J. Intern. Med.* **2012**, *271*, 204–212. [CrossRef] [PubMed]

163. Brown, B.; Huang, M.H.; Karlamangla, A.; Seeman, T.; Kado, D. Do the effects of APOE-epsilon4 on cognitive function and decline depend upon vitamin status? MacArthur Studies of Successful Aging. *J. Nutr. Health Aging* **2011**, *15*, 196–201. [CrossRef] [PubMed]

164. Kim, J.; Stewart, R.; Kim, S.; Shin, I.; Yang, S.; Shin, H.; Yoon, J. Changes in folate, vitamin B12 and homocysteine associated with incident dementia. *J. Neurol. Neurosurg. Psychiatry* **2008**, *79*, 864–868. [CrossRef] [PubMed]

165. Erickson, K.I.; Suever, B.L.; Prakash, R.S.; Colcombe, S.J.; McAuley, E.; Kramer, A.F. Greater intake of vitamins B6 and B12 spares gray matter in healthy elderly: A voxel-based morphometry study. *Brain Res.* **2008**, *1199*, 20–26. [CrossRef] [PubMed]

166. Moorthy, D.; Peter, I.; Scott, T.M.; Parnell, L.D.; Lai, C.; Crott, J.W.; Ordovas, J.M.; Selhub, J.; Griffith, J.; Rosenberg, I.H.; et al. Status of vitamins B-12 and B-6 but not of folate, homocysteine, and the methylenetetrahydrofolate reductase *C677T* polymorphism are associated with impaired cognition and depression in adults. *J. Nutr.* **2012**, *142*, 1554–1560. [CrossRef] [PubMed]

167. Mooijaart, S.P.; Gussekloo, J.; Frolich, M.; Jolles, J.; Stott, D.J.; Westendorp, R.G.J.; De Craen, A.J.M. Homocysteine, vitamin B-12, and folic acid and the risk of cognitive decline in old age: The Leiden 85-Plus study. *Am. J. Clin. Nutr.* **2005**, *82*, 866–871. [PubMed]

168. Kang, J.H.; Irizarry, M.C.; Grodstein, F. Prospective study of plasma folate, vitamin B12, and cognitive function and decline. *Epidemiology* **2006**, *17*, 650–657. [CrossRef] [PubMed]

169. Clarke, R.; Birks, J.; Nexo, E.; Ueland, P.M.; Schneede, J.; Scott, J.; Molloy, A.; Evans, J.G. Low vitamin B-12 status and risk of cognitive decline in older adults. *Am. J. Clin. Nutr.* **2007**, *86*, 1384–1391. [PubMed]

170. Haan, M.N.; Miller, J.W.; Aiello, A.E.; Whitmer, R.A.; Jagust, W.J.; Mungas, D.M.; Allen, L.H.; Green, R. Homocysteine, B vitamins, and the incidence of dementia and cognitive impairment: Results from the Sacramento Area Latino Study on Aging. *Am. J. Clin. Nutr.* **2007**, *85*, 511–517. [PubMed]

171. Lildballe, D.L.; Fedosov, S.; Sherliker, P.; Hin, H.; Clarke, R.; Nexo, E. Association of cognitive impairment with combinations of vitamin B12-related parameters. *Clin. Chem.* **2011**, *57*, 1436–1443. [CrossRef] [PubMed]

172. Tangney, C.C.; Tang, Y.; Evans, D.A.; Morris, M.C. Biochemical indicators of vitamin B12 and folate insufficiency and cognitive decline. *Neurology* **2009**, *72*, 361–367. [CrossRef] [PubMed]

173. Morris, M.S.; Selhub, J.; Jacques, P.F. Vitamin B-12 and folate status in relation to decline in scores on the mini-mental state examination in the Framingham heart study. *J. Am. Geriatr. Soc.* **2012**, *60*, 1457–1464. [CrossRef] [PubMed]

174. O'Leary, F.; Allman-Farinelli, M.; Samman, S. Vitamin B12 status, cognitive decline and dementia: A systematic review of prospective cohort studies. *Br. J. Nutr.* **2012**, *108*, 1948–1961. [CrossRef] [PubMed]

175. Kado, D.M.; Karlamangla, A.S.; Huang, M.; Troen, A.; Rowe, J.W.; Selhub, J.; Seeman, T.E. Homocysteine versus the vitamins folate, B6, and B12 as predictors of cognitive function and decline in older high-functioning adults: MacArthur Studies of Successful Aging. *Am. J. Med.* **2005**, *118*, 161–167. [CrossRef] [PubMed]

176. Riggs, K.M.; Spiro, A.; Tucker, K.; Rush, D. Relations of vitamin B-12, vitamin B-6, folate, and homocysteine to cognitive performance in the normative aging study. *Am. J. Clin. Nutr.* **1996**, *63*, 306–314. [PubMed]

177. Tucker, K.L.; Qiao, N.; Scott, T.; Rosenberg, I.; Spiro, A. High homocysteine and low B vitamins predict cognitive decline in aging men: The Veterans affairs normative aging study. *Am. J. Clin. Nutr.* **2005**, *82*, 627–635. [PubMed]

178. Corrada, M.M.; Kawas, C.H.; Hallfrisch, J.; Muller, D.; Brookmeyer, R. Reduced risk of Alzheimer's disease with high folate intake: The Baltimore Longitudinal Study of Aging. *Alzheimer's Dement. J. Alzheimer's Assoc.* **2005**, *1*, 11–18. [CrossRef] [PubMed]

179. Xiu, L.; Lee, M.; Wahlqvist, M.L.; Chen, R.C.; Huang, Y.; Chen, K.; Li, D. Low and high homocysteine are associated with mortality independent of B group vitamins but interactive with cognitive status in a free-living elderly cohort. *Nutr. Res.* **2012**, *32*, 928–939. [CrossRef] [PubMed]

180. Wald, D.S.; Kasturiratne, A.; Simmonds, M. Effect of folic acid, with or without other B vitamins, on cognitive decline: Meta-analysis of randomized trials. *Am. J. Med.* **2010**, *123*, 522–527. [CrossRef] [PubMed]

181. Clarke, R.; Bennett, D.; Parish, S.; Lewington, S.; Skeaff, M.; Eussen, S.J.P.M.; Lewerin, C.; Stott, D.J.; Armitage, J.; Hankey, G.J.; et al. Effects of homocysteine lowering with B vitamins on cognitive aging: Meta-analysis of 11 trials with cognitive data on 22,000 individuals. *Am. J. Clin. Nutr.* **2014**, *100*, 657–666. [CrossRef] [PubMed]

182. McCaddon, A.; Miller, J.W. Assessing the association between homocysteine and cognition: Reflections on Bradford Hill, meta-analyses, and causality. *Nutr. Rev.* **2015**, *73*, 723–735. [CrossRef] [PubMed]

183. Smith, D.; de Jager, C.; Refsum, H.; Rosenberg, I.H. B-vitamin trials meta-analysis: Less than meets the eye. *Am. J. Clin. Nutr.* **2015**, *101*, 415–416. [CrossRef] [PubMed]

184. Garrard, P.; Jacoby, R. Homocysteine lowering, B vitamins, and cognitive aging. *Am. J. Clin. Nutr.* **2015**, *101*, 414–415. [CrossRef] [PubMed]

185. Van der Zwaluw, N.L.; Dhonukshe-Rutten, R.A.M.; Van Wijngaarden, J.P.; Brouwer-Brolsma, E.M.; Van De Rest, O.; In't Veld, P.H.; Enneman, A.W.; Van Dijk, S.C.; Ham, A.C.; Swart, K.M.A.; et al. Results of 2-year vitamin B treatment on cognitive performance: Secondary data from an RCT. *Neurology* **2014**, *83*, 2158–2166. [CrossRef] [PubMed]

186. Durga, J.; Van Boxtel, M.P.J.; Schouten, E.G.; Kok, F.J.; Jolles, J.; Katan, M.B.; Verhoef, P. Effect of 3-year folic acid supplementation on cognitive function in older adults in the FACIT trial: A randomised, double blind, controlled trial. *Lancet* **2007** *369*, 208–216. [CrossRef]

187. Walker, J.G.; Batterham, P.J.; Mackinnon, A.J.; Jorm, A.F.; Hickie, I.; Fenech, M.; Kljakovic, M.; Crisp, D.; Christensen, H. Oral folic acid and vitamin B-12 supplementation to prevent cognitive decline in community-dwelling older adults with depressive symptoms—The beyond ageing project: A randomized controlled trial. *Am. J. Clin. Nutr.* **2012**, *95*, 194–203. [CrossRef] [PubMed]
188. Douaud, G.; Refsum, H.; de Jager, C.A.; Jacoby, R.; Nichols, T.E.; Smith, S.M.; Smith, A.D. Preventing Alzheimer's disease-related gray matter atrophy by B-vitamin treatment. *Proc. Natl. Acad. Sci. USA* **2013**, *110*, 9523–9528. [CrossRef] [PubMed]
189. Kwok, T.; Lee, J.; Law, C.B.; Pan, P.C.; Yung, C.Y.; Choi, K.C.; Lam, L.C. A randomized placebo controlled trial of homocysteine lowering to reduce cognitive decline in older demented people. *Clin. Nutr.* **2011**, *30*, 297–302. [CrossRef] [PubMed]
190. Kang, J.H.; Cook, N.; Manson, J.; Buring, J.E.; Albert, C.M.; Grodstein, F. A trial of B vitamins and cognitive function among women at high risk of cardiovascular disease. *Am. J. Clin. Nutr.* **2008**, *88*, 1602–1610. [CrossRef] [PubMed]
191. McMahon, J.A.; Green, T.J.; Skeaff, C.M.; Knight, R.G.; Mann, J.I.; Williams, S.M. A controlled trial of homocysteine lowering and cognitive performance. *N. Engl. J. Med.* **2006**, *354*, 2764–2772. [CrossRef] [PubMed]
192. Balk, E.M.; Raman, G.; Tatsioni, A.; Chung, M.; Lau, J.; Rosenberg, I.H. Vitamin B-6, B-12, and folic acid supplementation and cognitive function—A systematic review of randomized trials. *Arch. Intern. Med.* **2007**, *167*, 21–30. [CrossRef] [PubMed]
193. Brady, C.B.; Gaziano, J.M.; Cxypoliski, R.A.; Guarino, P.D.; Kaufman, J.S.; Warren, S.R.; Hartigan, P.; Goldfarb, D.S.; Jamison, R.L. Homocysteine lowering and cognition in CKD: The Veterans Affairs homocysteine study. *Am. J. Kidney Dis.* **2009**, *54*, 440–449. [CrossRef] [PubMed]
194. Ford, A.H.; Flicker, L.; Alfonso, H.; Thomas, J.; Clarnette, R.; Martins, R.; Almeida, O.P. Vitamins B(12), B(6), and folic acid for cognition in older men. *Neurology* **2010**, *75*, 1540–1547. [CrossRef] [PubMed]
195. De Jager, C.A.; Oulhaj, A.; Jacoby, R.; Refsum, H.; Smith, A.D. Cognitive and clinical outcomes of homocysteine-lowering B-vitamin treatment in mild cognitive impairment: A randomized controlled trial. *Int. J. Geriatr. Psychiatry* **2012**, *27*, 592–600. [CrossRef] [PubMed]
196. Smith, A.D.; Smith, S.M.; de Jager, C.A.; Whitbread, P.; Johnston, C.; Agacinski, G.; Oulhaj, A.; Bradley, K.M.; Jacoby, R.; Refsum, H. Homocysteine-lowering by B vitamins slows the rate of accelerated brain atrophy in mild cognitive impairment: A randomized controlled trial. *PLoS ONE* **2010**, *5*, e1224. [CrossRef] [PubMed]
197. Tsai, S.; Hong, C.; Yeh, H.; Liou, Y.; Yang, A.C.; Liu, M.; Hwang, J. Heterozygote advantage of the *MTHFR C677T* Polymorphism on specific cognitive performance in elderly Chinese males without dementia. *Dement. Geriatr. Cogn. Disord.* **2011**, *32*, 159–163. [CrossRef] [PubMed]
198. Ford, A.H.; Flicker, L.; Hankey, G.J.; Norman, P.; van Bockxmeer, F.M.; Almeida, O.P. Homocysteine, methylenetetrahydrofolate reductase *C677T* polymorphism and cognitive impairment: The health in men study. *Mol. Psychiatry* **2012**, *17*, 559–566. [CrossRef] [PubMed]
199. Rai, V. Methylenetetrahydrofolate Reductase (MTHFR) C677T Polymorphism and Alzheimer Disease Risk: A meta-analysis. *Mol. Neurobiol.* **2016**. [CrossRef] [PubMed]
200. Liu, H.; Yang, M.; Li, G.; Qiu, Y.; Zheng, J.; Du, X.; Wang, J.; Liu, R. The *MTHFR C677T* polymorphism contributes to an increased risk for vascular dementia: A meta-analysis. *J. Neurol. Sci.* **2010**, *294*, 74–80. [CrossRef] [PubMed]
201. Hua, Y.; Zhao, H.; Kong, Y.; Ye, M. Association between the *MTHFR* Gene and Alzheimer's Disease: A meta-analysis. *Int. J. Neurosci.* **2011**, *121*, 462–471. [CrossRef] [PubMed]
202. Hooshmand, B.; Mangialasche, F.; Kalpouzos, G.; Solomon, A.; Kareholt, I.; Smith, A.D.; Refsum, H.; Wang, R.; Muhlmann, M.; Ertl-Wagner, B.; et al. Association of vitamin B12, folate, and sulfur amino acids with brain magnetic resonance imaging measures in older adults: A longitudinal population-based study. *JAMA Psychiatry* **2016**, *73*, 606–613. [CrossRef] [PubMed]
203. Kobe, T.; Witte, A.V.; Schnelle, A.; Grittner, U.; Tesky, V.A.; Pantel, J.; Schuchardt, J.P.; Hahn, A.; Bohlken, J.; Rujescu, D.; et al. Vitamin B-12 concentration, memory performance, and hippocampal structure in patients with mild cognitive impairment. *Am. J. Clin. Nutr.* **2016**, *103*, 1045–1054. [CrossRef] [PubMed]
204. Vogiatzoglou, A.; Refsum, H.; Johnston, C.; Smith, S.M.; Bradley, K.M.; De Jager, C.; Budge, M.M.; Smith, A.D. Vitamin B12 status and rate of brain volume loss in community-dwelling elderly. *Neurology* **2008**, *71*, 826–832. [CrossRef] [PubMed]

205. Tangney, C.C.; Aggarwal, N.T.; Li, H.; Wilson, R.S.; Decarli, C.; Evans, D.A.; Morris, M.C. Vitamin B12, cognition, and brain *MRI* measures: A cross-sectional examination. *Neurology* **2011**, *77*, 1276–1282. [CrossRef] [PubMed]
206. De Lau, L.M.L.; Smith, A.D.; Refsum, H.; Johnston, C.; Breteler, M.M.B. Plasma vitamin B12 status and cerebral white-matter lesions. *J. Neurol. Neurosurg. Psychiatry* **2009**, *80*, 149–157. [CrossRef] [PubMed]
207. Gallucci, M.; Zanardo, A.; Bendini, M.; Di Paola, F.; Boldrini, P.; Grossi, E. Serum folate, homocysteine, brain atrophy, and auto-CM system: The Treviso Dementia (TREDEM) study. *J. Alzheimer's Dis.* **2014**, *38*, 581–587.
208. Maestu, F.; Campo, P.; Del Rio, D.; Moratti, S.; Gil-Gregorio, P.; Fernandez, A.; Capilla, A.; Ortiz, T. Increased biomagnetic activity in the ventral pathway in mild cognitive impairment. *Clin. Neurophysiol.* **2008**, *119*, 1320–1327. [CrossRef] [PubMed]
209. Lipton, S.A.; Kim, W.K.; Choi, Y.B.; Kumar, S.; DEmilia, D.M.; Rayudu, P.V.; Arnelle, D.R.; Stamler, J.S. Neurotoxicity associated with dual actions of homocysteine at the *N*-methyl-D-aspartate receptor. *Proc. Natl. Acad. Sci. USA* **1997**, *94*, 5923–5928. [CrossRef] [PubMed]
210. Kennedy, B.P.; Bottiglieri, T.; Arning, E.; Ziegler, M.G.; Hansen, L.A.; Masliah, E. Elevated *S*-adenosylhomocysteine in Alzheimer brain: Influence on methyltransferases and cognitive function. *J. Neural Transm.* **2004**, *111*, 547–567. [CrossRef] [PubMed]
211. Fuso, A.; Seminara, L.; Cavallaro, R.A.; D'Anselmi, F.; Scarpa, S. *S*-adenosylmethionine/homocysteine cycle alterations modify DNA methylation status with consequent deregulation of *PS1* and *BACE* and beta-amyloid production. *Mol. Cell. Neurosci.* **2005**, *28*, 195–204. [CrossRef] [PubMed]
212. Duthie, S.J.; Narayanan, S.; Brand, G.M.; Pirie, L.; Grant, G. Impact of folate deficiency on DNA stability. *J. Nutr.* **2002**, *132*, 2444S–2449S. [PubMed]
213. Kruman, I.I.; Kumaravel, T.S.; Lohani, A.; Pedersen, W.A.; Cutler, R.G.; Kruman, Y.; Haughey, N.; Lee, J.; Evans, M.; Mattson, M.P. Folic acid deficiency and homocysteine impair DNA repair in hippocampal neurons and sensitize them to amyloid toxicity in experimental models of Alzheimer's disease. *J. Neurosci.* **2002**, *22*, 1752–1762. [PubMed]
214. Kruman, I.I.; Culmsee, C.; Chan, S.L.; Mattson, M.P. Folic acid deficiency and homocysteine induce neuronal apoptosis. *Soc. Neurosci.* **2000**, *26*, 93.
215. Selhub, J.; Troen, A.; Rosenberg, I.H. B vitamins and the aging brain. *Nutr. Rev.* **2010**, *68*, S112–S118. [CrossRef] [PubMed]
216. Bernstein, A.L. Vitamin B6 in clinical neurology. *Ann. N. Y. Acad. Sci.* **1990**, *585*, 250–260. [CrossRef] [PubMed]
217. Tracy, R.P. Emerging relationships of inflammation, cardiovascular disease and chronic diseases of aging. *Int. J. Obes.* **2003**, *27*, S29–S34. [CrossRef] [PubMed]
218. Dik, M.; Ferrucci, L. Chronic inflammation and common geriatric syndromes: The longitudinal aging study Amsterdam. *Gerontologist* **2005**, *45*, 654–656.
219. Van Oijen, M.; de Jong, F.J.; Witteman, J.C.M.; Hofman, A.; Koudstaal, P.J.; Breteler, M.M.B. Atherosclerosis and risk for dementia. *Ann. Neurol.* **2007**, *61*, 403–410. [CrossRef] [PubMed]
220. Kim, G.; Kim, C.; Park, J.; Lee, K.; Park, C. Effects of vitamin B12 on cell proliferation and cellular alkaline phosphatase activity in human bone marrow stromal osteoprogenitor cells and UMR106 osteoblastic cells. *Metabolism* **1996**, *45*, 1443–1446. [CrossRef]
221. Masse, P.; Delvin, E.; Hauschka, P.; Donovan, S.; Grynpas, M.; Mahuren, J.; Watkins, B.; Howell, D. Perturbations in factors that modulate osteoblast functions in vitamin B6 deficiency. *Can. J. Physiol. Pharmacol.* **2000**, *78*, 904–911. [CrossRef] [PubMed]
222. Holstein, J.H.; Herrmann, M.; Splett, C.; Herrmann, W.; Garcia, P.; Histing, T.; Klein, M.; Kurz, K.; Siebel, T.; Pohlemann, T.; et al. High bone concentrations of homocysteine are associated with altered bone morphology in humans. *Br. J. Nutr.* **2011**, *106*, 378–382. [CrossRef] [PubMed]
223. Wei, I.L.; Huang, Y.H.; Wang, G.S. Vitamin B-6 deficiency decreases the glucose utilization in cognitive brain structures of rats. *J. Nutr. Biochem.* **1999**, *10*, 525–531. [CrossRef]
224. Fuso, A.; Nicolia, V.; Cavallaro, R.A.; Ricceri, L.; D'Anselmi, F.; Coluccia, P.; Calamandrei, G.; Scarpa, S. B-vitamin deprivation induces hyperhomocysteinemia and brain *S*-adenosylhomocysteine, depletes brain *S*-adenosylmethionine, and enhances *PS1* and *BACE* expression and amyloid-beta deposition in mice. *Mol. Cell. Neurosci.* **2008**, *37*, 731–746. [CrossRef] [PubMed]
225. Wang, B.B.; Jin, F.; Kan, R.; Ji, S.; Zhang, C.F.; Lu, Z.P.; Zheng, C.G.; Yang, Z.; Wang, L. Association of *MTHFR*

gene polymorphism *C677T* with susceptibility to late-onset Alzheimer's disease. *J. Mol. Neurosci.* **2005**, *27*, 23–27. [CrossRef]

226. Bi, X.; Zhao, H.; Zhang, Z.; Zhang, J. Association of *RFC1 A80G* and *MTHFR C677T* polymorphisms with Alzheimer's disease. *Neurobiol. Aging* **2009**, *30*, 1601–1607. [CrossRef] [PubMed]
227. Global Progress. Available online: http://ffinetwork.org/global_progress/index.php (accessed on 1 September 2016).
228. Williams, J.; Mai, C.T.; Mulinare, J.; Isenburg, J.; Flood, T.J.; Ethen, M.; Frohnert, B.; Kirby, R.S. Updated estimates of neural tube defects prevented by mandatory folic Acid fortification—United States, 1995–2011. *MMWR Morb. Mortal. Wkly. Rep.* **2015**, *64*, 1–5. [PubMed]
229. Jacques, P.F.; Selhub, J.; Bostom, A.G.; Wilson, P.W.F.; Rosenberg, I.H. The effect of folic acid fortification on plasma folate and total homocysteine concentrations. *N. Engl. J. Med.* **1999**, *340*, 1449–1454. [CrossRef] [PubMed]
230. Morris, M.S.; Jacques, P.F.; Rosenberg, I.H.; Selhub, J. Folate and vitamin B-12 status in relation to anemia, macrocytosis, and cognitive impairment in older Americans in the age of folic acid fortification. *Am. J. Clin. Nutr.* **2007**, *85*, 193–200. [PubMed]
231. Bailey, R.L.; Looker, A.C.; Lu, Z.; Fan, R.; Eicher-Miller, H.A.; Fakhouri, T.H.; Gahche, J.J.; Weaver, C.M.; Mills, J.L. B-vitamin status and bone mineral density and risk of lumbar osteoporosis in older females in the United States. *Am. J. Clin. Nutr.* **2015**, *102*, 687–694. [CrossRef] [PubMed]
232. Hoey, L.; McNulty, H.; Askin, N.; Dunne, A.; Ward, M.; Pentieva, K.; Strain, J.J.; Molloy, A.M.; Flynn, C.A.; Scott, J.M. Effect of a voluntary food fortification policy on folate, related B vitamin status, and homocysteine in healthy adults. *Am. J. Clin. Nutr.* **2007**, *86*, 1405–1413. [PubMed]
233. Hopkins, S.M.; Gibney, M.J.; Nugent, A.P.; McNulty, H.; Molloy, A.M.; Scott, J.M.; Flynn, A.; Strain, J.J.; Ward, M.; Walton, J.; et al. Impact of voluntary fortification and supplement use on dietary intakes and biomarker status of folate and vitamin B-12 in Irish adults. *Am. J. Clin. Nutr.* **2015**, *101*, 1163–1172. [CrossRef] [PubMed]
234. Institute of Medicine Panel. *Dietary Reference Intake: Thiamin, Riboflavin, Niacin, Vitamin B6, Vitamin B12, Pantothenic acid, Biotin and Choline*; National Academies Press: Washington, DC, USA, 2000; pp. 306–356.
235. EFSA NDA Panel. Scientific opinion on dietary reference values for cobalamin (Vitamin B12). *EFSA J.* **2015**, *13*, 4150.
236. Carmel, R.; Green, R.; Rosenblatt, D.S.; Watkins, D. Update on cobalamin, folate, and homocysteine. *Hematol. Am. Soc.* **2003**, *1*, 62–81. [CrossRef]
237. Mills, J.L.; Von Kohorn, I.; Conley, M.R.; Zeller, J.A.; Cox, C.; Williamson, R.E.; Dufour, D.R. Low vitamin B-12 concentrations in patients without anemia: The effect of folic acid fortification of grain. *Am. J. Clin. Nutr.* **2003**, *77*, 1474–1477. [PubMed]
238. Mills, J.L.; Carter, T.C.; Scott, J.M.; Troendle, J.F.; Gibney, E.R.; Shane, B.; Kirke, P.N.; Ueland, P.M.; Brody, L.C.; Molloy, A.M. Do high blood folate concentrations exacerbate metabolic abnormalities in people with low vitamin B-12 status? *Am. J. Clin. Nutr.* **2011**, *94*, 495–500. [CrossRef] [PubMed]
239. Qi, Y.; Hamner, H.; Pfeiffe, C.; Berry, R. The prevalence of low serum vitamin B-12 status in the absence of anemia or macrocytosis did not increase among older U.S. adults after mandatory folic acid fortification. *J. Nutr.* **2014**, *144*, 170–176. [CrossRef] [PubMed]
240. Selhub, J.; Morris, M.S.; Jacques, P.F.; Rosenberg, I.H. Folate-vitamin B-12 interaction in relation to cognitive impairment, anemia, and biochemical indicators of vitamin B-12 deficiency. *Am. J. Clin. Nutr.* **2009**, *89*, 702s–706s. [CrossRef] [PubMed]
241. Moore, E.M.; Ames, D.; Mander, A.G.; Carne, R.P.; Brodaty, H.; Woodward, M.C.; Boundy, K.; Ellis, K.A.; Bush, A.I.; Faux, N.G.; et al. Among vitamin B12 deficient older people, high folate levels are associated with worse cognitive function: Combined data from three cohorts. *J. Alzheimer's Dis.* **2014**, *39*, 661–668.
242. Clarke, R.; Sherliker, P.; Hin, H.; Molloy, A.M.; Nexo, E.; Ueland, P.M.; Emmens, K.; Scott, J.M.; Evans, J.G. Folate and vitamin B12 status in relation to cognitive impairment and anaemia in the setting of voluntary fortification in the UK. *Br. J. Nutr.* **2008**, *100*, 1054–1059. [CrossRef] [PubMed]
243. Doets, E.L.; Ueland, P.M.; Tell, G.S.; Vollset, S.E.; Nygard, O.K.; Van't Veer, P.; De Groot, L.C.P.G.M.; Nurk, E.; Refsum, H.; Smith, A.D.; et al. Interactions between plasma concentrations of folate and markers of

vitamin B(12) status with cognitive performance in elderly people not exposed to folic acid fortification: The Hordaland Health Study. *Br. J. Nutr.* **2014**, *111*, 1085–1095. [CrossRef] [PubMed]
244. National Toxicology Program. Identifying Research Needs for Safe Use of High Intakes of Folic Acid. 2015. Available online: https://ntp.niehs.nih.gov/ntp/ohat/folicacid/ntpfolicacid_approach_508.pdf (accessed on 1 August 2016).
245. Ebbing, M.; Bonaa, K.H.; Nygard, O.; Arnesen, E.; Ueland, P.M.; Nordrehaug, J.E.; Rasmussen, K.; Njolstad, I.; Refsum, H.; Nilsen, D.W.; et al. Cancer incidence and mortality after treatment with folic acid and vitamin B-12. *JAMA* **2009**, *302*, 2119–2126. [CrossRef] [PubMed]
246. Figueiredo, J.C.; Grau, M.V.; Haile, R.W.; Sandler, R.S.; Summers, R.W.; Bresalier, R.S.; Burke, C.A.; McKeown-Eyssen, G.E.; Baron, J.A. Folic acid and risk of prostate cancer: Results from a randomized clinical trial. *J. Natl. Cancer Inst.* **2009**, *101*, 432–435. [CrossRef] [PubMed]
247. Mason, J.B. Folate consumption and cancer risk: A confirmation and some reassurance, but we're not out of the woods quite yet. *Am. J. Clin. Nutr.* **2011**, *94*, 965–966. [CrossRef] [PubMed]
248. Report to CMO on Folic Acid and Colorectal Cancer. Available online: https://www.gov.uk/government/publications/sacn-report-to-cmo-on-folic-acid-and-colorectal-cancer-risk (accessed on 24 August 2016).
249. Troen, A.M.; Mitchell, B.; Sorensen, B.; Wener, M.H.; Johnston, A.; Wood, B.; Selhub, J.; McTiernan, A.; Yasui, Y.; Oral, E.; et al. Unmetabolized folic acid in plasma is associated with reduced natural killer cell cytotoxicity among postmenopausal women. *J. Nutr.* **2006**, *136*, 189–194. [PubMed]

Permissions

All chapters in this book were first published by MDPI; hereby published with permission under the Creative Commons Attribution License or equivalent. Every chapter published in this book has been scrutinized by our experts. Their significance has been extensively debated. The topics covered herein carry significant findings which will fuel the growth of the discipline. They may even be implemented as practical applications or may be referred to as a beginning point for another development.

The contributors of this book come from diverse backgrounds, making this book a truly international effort. This book will bring forth new frontiers with its revolutionizing research information and detailed analysis of the nascent developments around the world.

We would like to thank all the contributing authors for lending their expertise to make the book truly unique. They have played a crucial role in the development of this book. Without their invaluable contributions this book wouldn't have been possible. They have made vital efforts to compile up to date information on the varied aspects of this subject to make this book a valuable addition to the collection of many professionals and students.

This book was conceptualized with the vision of imparting up-to-date information and advanced data in this field. To ensure the same, a matchless editorial board was set up. Every individual on the board went through rigorous rounds of assessment to prove their worth. After which they invested a large part of their time researching and compiling the most relevant data for our readers.

The editorial board has been involved in producing this book since its inception. They have spent rigorous hours researching and exploring the diverse topics which have resulted in the successful publishing of this book. They have passed on their knowledge of decades through this book. To expedite this challenging task, the publisher supported the team at every step. A small team of assistant editors was also appointed to further simplify the editing procedure and attain best results for the readers.

Apart from the editorial board, the designing team has also invested a significant amount of their time in understanding the subject and creating the most relevant covers. They scrutinized every image to scout for the most suitable representation of the subject and create an appropriate cover for the book.

The publishing team has been an ardent support to the editorial, designing and production team. Their endless efforts to recruit the best for this project, has resulted in the accomplishment of this book. They are a veteran in the field of academics and their pool of knowledge is as vast as their experience in printing. Their expertise and guidance has proved useful at every step. Their uncompromising quality standards have made this book an exceptional effort. Their encouragement from time to time has been an inspiration for everyone.

The publisher and the editorial board hope that this book will prove to be a valuable piece of knowledge for researchers, students, practitioners and scholars across the globe.

List of Contributors

Peter Lyon, Victoria Strippoli, Byron Fang and Luisa Cimmino
Department of Biochemistry and Molecular Biology, Miller School of Medicine, University of Miami, Miami, FL 33136, USA
Sylvester Comprehensive Cancer Center, Miller School of Medicine, University of Miami, Miami, FL 33136, USA

Christine Tara Peterson
Center of Excellence for Research and Training in Integrative Health, Department of Family Medicine and Public Health, UC San Diego, School of Medicine, La Jolla, CA 92093, USA

Dmitry A. Rodionov
Bioinformatics and Structural Biology Program, Sanford Burnham Prebys Medical Discovery Institute, La Jolla, CA 92037, USA
A.A. Kharkevich Institute for Information Transmission Problems, Russian Academy of Sciences, 119991 Moscow, Russia

Andrei L. Osterman
Immunity and Pathogenesis Program, Infectious and Inflammatory Diseases Center, Sanford Burnham Prebys Medical Discovery Institute, La Jolla, CA 92037, USA

Scott N. Peterson
Tumor Microenvironment and Cancer Immunology Program, Sanford Burnham Prebys Medical Discovery Institute, La Jolla, CA 92037, USA

Elisa J. de Koning, Evelien Sohl, Karin M. A. Swart and Natasja M. van Schoor
EMGO Institute for Health and Care Research, VU University Medical Center, 1007 MB Amsterdam, The Netherlands
Department of Epidemiology and Biostatistics, VU University Medical Center, 1007 MB Amsterdam, The Netherlands

Nikita L. van der Zwaluw, Janneke P. van Wijngaarden, Elske M. Brouwer-Brolsma, Rosalie A. M. Dhonukshe-Rutten and Lisette C. P. G. M. de Groot
Division of Human Nutrition, Wageningen University, 6700 EVWageningen, The Netherlands

Harm W. J. van Marwijk
EMGO Institute for Health and Care Research, VU University Medical Center, 1007 MB Amsterdam, The Netherlands
Department of General Practice and Elderly Care Medicine, VU University Medical Center, 1007 MB Amsterdam, The Netherlands
Primary Care Research Center, Institute of Population Health, University of Manchester, Oxford Road, M13 9PL Manchester, UK

Anke W. Enneman, Suzanne C. van Dijk, Annelies C. Ham, Nathalie van der Velde and André G. Uitterlinden
Department of Internal Medicine, Erasmus University Medical Center, 3000 CA Rotterdam, The Netherlands

Brenda W. J. H. Penninx
EMGO Institute for Health and Care Research, VU University Medical Center, 1007 MB Amsterdam, The Netherlands
Department of Psychiatry, VU University Medical Center/GGZ inGeest, 1007 MB Amsterdam, The Netherlands

Petra J. M. Elders
Department of General Practice and Elderly Care Medicine, VU University Medical Center, 1007 MB Amsterdam, The Netherlands

Paul Lips
EMGO Institute for Health and Care Research, VU University Medical Center, 1007 MB Amsterdam, The Netherlands
Department of Internal Medicine/Endocrinology, VU University Medical Center, 1007 MB Amsterdam, The Netherlands

Gianluca Rizzo
Vico Sant'andrea 5, Ritiro, Messina 98152, Italy

Antonio Simone Laganà and Salvatore Giovanni Vitale
Unit of Gynecology and Obstetrics, Department of Human Pathology in Adulthood and Childhood, "G. Barresi", University of Messina, Via Consolare Valeria 1, Messina 98125, Italy

Agnese Maria Chiara Rapisarda, Gaetano Valenti, Fabrizio Sapia, Giuseppe Sarpietro and Micol Zigarelli
Department of General Surgery and Medical Surgical Specialties, University of Catania, Via S. Sofia 78, Catania 95124, Italy

Gioacchina Maria Grazia La Ferrera
Department of Gastroenterology and Digestive Endoscopy Maddalena Raimondi San Cataldo, Via Forlanini 5, San Cataldo, Caltanissetta 93017, Italy

Massimo Buscema, Paola Rossetti, Angela Nigro and Vincenzo Muscia
Unit of Diabetology and Endocrino-Metabolic Diseases, Hospital for Emergency Cannizzaro, Via Messina 829, Catania 95126, Italy

Jill A. McKay
Human Nutrition Research Centre, Institute for Health & Society, Newcastle University, Sir James Spence Institute, Royal Victoria Infirmary, Queen Victoria Road, Newcastle upon Tyne NE1 4LP, UK

Long Xie and John C. Mathers
Human Nutrition Research Centre; Institute of Cellular Medicine, Newcastle University, Newcastle upon Tyne NE4 5PL, UK

Michiel Adriaens
Maastricht Centre for Systems Biology, MaCSBio, Maastricht University, Maastricht 6200 MD, The Netherlands

Chris T. Evelo
Department of Bioinformatics, BiGCaT, Maastricht University, Maastricht 6200 MD, The Netherlands

Dianne Ford
Faculty of Health and Life Sciences, Northumbria University, Newcastle upon Tyne NE1 8ST, UK

Anne-Lise Bjørke-Monsen
Laboratory of Clinical Biochemistry, Haukeland University Hospital, 5021 Bergen, Norway

Arve Ulvik and Øivind Midttun
Bevital AS, 5021 Bergen, Norway

Roy M. Nilsen
Centre for Clinical Research, Haukeland University Hospital, 5021 Bergen, Norway

Christine Roth
The Norwegian Institute of Public Health, 0403 Oslo, Norway
Nic Waals Institute, Lovisenberg Hospital, Oslo 0456, Norway

Per Magnus
The Norwegian Institute of Public Health, 0403 Oslo, Norway

Camilla Stoltenberg and Stein Emil Vollset
The Norwegian Institute of Public Health, 0403 Oslo, Norway
Department of Public Health and Primary Health Care, University of Bergen, 5007 Bergen, Norway

Ted Reichborn-Kjennerud
The Norwegian Institute of Public Health, 0403 Oslo, Norway
Institute of Clinical Medicine, University of Oslo, 0313 Oslo, Norway

Per Magne Ueland
Laboratory of Clinical Biochemistry, Haukeland University Hospital, 5021 Bergen, Norway
Department of Clinical Science, University of Bergen, 5007 Bergen, Norway

Qianying Zhang, Sheyu Li, Qianrui Li, Kaiyun Ren and Jianwei Li
Department of Endocrinology and Metabolism, West China Hospital, Sichuan University, Chengdu 610041, China

Ling Li and Xin Sun
Chinese Evidence-based Medicine Center, West China Hospital, Sichuan University, Chengdu 610041, China

Marta Jeruszka-Bielak, Carly Isman and Wangyang Li
Food Nutrition and Health Program, Faculty of Land and Food Systems, The University of British Columbia, Vancouver, BC V6T 1Z4, Canada

Theresa H. Schroder and Yvonne Lamers
Food Nutrition and Health Program, Faculty of Land and Food Systems, The University of British Columbia, Vancouver, BC V6T 1Z4, Canada
BC Children's Hospital Research Institute, Vancouver, BC V5Z 4H4, Canada

Tim J. Green
Food Nutrition and Health Program, Faculty of Land and Food Systems, The University of British Columbia, Vancouver, BC V6T 1Z4, Canada
South Australian Health Medical Research Institute, Adelaide 5000, Australia

Zheng Zhou, Mario Vailati-Riboni and Juan J. Loor
Mammalian NutriPhysioGenomics, Department of Animal Sciences and Division of Nutritional Sciences, University of Illinois, Urbana, IL 61801, USA

Daniel N. Luchini
Adisseo North America, Alpharetta, GA 30022, USA

Jose M. Colomina, Sílvia Fernàndez-Roig, Pol Solé-Navais and Joan D. Fernandez-Ballart
Area of Preventive Medicine and Public Health, Faculty of Medicine and Health Sciences, Universitat Rovira i Virgili, IISPV, C/Sant Llorenç 21, Reus 43201, Spain
Ciberobn Fisiopatología de la Obesidad y Nutrición (CB06/03), Instituto Carlos III, Madrid 28029, Spain

Pere Cavallé-Busquets
Ciberobn Fisiopatología de la Obesidad y Nutrición (CB06/03), Instituto Carlos III, Madrid 28029, Spain
Area of Obstetrics and Gynaecology, Hospital Universitari Sant Joan, Reus and Universitat Rovira i Virgili, Reus 43204, Spain

Mónica Ballesteros
Area of Obstetrics and Gynaecology, Hospital Universitari Joan XXIII, Tarragona and Universitat Rovira I Virgili, Tarragona 43005, Spain

Per M. Ueland
Section for Pharmacology, Department of Internal Medicine, University of Bergen, Bergen N-5020, Norway

Klaus Meyer
Bevital A/S, Laboratory building, 9th floor, Bergen N-5021, Norway

Michelle M. Murphy
Area of Preventive Medicine and Public Health, Faculty of Medicine and Health Sciences, Universitat Rovira i Virgili, IISPV, C/Sant Llorenç 21, Reus 43201, Spain
Ciberobn Fisiopatología de la Obesidad y Nutrición (CB06/03), Instituto Carlos III, Madrid 28029, Spain

Sophie Lefèvre-Arbogast, Catherine Féart, Jean-François Dartigues, Catherine Helmer, Luc Letenneur and Cécilia Samieri
University Bordeaux, Institut de Santé Publique d'Epidémiologie et de Développement (ISPED), Centre INSERM U1219-Bordeaux Population Health, Bordeaux 33076, France
Institut National de la Santé et de la Recherche Médicale (INSERM), Institut de Santé Publique d'Epidémiologie et de Développement (ISPED), Centre INSERM U1219-Bordeaux Population Health, Bordeaux 33076, France

Nasser M. Al-Daghri, Shakilur Rahman, Shaun Sabico, Sobhy Yakout, Kaiser Wani, Omar S. Al-Attas and Majed S. Alokail
Biomarkers Research Program, Biochemistry Department, College of Science, King Saud University, Riyadh 11451, Saudi Arabia
Prince Mutaib Chair for Biomarkers of Osteoporosis, Biochemistry Department, College of Science, King Saud University, Riyadh 11451, Saudi Arabia

Ponnusamy Saravanan
Division of Health Sciences, Warwick Medical School, University of Warwick, Coventry CV4 7AL, UK

Gyanendra Tripathi
Biomarkers Research Program, Biochemistry Department, College of Science, King Saud University, Riyadh 11451, Saudi Arabia
Prince Mutaib Chair for Biomarkers of Osteoporosis, Biochemistry Department, College of Science, King Saud University, Riyadh 11451, Saudi Arabia
Division of Biomedical Sciences, Warwick Medical School, University of Warwick, UHCW Trust, Clifford Bridge Road, Walsgrave, Coventry CV2 2DX, UK
Department of Biomedical Sciences, University of Westminster, London W1W 6UW, UK

Philip G. Mc Ternan
Division of Biomedical Sciences, Warwick Medical School, University of Warwick, UHCW Trust, Clifford Bridge Road, Walsgrave, Coventry CV2 2DX, UK

Kirsty Porter, Leane Hoey, Catherine F. Hughes, Mary Ward and Helene McNulty
Northern Ireland Centre for Food and Health, Ulster University, Cromore Road, Coleraine BT52 1SA, UK

Index

www.ingramcontent.com/pod-product-compliance
Lightning Source LLC
LaVergne TN
LVHW060545210926
848485LV00005B/1263